STRATEGIES IN ADJUVANT THERAPY

STRATEGIES IN ADJUVANT THERAPY

Edited by

JOHN M KIRKWOOD, MD
Professor and Vice Chairman for Clinical Research
Department of Medicine
University of Pittsburgh School of Medicine
Director, Melanoma Center
University of Pittsburgh Cancer Institute
Pittsburgh, PA 15232
USA

MARTIN DUNITZ

© Martin Dunitz 2000

First published in the United Kingdom in 2000 by:
Martin Dunitz Ltd
The Livery House
7–9 Pratt Street
London NW1 0AE

Tel: +44-(0)20-7482-2202
Fax: +44-(0)20-7267-0159
E-mail: info@mdunitz.globalnet.co.uk
Website: http://www.dunitz.co.uk

A CIP catalogue record for this book is available from the British Library

ISBN 1-85317-317-7

Distributed in the United States by:
Blackwell Science Inc.
Commerce Place, 350 Main Street
Malden MA 02148, USA
Tel: 1 800 215 1000

Distributed in Canada by:
Login Brothers Book Company
324 Salteaux Crescent
Winnipeg, Manitoba R3J 3T2
Canada
Tel: 1 204 224 4068

Distributed in Brazil by:
Ernesto Reichmann Distribuidora de Livros, Ltda
Rua Coronel Marques 335, Tatuape 03440-000
Sao Paulo,
Brazil

Composition by Wearset, Boldon, Tyne and Wear
Printed and bound in Great Britain by Biddles Ltd, Guildford and King's Lynn

Contents

Preface

Adjuvant approaches have given us multiple new insights into cancer in the past generation. Indeed, the application of biologic therapies on the basis of fundamental principles of tumor immunology has moved from advanced disease to the setting of earlier disease, where the efficacy of several biologic agents have first been demonstrated. To date, these same agents have had only marginal impact when applied in advanced disease settings. As our understanding of the area of vaccine immunotherapy and antibody therapies increases, this trend is likely to grow dramatically. The advent of molecular techniques for the detection of markers of cancer and its precursors, and for quantitation of cancer burden in several diseases, offers new means to more precisely guide the application of adjuvant interventions, and the measurement of therapeutic efficacy.

One of the most attractive new options arises from increased understanding of the mechanisms of action for biologic agents, and for anticancer drugs in general. This will provide a foundation for the more rational evaluation of these agents in terms of these mechanisms. Based upon an understanding of molecular events associated with tumor progression, and the immunologic responses that are associated with it, our strategies of adjuvant therapy are likely to evolve considerably in the next decade. This undestanding, coupled with increasing knowledge of the specific antigenic composition of many tumors, as well as of the role of antigen processing and host cellular/humoral immune responses, is most reasonably applied to the adjuvant therapy of cancer. The underlying principles of adjuvant therapy are based on the observation that host immune competence and tumor cell susceptibility to immunologic interventions is greatest in the earlier stages of disease.

For many solid tumors, the presence of lymph node metastasis is one of the most powerful predictors of prognosis. Adjuvant therapy has been directed at patients with regional node metastasis, and from this beachhead, effective interventions have been extended to earlier and/or later stages of disease. Sentinel node mapping has radically improved the precision with which lymph node involvement can be identified in patients with melanoma, breast carcinoma, and other solid tumors, and has also refined patient selection for adjuvant therapy. The pivotal unanswered questions in the context of adjuvant therapy relate to the molecular and/or immunologic basis(es) of response to new biologic interventions. This volume discusses the current status of adjuvant therapy for cancer from an international viewpoint, and provides the foundations for future interventions.

JMK

Contributors

Sanjiv S Agarawala, MD
Department of Medicine
Division of Hematology/Oncology
University of Pittsburgh Cancer Institute
200 Lothrop Street
Pittsburgh, PA 15232
USA

Robert J Amdur, MD
The Uro-Oncology Group
Norris Cotton Cancer Center
Dartmouth-Hitchcock Medical Center
1 Medical Center Drive
Lebanon, NH 03756-0001
USA

Jens Atzpodien, MD, PhD
Robert-Janker-Klinik
Villenstrasse 4
30623 Bonn
Germany

Michael R Curtis, MD
The Uro-Oncology Group
Norris Cotton Cancer Center
Dartmouth-Hitchcock Medical Center
1 Medical Center Drive
Lebanon, NH 03756-0001
USA

Alexander M M Eggermont, MD, PhD
Professor of Surgical Oncology
Department of Surgical Oncology
University Hospital Rotterdam
Daniel den Hoed Cancer Center
3008 AE Rotterdam
The Netherlands

Marc S Ernstoff, MD
The Uro-Oncology Group
Norris Cotton Cancer Center
Dartmouth-Hitchcock Medical Center
1 Medical Center Drive
Lebanon, NH 03756-0001
USA

Jean-Jacques Grob, MD
Service de Dermatologie
Hôpital Ste Marguerite
270 Blvd St Marguerite
13009 Marseille
France

Robert Harris, MD
The Uro-Oncology Group
Norris Cotton Cancer Center
Dartmouth-Hitchcock Medical Center
1 Medical Center Drive
Lebanon, NH 03756-0001
USA

John A Heaney, MD
The Uro-Oncology Group
Norris Cotton Cancer Center
Dartmouth-Hitchcock Medical Center
1 Medical Center Drive
Lebanon, NH 03756-0001
USA

Waun Ki Hong, MD
Professor and Chairman
Department of Thoracic/Head and Neck
Medical Oncology
UTMD Anderson Cancer Center
1515 Holcombe Boulevard
Houston, TX 77030
USA

Julie G Izzo, MD
Assistant Professor of Medicine
Department of Experimental Therapeutics
UTMD Anderson Cancer Center
1515 Holcombe Boulevard
Houston, TX 77030
USA

Ulrich Keilholz, MD
Professor
Medizinische Klinik III
Frei Universität Berlin
Hindenburgdamm 30
12200 Berlin
Germany

Fadlo R Khuri, MD
Assistant Professor of Medicine
Department of Thoracic/
Head and Neck Medical Oncology
UTMD Anderson Cancer Center
1515 Holcombe Boulevard
Houston, TX 77030
USA

John M Kirkwood, MD
Professor and Vice Chairman for Clinical Research
Department of Medicine
University of Pittsburgh School of Medicine
Director, Melanoma Center
University of Pittsburgh Cancer Institute
200 Lothrop Street
Pittsburgh, PA 15232
USA

Timothy M Kuzel, MD
Division of Hematology/Oncology
Northwestern University Medical School
Robert H Lurie Comprehensive Cancer Center
Northwestern University
676 N St Clair, Suite 850
Chicago, IL 60611-3008
USA

Karin V Mattson, MD
Department of Internal Medicine
Division of Pulmonary Medicine and
Allergology
Helsinki University Central Hospital
Haartmaninkatu 4
FIN 00290 Helsinki
Finland

Nicole Max, MD
Medizinische Klinik III
Frei Universität Berlin
Hindenburgdamm 30
12200 Berlin
Germany

Margaret von Mehren, MD
Associate Member
Department of Medical Oncology
Fox Chase Cancer Center
7701 Burholme Avenue
Philadelphia, PA 19111
USA

Steven T Rosen, MD
Director
Robert H Lurie Comprehensive Cancer Center
Northwestern University
303 E Chicago Avenue, Suite 8524
Chicago, IL 60611-3008
USA

Alan R Schned, MD
The Uro-Oncology Group
Norris Cotton Cancer Center
Dartmouth-Hitchcock Medical Center
1 Medical Center Drive
Lebanon, NH 03756-0001
USA

Thomas Schwaab, MD
Department of Urology
Dartmouth-Hitchcock Medical Center
1 Medical Center Drive
Lebanon, NH 03756-0001
USA

Benjamin Spike, MD
Medizinische Klinik III
Frei Universität Berlin
Hindenburgdamm 30
12200 Berlin
Germany

Ann E Traynor, MD
Assistant Professor of Medicine
Division of Hematology/Oncology
Northwestern University Medical School
Robert H Lurie Comprehensive Cancer Center
Northwestern University
303 E Chicago Avenue, Suite 8524
Chicago, IL 60611-3008
USA

Scott Wadler, MD, FACP
Associate Chairman
Department of Oncology
Montefiore Medical Center
Associate Director (Acting) for Clinical Research
Albert Einstein Cancer Center
Albert Einstein College of Medicine
1300 Morris Park Avenue
Bronx, NY 10467
USA

Louis M Weiner, MD
Chairman, Department of Medical Oncology
Fox Chase Cancer Center
7701 Burholme Avenue
Philadelphia, PA 19111
USA

Martina Willhauk, MD
Medizinische Klinik V
Universität Heidelberg
Hospitalstrasse 3
69115 Heidelberg
Germany

1

PCR-based detection of malignant cells: Towards molecular staging?

Ulrich Keilholz, Nicole Max, Benjamin Spike, Martina Willhauk

CONTENTS • **Introduction** • **Principal PCR detection methods** • **Quality assurance** • **Survey of clinical data** • **Future prospects**

INTRODUCTION

The current understanding of the process of metastasis is that single neoplastic cells leave the primary tumour and travel to distant sites in the body via the lymphatic system and the bloodstream. If single neoplastic cells or small aggregates travel via the lymphatic ducts, they may find a suitable environment for survival, and possibly expansion and further spread, in the first draining lymph node, also called the sentinel lymph node. If the tumour cells spread haematogenously, multiple factors may influence which tissues are invaded and whether invading tumour cells survive and give rise to further metastases. Many details of the metastatic process, especially the kinetics, are still under investigation. Oncologists have long sought to accurately monitor lymphatic and haematogenous spread of neoplastic cells. Single tumour cells, in the bone marrow for instance, can be detected by immunohistological techniques. However, this method is not sufficiently sensitive to reliably monitor early metastasis or minimal residual disease, since only a very limited number of cells can be assayed at one time. Recently, polymerase chain reaction (PCR)-based methods capable of detecting single neoplastic cells in much larger samples have been developed (Table 1.1).

Immunohistological methods of tumour detection are based on the recognition of tumour-specific or tumour-associated proteins by highly specific monoclonal antibodies. However, several studies have confirmed that regional lymph nodes that appear free of disease macroscopically and by routine light microscopy may still harbour tumour cells. Single tumour cells have been detected in some patients with colon carcinoma, carcinoma of the breast and sarcoma in the bone marrow, and occasionally in the peripheral blood, using immunohistological techniques.[1-5] However, the prognostic value of these techniques remains limited, since tumour cells can only be detected if the expression of the target protein is sufficiently high to promote visible antibody binding. Moreover, because the number of cells that can be efficiently screened by light microscopy is limited, confidence in a 'tumour-negative' result using these techniques, especially in the case of tissue biopsies, is not statistically sound.

PCR allows exponential amplification of spe-

Table 1.1 Limits of detection for tumour cells in peripheral blood and bone marrow	
Technique	**Limit of detection**
Light microscopy	1 tumour cell in 100–1000 normal cells
Immunohistology	1 tumour cell in 10^5–10^6 normal cells
PCR	1 tumour cell in 10^7–10^8 normal cells

cific regions of DNA and RNA molecules using repeated cycles of helix denaturation, primer annealing and strand extension. Specificity is achieved by designing the oligonucleotide primers with nucleotide sequences specific for a gene of interest. With this technique, the expression of tumour-specific or tumour-associated genes as well as the presence of genetic abnormalities can be detected in a clinical specimen with very high sensitivity. Because the total genomic DNA or RNA from an entire clinical sample can be extracted and tested in a single reaction, PCR-based analysis also offers a high level of efficiency. Over the past five years, PCR assays have been developed for various types of neoplastic cells, and initial results describing the possible clinical usefulness of these techniques have accumulated. This chapter describes the principles of occult tumour cell detection using PCR, and summarizes the currently available clinical data from trials utilizing PCR-based techniques.

PRINCIPAL PCR DETECTION METHODS

The best markers for detection of tumour cells by PCR are well-characterized DNA abnormalities or consistently expressed tumour-specific RNA sequences.

Genomic DNA level

Structural abnormalities (translocations, deletions and insertions) as well as specific point mutations in proto-oncogenes are the genetic alterations that are usually present in the DNA of tumour cells, but not in normal cells of the organism. As such, these alterations represent specific indicators of tumour cells that can be detected using DNA-based PCR. The most important advantages of DNA-based techniques are the ease of extracting sufficient DNA from all kinds of clinical material, including paraffin-embedded tissue, the stability of DNA, and the independence of DNA abnormalities from the transcriptional activity of the tumour cells. One disadvantage of DNA-based techniques is sensitivity, since one tumour cell usually contains only a single copy of the gene of interest. However, many of the genetic abnormalities in tumour cells detectable by DNA techniques can also be detected on the RNA level, which may improve sensitivity.

RNA level

The major application of RNA techniques in tumour detection is in detecting differentiation antigens that are expressed only in tumour cells and their parent tissues. For this type of assay, it is essential that the target gene be expressed only by tumour cells in the sample studied, and that normal counterparts of the tumour are not present in this sample. Carefully chosen target genes can be exploited for the detection of almost all solid malignancies by assaying for transcripts of these genes in the peripheral blood or perhaps in the bone marrow.

RNA-based methods do require active transcription of the gene of interest. Fortunately, a high transcript number from the gene of

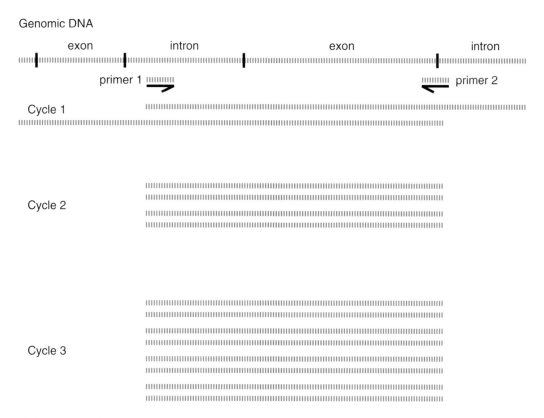

Figure 1.1 Principle of PCR assays from genomic DNA.

interest is usually present in a tumour cell. RNA-based detection therefore has the advantage of high sensitivity and of detecting primarily viable cells, although detection of unviable cells in the early stages of apoptosis is theoretically possible. The number of RNA copies of a gene in any particular tumour cell may, however, vary during the cell's life cycle or as a result of de-differentiation.

DNA amplification

In the case of a tumour-specific translocation, two gene fragments are joined, commonly leading either to the activation of a proto-oncogene or the inactivation of a tumour suppressor gene. By choosing a pair of primers that flank the breakpoint of such a fusion gene, a DNA

fragment can be amplified specifically from neoplastic cells (Figure 1.1). In the case of B- or T-cell malignancies, the rearranged immunoglobulin or T-cell receptor gene can be utilized for the purpose of tumour-specific amplification, if the hypervariable (e.g. CDR3) region has been sequenced and at least one primer is located in this region, or by using consensus primers flanking the CDR3 region and probing with a CDR3-specific probe.

DNA amplification has been utilized for the detection of minimal residual disease in haematological malignancies, such as lymphoma, in which the tumour cells have clonally rearranged immunoglobulin genes or T-cell receptor genes. DNA amplification has also been employed for chromosomal translocations, such as the frequently occurring t(14;18) or the *bcr–abl* fusion gene (the Philadelphia

Table 1.2 Markers utilized for detection of tumour cells

Tumour type	Tumour markers[a]
Melanoma	Tyrosinase, p97, MUC18, MAGE-3
Prostate cancer	PSA, PSM
Gastrointestinal cancer:	
Stomach	CEA
Pancreatic	Mutated K-ras
Colorectal	CEA, CK20, mutated K-ras
Breast carcinoma	CK19, CK20, CEA
Neuroblastoma	Tyrosine hydroxylase, N-CAM, PGP9.5, MAGE
Head and neck carcinoma	Mutated p53
Ewing's sarcoma	t(11;22)(q24;q12)
Hepatocellular carcinoma	AFP
Lung cancer	NSE, bombesin

[a]PSA, prostate-specific antigen; PSM, prostate-specific membrane antigen; CEA, carcinoembryonic antigen; CK, cytokeratin; AFP, α-fetoprotein; NSE, neuron-specific enolase.

chromosome) of chronic myeloid leukemia (CML). For solid tumours, not many specific and frequent translocations or mutations have been described thus far, the best known exception being the well-characterized mutations of the *ras* proto-oncogene, which are especially prevalent in gastrointestinal carcinomas.

RNA amplification

Gene transcripts encoding tissue- or tumour-specific proteins can be used to detect the vast majority of solid tumours. The most commonly used examples are listed in Table 1.2. These genes are not normally transcribed by cells of the peripheral blood and bone marrow, nor are they likely to be expressed in lymphatic tissue. Further, non-neoplastic cells of the tumour's parent tissue are not normally found outside the organs in which they originate.

Some of these genes, such as those encoding the oncofetal proteins CEA and AFP, are highly expressed in tumour cells, although they are expressed at very low or even undetectable levels in normal cells from the same tissue. On the other hand, expression of some genes that encode proteins of functional importance for normal cells may be reduced or lost in tumour cells as a consequence of de-differentiation or selection during tumour progression. Stable expression of the target gene is thus an important parameter in marker gene choice. An ideal marker gene would be one whose expression is

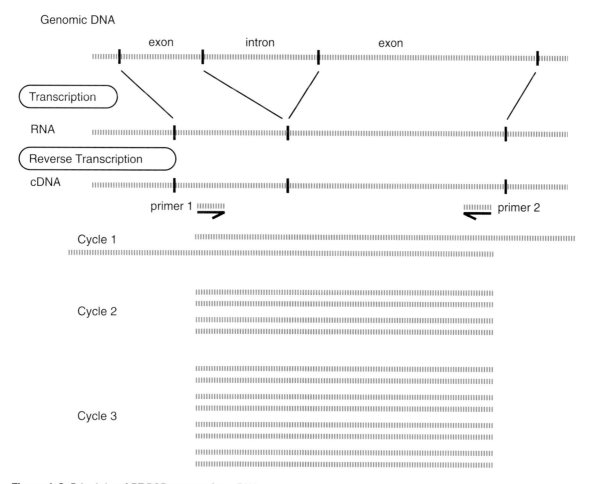

Figure 1.2 Principle of RT-PCR assays from RNA.

essential for the survival of the neoplastic cell. And, while the targets listed in Table 1.2 have proven valuable as indicators of circulating tumour cells, none of them has turned out to be absolutely essential for tumour survival.

Reverse-transcription PCR (RT-PCR)
First, the RNA is extracted from the sample and reverse-transcribed into cDNA (Figure 1.2). The gene of interest is then amplified using primers specific for that gene. Ideally, these primers should not amplify genomic DNA, which often contaminates the cDNA preparation. Amplification of a cDNA sequence without amplification of the genomic counterpart of this

sequence can be achieved if one primer is interrupted by an intron in the genomic DNA. The intron will have been deleted during RNA processing and therefore will not interrupt the primer sequence in the cDNA version of the gene. Alternatively, primers can be chosen that flank an intron in the genomic sequence, thereby facilitating easy differentiation between a PCR product derived from genomic DNA and one derived from cDNA based on the size of the product.

To increase sensitivity, a second round of PCR can be performed using primers located between the first-round primer pair (nested PCR). These internal primers should specifically amplify a portion of the internal sequences from the first-round PCR product. Besides increased sensitivity, the nested PCR also has increased specificity, because a non-specific product generated during the first round of PCR will not be further amplified in the second round.

After PCR amplification, the product is usually detected on an agarose gel, or specifically hybridized on a Southern blot. In addition, the PCR product can be sequenced to verify that the sequence of the PCR product corresponds to the gene of interest.

Sample preparation for RT-PCR

If a cell is disrupted, ubiquitous RNases rapidly degrade the cell's RNA. For these reasons, rapid processing of the clinical samples is crucial, and certain general precautions must be taken to prevent RNA degradation.

Tissue samples should be frozen in liquid nitrogen as soon as possible after resection and minced while frozen. The sample is then admixed with RNA extraction buffer, which inhibits RNases. Bone marrow and blood samples can be admixed with RNA extraction buffer directly. Prolonged storage of blood samples should be strictly avoided.

Methods that call for lysis of erythrocytes during sample preparation should be avoided, since lysis may release RNases and because tumour cells may themselves be subject to lysis under these conditions. Further, if gradient separation techniques are to be employed to separate red blood cells in peripheral blood from leukocytes, it must be ensured that the tumour cells remain above the separation fluid. If regular Ficoll with specific gravity of $1.077\,\mathrm{g}/1$ is used, tumour cells may sediment with the granulocytes and erythrocytes. Split-sample analyses from melanoma patients have revealed that the majority of melanoma cells in the peripheral blood can only be separated from red blood cells if a separation medium of $1.09\,\mathrm{g}/1$ is used, which yields separation of all peripheral blood leukocytes from erythrocytes.[6] However, it is uncertain whether or not some tumour cells are still trapped in the erythrocyte pellet. Because of these observations, we recommend the use of whole blood samples or separation medium of sufficient density.

RNA extraction/cDNA synthesis

Various protocols are available for extraction of RNA. Guanidinium isothiocyanate/phenol–chloroform-based extraction methods, as first described by Chomczynski and Sacchi,[7] are most commonly employed. Alternatively, commercial kits for RNA extraction based on ion-exchange columns can be used. Caesium chloride gradient separation techniques require long-term ultracentrifugation, and therefore are less suitable for routine analysis; however, this method yields the purest RNA. Probably all of these methods are suited to RNA extraction; however, the efficiency of RNA extraction from sample to sample and between methods varies considerably and is somewhat unpredictable. Therefore, in order to carry out quantitative assessments of RNA using PCR, controls must be employed during both the RNA extraction and the cDNA synthesis steps.

Various protocols and reverse transcriptases may be used for cDNA synthesis, and most protocols yield adequate cDNA.

PCR

Several different DNA polymerases are available for PCR. For all primers and enzymes, the optimal PCR conditions must first be established. With reliable thermal cycles, the variations in PCR efficiency are considerably smaller than the variations in RNA extraction and cDNA synthesis.

QUALITY ASSURANCE

Figure 1.3(a) depicts the standard controls that are routinely used to ensure accuracy of each step from RNA extraction to visualization of the PCR product.

RNA yield can be determined photometrically at a wavelength of 260 nm; however, contaminating DNA can lead to inflated RNA yields. The purity of the RNA preparation can be assessed using an ethidium bromide-stained MOPS agarose gel, which also allows rough

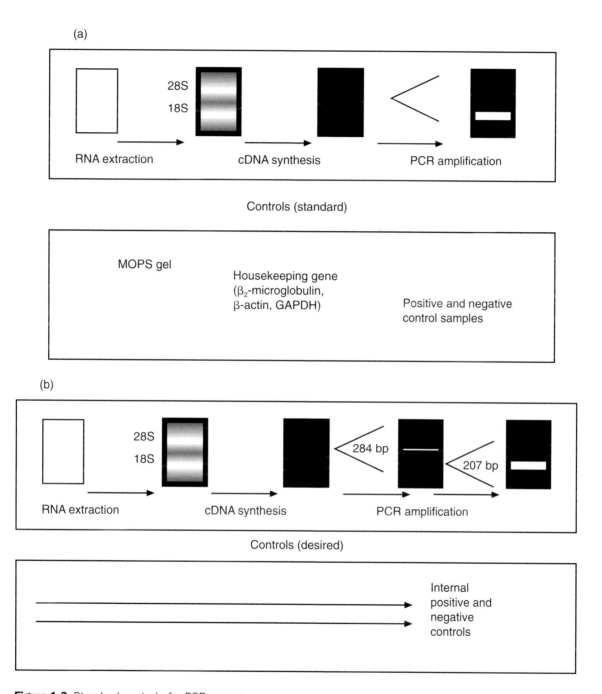

Figure 1.3 Standard controls for PCR assays.

(a) After extraction of total RNA from a homogenized sample, the extract can be run on a MOPS or $1 \times$ TBE agarose gel and stained with ethidium bromide. The 28S and 18S ribosomal RNA (rRNA) bands indicate the amount of intact RNA. The amount can be quantified photometrically.

(b) The subsequent cDNA synthesis cannot be controlled directly. To determine, whether amplifiable cDNA has been synthesized, a 'housekeeping' gene, translated in every viable cell, can be amplified by PCR and detected. If with a limited number of PCR cycles (usually between 22 and 26) no signal is visible for the housekeeping gene, the cDNA or the RNA is of insufficient quality for analysis.   (*Continued*)

(c)

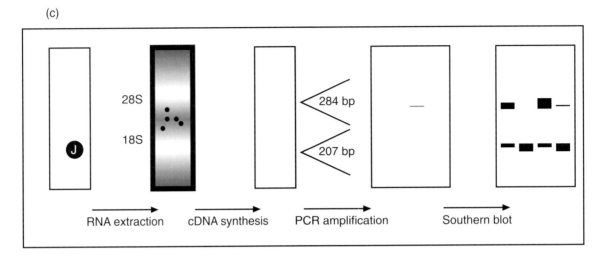

Figure 1.3 *Continued*

(c) After PCR amplification of the target gene, the product can be run on an agarose gel and visualized by ethidium bromide staining. Simultaneously processed positive and negative control samples can exclude contamination of the reagents (but not sporadic contamination) and give an estimate of the PCR sensitivity. The identity of the RT-PCR product should be confirmed by Southern blot.

assessment of the RNA quantity and the detection of any significant degradation.

One problem in assessing the integrity of cDNA is that it cannot be visualized directly – instead, indirect methods must be used. Such an assessment is usually accomplished by PCR-amplification of a 'housekeeping' gene, for example β$_2$-microglobulin, β-actin or GAPDH. However, the value of this type of assessment for reverse-transcription efficiency should not be overestimated, since housekeeping genes are so abundantly expressed that they are often detected even in cDNAs of rather poor quality. Thus they do not reliably indicate whether the cDNA quality is sufficient to detect a gene of interest expressed on a level several orders of magnitude lower than that of the housekeeping gene itself. This problem can be reduced by limiting the number of cycles used to detect the housekeeping gene. Approximately 18–20 cycles for tumour tissue and cell lines and up to 26 cycles for peripheral blood should lead to exponential amplification of housekeeping genes only in cDNAs of sufficient quality

for tumour marker detection. Under these circumstances, the cDNA quality can be semiquantitatively assessed using a 2% agarose gel.

It would be more desirable to develop a single system that controls for variations throughout the process (Figure 1.3b). The following is one proposal (Figure 1.3c). A small number of cells expressing a gene not usually present in the sample is admixed with the sample prior to processing. The number of transcripts from the control gene should be of the same order of magnitude as the expected transcript number from the gene of interest in tumour cells, so that addition of control cells per test would approximate the number of tumour cells expected in an average sample (i.e. 100–1000 cells). The control gene transcript is then carried throughout the whole process, extracted, reverse-transcribed and coamplified with the tumour cell gene in the PCR. The primers must be designated such that the PCR product from the control gene is approximately 100 bases larger than the PCR product from the

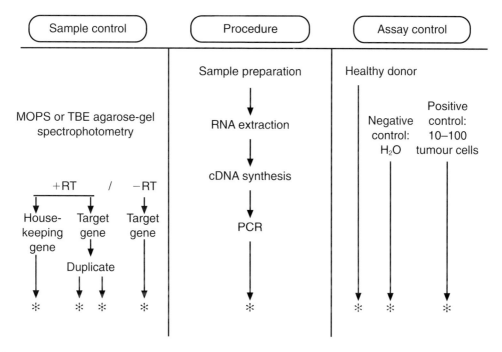

Figure 1.4 Extended set of controls recommended for diagnostic PCR.

Contamination and low sensitivity can result from any step in the process of sample preparation, RNA extraction, cDNA synthesis, and PCR (centre lane); therefore all steps need to be controlled.

Sample control: The suitability of an RNA for analysis should be verified on a gel, and quantitation done by spectrophotometry. The cDNA synthesis should be performed in parallel with and without reverse transcriptase (RT) to exclude systematic and sporadic contamination at the level of sample handling and RNA extraction. In the sample without RT, a positive PCR signal would indicate contamination. The cDNA of the sample with RT should be checked by amplification of a housekeeping gene. The results of the duplicate PCR for the marker gene should give identical results.

Assay control: At least one sample from a healthy donor should be analysed in parallel to a series of patient samples. For the PCR, a negative water control is suitable to rule out contamination of reagents, while a positive control of an mRNA from a blood sample spiked with a low number (10–100) of tumour cells will assess efficiency of the PCR.

tumour marker gene. For this assay, it must be ensured that neither primer completely outcompetes the other. If 30 PCR cycles are employed, followed by subsequent Southern blotting and specific hybridization of the tumour cell gene and the control gene, the PCR product for the control gene should be clearly visible for every sample.

As a negative control, the whole process should be duplicated with a sample lacking reverse transcriptase to control for contaminat-

ing DNA and a deionized water sample to control for contaminating RNA.

The importance of positive and negative controls for the PCR assay cannot be overemphasized.[6,8–11] Before widespread, and possibly commercial, application may start, it is of the utmost importance to establish very rigid quality assurance systems. Otherwise, it will not be possible to compare results of different groups and accurately determine the usefulness of this method in the clinical setting. Figure 1.4

summarizes a set of positive and negative controls ensuring the detection of any systematic and/or sporadic contamination and indicating differences in sensitivity.

SURVEY OF CLINICAL DATA

For solid malignancies, the expression of tissue-specific genes has most frequently been utilized to detect occult disease (see Table 1.2). In contrast, defined genetic abnormalities are most commonly used for monitoring minimal residual disease in lymphomas and leukaemias (not described in this chapter).

Melanoma

A number of genes encoding melanosomal proteins are expressed specifically in melanocytes and melanomas. Tyrosinase is the first enzyme in the melanin biosynthesis pathway. It is a monooxygenase that catalyses the conversion of tyrosine to DOPA and of DOPA to dopaquinone. Tyrosinase is therefore one of the most specific markers of melanocytes, and it is conserved in most amelanotic melanoma metastases. Expression of the tyrosinase gene is the most widely used indicator for the detection of circulating melanoma cells. Other melanocyte-specific proteins include gp100, which is recognized by the diagnostic antibodies HMB45 and NKI-beteb,[12] Melan-A/MART1[13,14] and a family of tyrosinase-related proteins. gp100 is less suited for monitoring of melanoma, since it is known to be frequently lost during tumour progression.[15,16] The expression of Melan-A/MART1 and tyrosinase-related proteins has been less well studied, but it has been shown that their expression is also lost in a significant percentage of metastatic lesions as detected by specific monoclonal antibodies.[17,18] Melanomas also express tumour-associated genes such as the MAGE family: about 60% of metastatic lesions are positive for MAGE-1 and 80% for MAGE-3 as detected by PCR.[19-22] The family of proteins encoded by these genes may therefore represent another useful marker for metastatic melanoma.

Smith et al[23] reported in 1991 that circulating melanoma cells can be detected by PCR amplification of tyrosinase RNA. Their PCR assay is used most frequently today because of its optimal primer design. The primers, designated as HTYR1 to HTYR4, exploit the presence of two introns in the tyrosinase gene. HTYR1 spans an intron, and another intron is located between the nested primers HTYR3 and -4. This primer design virtually excludes amplification of genomic DNA.

The initial report led to a number of more detailed investigations on the presence of tyrosinase RNA in the peripheral blood of melanoma patients.[24-30] Non-melanoma controls were always negative for expression of tyrosinase using this technique, suggesting that normal melanocytes do not circulate in blood, and that the presence of tyrosinase RNA can be considered evidence of circulating melanoma cells. Hoon et al[28] also described a multiple-marker PCR, where no false positives occurred, except in the case of two healthy controls expressing the MUC18 gene. This gene, however, is not specific for melanoma, and these two controls expressed none of the other markers tested.

Subsequent investigations have attempted to quantify tyrosinase expression using two different approaches. Curry et al[31] developed a competitive PCR assay with a heterologous DNA (PCR MIMIC), while Brossart et al[32] used Southern blotting of the PCR product and standardization to the expression of a housekeeping gene. In the first approach, several PCR reactions per sample are necessary, but the PCR results are truly quantitative. In the second approach, the PCR assay is semiquantitative, but the comparison with a housekeeping gene corrects for the sometimes considerable differences in efficacy of RNA extraction and cDNA synthesis.

The results reported in melanoma patients vary considerably between different laboratories. This is most obvious in stage IV patients, where the percentage with evidence for circulating melanoma cells ranges between 23% and 100%. The most likely explanation for the discrepancies is methodological differences between laboratories. Sample processing affect-

Table 1.3 Detection of circulating melanoma cells in patients with distant metastases (stage IV)

Ref	Sample processing	Marker gene	Tyrosinase mRNA-positive samples/ number of patients
23	Whole blood	Tyrosinase	4/7
26	Whole blood	Tyrosinase	21/21
27	Ficoll 1.077	Tyrosinase	25/73
29	Whole blood	Tyrosinase	0/6[a]
28	Ficoll 1.077	Multiple	46/48[b]
30	Whole blood	Tyrosinase	9/32
33	Whole blood	Tyrosinase	33/35
8	Whole blood	Tyrosinase	30/35[c] 65/81[d]

[a]Storage of blood samples without buffer at $-70°C$ prior to processing.
[b]Two of 39 healthy control samples tested positive.
[c]Untreated patients.
[d]After treatment.

ing efficacy of RNA extraction and cDNA synthesis may play a major role in these discrepancies (Table 1.3). In particular, the use of Ficoll-Hypaque density-gradient separation prior to RNA extraction may significantly decrease the number of positive results in stage IV patients. Quality-assurance initiatives have recently been undertaken in Europe and the USA to assess and ultimately resolve the methodological differences, thus facilitating the comparison of results from different laboratories.

The detection of circulating melanoma cells could be particularly useful in earlier stages of the disease, and could ultimately guide decisions concerning adjuvant treatment strategies. To date, however, the percentage of patients with stages I, II and III melanoma and the PCR evidence for circulating melanoma cells in these patients also varies considerably from one report to the next. This may be due not only to differences in methodology but also to differences in patient selection. Two analyses, however, have already suggested that PCR results are of prognostic value in melanoma: Battyani et al[27] described, that after resection of regional lymph node metastasis, the likelihood of recurrence within four months was significantly higher in patients with a positive tyrosinase signal using PCR, and that patients with stage IV disease and a positive PCR signal were significantly more likely to experience rapid disease progression within four months than patients who tested negative for tyrosinase expression in the PCR assay (Table 1.4). Mellado et al[33] reported, in a prospective investigation of stage II and III melanoma, that the presence of tyrosinase transcripts in the peripheral blood was associated with significantly shorter disease-free survival. Larger prospective investigations are necessary, and are currently under way, to confirm the prognostic value of the PCR assay, especially in melanoma patients with disease stages I through III who

Table 1.4 Tyrosinase PCR (TYR-PCR) in (a) stage II melanoma prior to lymph node dissection and (b) melanoma patients with distant metastases

(a)	Development of metastases within 6 months		
	TYR-PCR$^+$	TYR-PCR$^-$	Total
No recurrence	6	37	43
Recurrence	8 (57%)	7 (16%)	15 (26%)
Total	14	44	58
(b) **Evaluation within 4 months of PCR**	**TYR-PCR$^+$**	**TYR-PCR$^-$**	**Total**
Rapid progression	15 (60%)	7 (15%)	22 (30%)
Slow progression	5	20	25
Stable disease	5	21	26
Total	25	48	73

Modified from Battyani et al.[28]

have been rendered disease-free by surgery. These studies will also address the value of adjuvant treatment strategies (e.g. interferon-α, IFN-α) in PCR-positive and PCR-negative patients in the setting of large controlled clinical trials, and thereby investigate the possibility of guiding treatment decisions based on PCR results.

In melanoma patients with stage IV disease who have entered long-term complete remission upon treatment with IFN-α and interleukin-2 (IL-2) with or without resection of residual metastases, tyrosinase transcripts could still be detected in most patients after five years without clinical evidence of recurrence. Quantitative assessment revealed a very low number of tyrosinase transcripts, equivalent to less than 100 SK mel 28 melanoma cells.[32] It is not known whether a rise in signal intensity may serve as an early indicator of relapse.

The value of PCR for examination of solid tissue has been investigated. Lymph node preparations from patients with stage I or II melanoma were analysed pathologically and by PCR in one series of experiments.[34] Of 29 regional lymph node samples, 38% had pathological evidence of melanoma cells, whereas 66% including all pathologically positive nodes, were RT-PCR-positive as assessed by detection of tyrosinase RNA. The results of lymph node investigation are very encouraging, but larger studies are necessary to discern the clinical value of this procedure.[11]

It is important to strictly avoid contact with skin when processing tissue samples to avoid contamination of the sample with melanocytes. For peripheral blood samples, the risk of contamination with skin melanocytes is lower, and may be further reduced by discarding the first syringe of blood drawn after venipuncture and using a second syringe to draw the sample for the PCR assay.

Table 1.5 RT-PCR for prostate-specific markers in patients with prostate cancer

Ref	Target gene[a]	No. of positive samples/no. of patients	
		Localized cancer	Distant metastases
35	PSA	4/12	—
39	PSA	5/65	1/14
37	PSA	1/33	4/24
	PSM	22/33	16/24
42	PSM	40/60	—
	PSA	20/60	—
40	PSA	4/25	25/72
41	PSA	0/7	9/18

[a]PSA, prostate-specific antigen; PSM, prostate-specific membrane antigen.

Prostate cancer

Cancer of the prostate, one of the most common malignancies in older men, has a highly variable course. It may progress and metastasize rapidly or remain indolent, impairing neither survival nor quality of life. It would therefore be desirable to assess the metastatic potential of prostate cancer early. Two marker proteins have been used for serological screening purposes: prostate-specific antigen (PSA) and more recently prostate-specific membrane antigen (PSM). While PSA can be downregulated or lost during tumour progression, the expression level of PSM increases with tumour progression. Therefore PSM is an excellent candidate gene for detection of prostate cancer cells.

RT-PCR assays for both genes have been established.[35–39] No false-positive results have yet been reported from healthy controls or patients with benign prostate disease and elevated serum PSA levels. Table 1.5 summarizes the PCR results from various groups testing patients with localized or advanced prostate cancer.[35–42] The assay appears to be more sensitive for the expression of PSM than for that of PSA.[38] The frequency of positive results for either antigen increases with increasing stage of invasion.[37] Positive PCR results have been reported by several groups for patients with distant metastases but normal serum levels of PSA or PSM protein, suggesting increased sensitivity with the PCR assay as compared with serological assays. Prospective clinical investigations still have to be carried out in order to establish the clinical usefulness of PCR results in assessing prostate cancer.

Gastrointestinal cancer

Many cancers of the gastrointestinal system, such as colorectal, pancreatic and gastric carcinomas, express carcinoembryonic antigen (CEA). CEA is also expressed at a low level in normal gastrointestinal mucosa. The serological detection of CEA is well established as a method for monitoring patients with gastrointestinal cancers, though it is not completely specific. Several investigations have utilized expression of CEA to detect minimal cancer,[43] and have suggested a correlation between PCR-results and the extent of disease. Other approaches are based on the finding that many gastrointestinal carcinomas are associated with specific mutations in the K-*ras* proto-oncogene. A specific mutation in codon 12 has been detected by PCR of stool samples from patients with colorectal carcinoma[44] and in the excretory product of the pancreatic juice of patients with pancreatic carcinoma.[45,46] Current studies are testing the usefulness of this technique in screening patients for pancreatic cancer. Cell structural proteins, especially cytokeratins, have also been used as target genes to detect tumour cells.[47] Cytokeratin-18 (CK18) has long been used as target protein for immunohistological techniques, and is well established in its prognostic usefulness. Using PCR, the CK18 gene is readily detected in the blood of normal individuals, probably owing to the presence of pseudogenes.[48] Another isoform, cytokeratin-19, has led to false-positive results, even when nested PCR was employed.[49] CK20 seems to be more specific.[47] A more recent report describes the use of CD44 splice variants to detect colon carcinoma cells.[50] Further studies are required to investigate the value of these different approaches in the clinical setting.

Carcinoma of the breast

As in gastrointestinal cancers, CEA and cytokeratins have been used as target genes for detection of breast carcinoma cells.[51–53] However, because of the limited size of the studies carried out so far, the clinical utility of these approaches has not yet been established.

Neuroblastoma

Neuroblastoma, the fourth most frequent paediatric malignancy, derives from the embryonic neural crest and possesses various features of the autonomic nervous system. Although great progress has been made in the understanding of the chromosomal abnormalities involved, no specific structural abnormality has been defined suitable for detection of circulating neuroblastoma cells. Tyrosine hydroxylase, however, is frequently expressed as a tissue-specific gene suitable for detection of neuroblastoma cells.[54–57] The percentage of positive findings in bone marrow samples has been shown to increase with stage, reaching 100% (in a small series of 11 patients) in stage IV.[57] After cytotoxic treatment, tyrosinase hydroxylase mRNA disappears from peripheral blood, but it frequently resurfaces at the time of clinical relapse, and may be an early indicator of relapse.[56]

Other candidate genes for the detection of neuroblastoma include members of the *MAGE* family, *PGP9.5*, and an isoform of the adhesion molecule N-*CAM*, which utilizes exons 17 and 19. However, the investigations are so far inconclusive, and false positives have been reported.[58]

Carcinoma of the head and neck

Local recurrence of head and neck cancer occurs in up to half of the patients with microscopically negative surgical margins. Mutations in the *p53* tumour suppressor gene are the most common specific genetic alterations in carcinomas of the head and neck. Brennan et al[59] have investigated *p53* in resection margins of patients who appeared to have had complete tumour resection as determined by histopathology. The *p53* gene was amplified from DNA extracted from margins of the surgical resection specimen. The PCR products were then cloned into *E. coli*, and each clone was hybridized with a probe prepared from the patient's original tumour. This approach facilitated a semiquantitative assessment of the amount of mutated *p53* in the tissue sample. The presence of the tumour-specific *p53* mutations in the resection margins in 13 of 25 patients was associated with a significant increase in the probability of local recurrence, which is typically difficult to treat. This semiquantitative approach is labour-intensive and time-consuming, but may contribute to improving treatment strategies for this tumour.

Ewing's sarcoma

Ninety percent of reported Ewing's sarcoma cases are characterized by the chromosomal translocation t(11;22)(q24;q12). This rearrangement juxtaposes the 5' portion from a newly described gene, termed *EWS*, to the 3' part of the *FLI-1* oncogene, and is thought to represent the genetic basis of Ewing's sarcoma. RNA transcripts from this fusion gene have been utilized by several investigators[60–63] to successfully detect sarcoma cells in peripheral blood and bone marrow.

Lung cancer

Several genes have been used to detect haematogenous dissemination of lung cancer, including several that encode cell structural proteins.[64] In one study involving 40 patients with advanced small cell lung cancer, 60% of blood samples and 60% of sputum samples tested positive for bombesin mRNA, which was not detected in healthy controls (Knebel-Doeberitz, personal communication). Mutated *ras* and mutated *p53* have also been used for detection of occult lung cancer cells in sputum and blood.[65]

FUTURE PROSPECTS

Detection of tumour cells with PCR can be a very powerful and valuable tool, and we are just beginning to explore the reliability and clinical usefulness of this technology for detecting minimal cancer. A rapidly increasing number of candidate marker genes are being identified for a variety of tumours. In several instances, the presence of circulating tumour cells in the peripheral blood has been shown to correlate well with the extent of disease and therefore to be of prognostic value. This technique may be helpful in studying tumour biology and in defining risk populations. This would be especially important for tumour types that are susceptible to known adjuvant treatment strategies, since it may then be possible to base treatment decisions on 'molecular staging' in addition to conventional parameters.

It is, however, extremely important to develop this field with great caution. PCR is very susceptible to contamination. It has not been thoroughly investigated whether rare illegitimate transcription of tumour-specific genes in normal cells may cause false-positive results.[66] Prior to widespread application of these methods, it is important to establish very rigid quality assurance systems for academic centres and, in the future, for commercial laboratories. Detection of molecular signals of potential occult tumour cells by PCR cannot automatically be viewed as defining tumour cell presence and competence for further metastasis, or a disease stage warranting systemic treatment. To establish clinical utility and test the prognostic value of PCR results, large prospective studies are needed, in association with state-of-the-art clinical and pathological evaluation.[10,11]

REFERENCES

1. Osborne M, Wong GY, Asina S et al, Sensitivity on immunocytochemical detection of breast cancer cells in human bone marrow. *Cancer Res* 1991; **51:** 2706–9.

2. Lindemann F, Schlimok G, Dirschedl P et al, Prognostic significance of micrometastatic tumor cells in bone marrow of colorectal cancer patients. *Lancet* 1992; **340:** 685–9.

3. Cote RJ, Rosen PP, Lesser ML et al, Prediction of early relapse in patients with operable breast cancer by detection of occult bone marrow micrometastases. *J Clin Oncol* 1991; **9:** 1749–56.

4. Harbeck N, Untch M, Pache L, Eiermann W, Tumour cell detection in the bone marrow of breast cancer patients at primary therapy – results of a 3 year median follow-up. *Br J Cancer* 1994; **69:** 566–71.

5. Manni JL, Easton D, Berger U et al, Bone marrow micrometastases in primary breast cancer: prognostic significance after 6 years follow-up. *Eur J Cancer* 1991; **27:** 1552–5.

6. Keilholz U (for the EORTC Melanoma Cooperative Group), Diagnostic PCR in melanoma: methods and quality assurance. *Eur J*

Cancer 1996; **32**: 1661–3.

7. Chomczynski P, Sacchi N, Single step method of RNA isolation by acid guanidinium thiocyanate-phenol-chloroform extraction. *Anal Biochem* 1987; **162**: 156–9.

8. Keilholz U, Willhauke M, Scheibenbogen C et al, Polymerase chain reaction detection of circulating tumor cells. EORTC Melanoma Cooperative Group, Immunotherapy Subgroup. *Melanoma Res* 1997; **7**(Suppl 2): S133–41.

9. Kwok S, Higuchi R, Avoiding false positives with PCR. *Nature* 1989; **339**: 237–8.

10. Johnson PWM, Burchill SA, Selby PJ, The molecular detection of circulating tumour cells. *Br J Cancer* 1995; **72**: 268–76.

11. Buzaid AC, Balch CM, Polymerase chain reaction of melanoma in peripheral blood: too early to assess clinical value. *J Natl Cancer Inst* 1996; **88**: 569–70.

12. Adema G, de Boer AJ, van't Hullenaar R et al, Melanocyte lineage-specific antigens recognized by monoclonal antibodies NKI-beteb, HMB-50, and HMB-45 are encoded by a single cDNA. *Am J Pathol* 1993; **143**: 1579–85.

13. Adema GJ, de Boer AJ, Vogel AM et al, Molecular characterization of the melanoma linage specific antigen gp100. *J Biol Chem* 1994; **269**: 20126–33.

14. Kawakami Y, Eliyahu S, Delgado CH et al, Cloning the gene coding for a shared human melanoma antigen recognized by autologous T cells infiltrating into tumor. *Proc Natl Acad Sci USA* 1994; **91**: 3515–19.

15. Carrel S, Dore JF, Ruiter D et al, The EORTC melanoma group exchange program: evaluation of a multicenter monoclonal antibody study. *Int J Cancer* 1991; **48**: 836–47.

16. Scheibenbogen C, Weyers I, Ruiter D et al, Expression of the melanocyte lineage specific antigen gp100 in melanoma metastases prior to and following immunotherapy with IFN-α and IL-2. *Proc Am Soc Clin Oncol* 1996; **15**: 440.

17. Chen YT, Stockert E, Tsang S et al, Immunophenotyping of melanomas for tyrosinase: implications for vaccine development. *Proc Natl Acad Sci USA* 1995; **92**: 8125–9.

18. Marincola FM, Hijazi YM, Fetsch P et al, Analysis of expression of the melanoma-associated antigens MART-1 and gp100 in metastatic melanoma cell lines and in situ lesions. *J Immunother Emphasis Tumor Immunol* 1996; **19**: 192–205.

19. Coulie PG, Brichard V, van Pel A et al, A new gene coding for a differentiation antigen recognized by autologous cytoloytic T lymphocytes on HLA-A2 melanomas. *J Exp Med* 1994; **180**: 35–42.

20. Gaugler B, van den Eynde B, van der Bruggen P et al, Human gene MAGE-3 codes for an antigen recognized on a melanoma by autologous cytoloytic T lymphocytes. *J Exp Med* 1994; **179**: 921–30.

21. Brasseur F, Rimoldi D, Lienard D et al, Expression of MAGE genes in primary and metastatic cutaneous melanoma. *Int J Cancer* 1995; **63**: 375–80.

22. De Plaen E, Arden K, Traversari C et al, Structure, chromosomal localization and expression of twelve genes of the MAGE family. *Immunogenetics* 1994; **40**: 360–9.

23. Smith B, Selby P, Southgate J et al, Detection of melanoma cells in peripheral blood by means of reverse transcriptase and polymerase chain reaction. *Lancet* 1991; **338**: 1227–9.

24. Brossart P, Keilholz U, Willhauck M et al, Hematogenous spread of malignant melanoma cells in different stages of disease. *J Invest Dermatol* 1993; **101**: 887–9.

25. Tobal K, Sherman LS, Foss AJ, Lightman SL, Detection of melanocytes fron uveal melanoma in peripheral blood using the polymerase chain reaction. *Invest Opthalmol Vis Sci* 1993; **34**: 2622–5.

26. Brossart P, Keilholz U, Scheibenbogen C et al, Detection of residual tumor cells in patients with malignant melanoma responding to immunotherapy. *J Immunother* 1994; **15**: 38–41.

27. Battyani Z, Grob J, Xerri L et al, PCR detection of circulating melanocytes as a prognostic marker in patients with melanoma. *Arch Dermatol* 1995; **131**: 443–7.

28. Hoon DSB, Wang Y, Dale PS et al, Detection of occult melanoma cells in blood with a multiple-marker polymerase chain reaction assay. *J Clin Oncol* 1995; **13**: 2109–16.

29. Foss AJ, Guille MJ, Occleston NL et al, The detection of melanoma cells in peripheral blood by reverse transcription–polymerase chain reaction. *Br J Cancer* 1995; **72**: 155–9.

30. Kunter U, Buer J, Probst M et al, Peripheral blood tyrosinase messanger RNA detection and survival in malignant melanoma. *J Natl Cancer Inst* 1996; **88**: 590–4.

31. Curry BJ, Smith MJ, Hersey P, Detection and quantitation of melanoma cells in the circulation of patients. *Melanoma Res* 1996; **6**: 45–54.

32. Brossart P, Schmier J, Krüger S et al, A PCR-based semiquantitative assessment of malignant melanoma cells in peripheral blood. *Cancer Res* 1995; **55:** 4065–8.

33. Mellado B, Colomer D, Castel T et al, Detection of circulating neoplastic cells by reverse-transcriptase polymerase chain reaction (RT-PCR) correlates with stage and prognosis in malignant melanoma. *Proc Am Soc Clin Oncol* 1996; **15:** 433.

34. Wang X, Heller R, VanVoorhis N et al, Detection of submicroscopic lymph node metastases with polymerase chain reaction in patients with malignant melanoma. *Ann Surg* 1994; **220:** 768–74.

35. Moreno JG, Croce CM, Fischer R et al, Detection of hematogenous micrometastisis in patients with prostate cancer. *Cancer Res* 1992; **52:** 6110–12.

36. Deguchi T, Doi T, Ehara H et al, Detection of micrometastatic prostate cancer cells in lymph nodes by reverse transcriptase polymerase chain reaction. *Cancer Res* 1993; **53:** 5350–4.

37. Israeli RS, Miller WH, Su SL et al, Sensitive nested reserve transcription polymerase chain reaction detection of circulating prostatic tumor cells: comparison of prostate-specific membrane antigen and prostate-specific antigen-based assays. *Cancer Res* 1994; **54:** 6306–10.

38. Katz AE, Olsson CA, Raffo AJ et al, Molecular staging of prostate cancer with the use of an enhanced reverse transcriptase–PCR assay. *Urology* 1994; **43:** 765–75.

39. Seiden MV, Kantoff PW, Krithivas K et al, Detection of circulating tumor cells in men with localized prostate cancer. *J Clin Oncol* 1994; **12:** 2634–9.

40. Ghossein RA, Scher HI, Gerald WI et al, Detection of circulating tumor cells in patients with localized and metastatic prostatic carcinoma: clinical implications. *J Clin Oncol* 1995; **13:** 1195–200.

41. Jaakkola S, Vornanen T, Leinonen J et al, Detection of prostatic cells in peripheral blood: correlation with serum concentrations of prostate-specific antigen. *Clin Chem* 1995; **41:** 182–6.

42. Loric S, Dumas F, Eschwege P et al, Enhanced detection of hematogenous circulating prostatic cells in patients with prostate adenocarcinoma by using nested transcription polymerase chain reaction assay based on prostate-specific membrane antigen. *Clin Chem* 1995; **41:** 1698–704.

43. Gerhard M, Juhl H, Kaltoff H et al, Specific detection of carcinoembryonic antigen-expressing tumor cells in bone marrow aspirates by polymerase chain reaction. *J Clin Oncol* 1994; **12:** 725–9.

44. Sidransky D, Tokino T, Hamilton SR et al, Identification of ras oncogene mutations in the stool of patients with curable colorectal tumours. *Science* 1992; **256:** 102–5.

45. Almoguera C, Shibata D, Forrester K et al, Most human carcinomas of the exocrine pancreas contain mutant c-K-Ras genes. *Cell* 1988; **53:** 549–54.

46. Tada M, Omata M, Kawai S et al, Detection of ras gene mutations in pancreatic juice and peripheral blood of patients with pancreatic adenocarcinoma. *Cancer Res* 1993; **53:** 2472–4.

47. Burchill SA, Bradbury MF, Pittman K et al, Detection of epithelial cancer cells in peripheral blood by reverse transcriptase polymerase chain reaction. *Br J Cancer* 1994; **71:** 278–81.

48. Neumaier M, Gerhard M, Wagener C, Diagnosis of micrometastases by the amplification of tissue-specific genes. *Gene* 1995; **159:** 43–7.

49. Datta YH, Adams PT, Drobyski WR et al, Sensitive detection of occult breast cancer by the reverse transcriptase polymerase chain reaction. *J Clin Oncol* 1994; **12:** 475–82.

50. Matsumura Y, Tarin D, Significance of CD44 gene products for cancer diagnosis and disease evaluation. *Lancet* 1992; **340:** 1053–8.

51. Krismann M, Todt B, Schroder J et al, Low specificity of cytokeratin 19 reverse transcriptase–polymerase chain reaction analyses for detection of hematogenous lung cancer dissemination. *J Clin Oncol* 1995; **13:** 2769–75.

52. Schoenfeld A, Luqmani E, Smith D et al, Detection of breast cancer micrometastases in axillary lymph-nodes by using polymerase chain reaction. *Cancer Res* 1994; **54:** 2986–90.

53. Brown DC, Purushotham AD, Birnie GD, George WD, Detection of intraoperative tumor cell dissemination in patients with breast cancer by use of reverse transcription and polymerase chain reaction. *Surgery* 1995; **117:** 95–101.

54. Naito H, Kuzumaki N, Uchino J-I et al, Detection of tyrosine hydroxylase mRNA and minimal neuroblastoma cells by the reverse transcription–polymerase chain reaction. *Eur J Cancer* 1991; **27:** 762–5.

55. Mattano LA, Moss TJ, Emerson SG, Sensitive detection of rare circulating neuroblastoma cells by the reverse transcriptase-polymerase chain reaction. *Cancer Res* 1992; **52:** 4701–5.

56. Burchill SA, Bradbury FM, Smith B et al, Neuroblastoma cell detection by reverse transcriptase polymerase chain reaction (rt-PCR) for tyrosine hydroxylase messenger RNA. *Int J Cancer* 1994; **57:** 671–5.

57. Miyajima Y, Kato K, Numata S et al, Detection of neuroblastoma cells in bone marrow and peripheral blood at diagnosis by the reverse transcriptase–polymerase chain reaction for tyrosine hydroxylase mRNA. *Cancer* 1995; **75:** 2757–61.

58. Butturini A, Chen RL, Tang SQ et al, Detection of bone marrow (BM) metastases in neuroblastoma (NBL) by RT-PCR for neural and tumor associated genes. *Proc Am Soc Clin Oncol* 1996; **15:** 468.

59. Brennan JA, Mao L, Hruban RH et al, Molecular assessment of histopathological staging in squamous cell carcinoma of the head and neck. *N Engl J Med* 1995; **332:** 429–35.

60. Pfleiderer C, Zoubek A, Gruber B et al, Detection of tumour cells in peripheral blood and bone marrow from Ewing tumour patients by RT-PCR. *Int J Cancer* 1995; **64:** 135–9.

61. Delattre O, Zucman J, Melot T et al, The Ewing family of tumors – a subgroup of small round cell tumors defined by specific chimeric transcripts. *N Engl J Med* 1994; **331:** 294–9.

62. Peter M, Magdelenat H, Michon J et al, Sensitive detection of occult Ewing's cells by the reverse transcriptase–polymerase chain reaction. *Br J Cancer* 1995; **72:** 96–100.

63. Zoubek A, Pfleiderer C, Ambros PF et al, Minimal metastatic and minimal residual disease in patients with Ewing tumours. *Klin Pädiatr* 1995; **207:** 242–7.

64. Krismann M, Todt B, Gareis D et al, Low specificity of cytokeratin 19 reverse transcriptase–polymerase chain reaction analyses for detection of hematogenous lung cancer detection. *J Clin Oncol* 1995; **13:** 2769–75.

65. Mao L, Hruban RH, Boyle JO et al, Detection of oncogene mutations in sputum precedes the diagnosis of lung cancer. *Cancer Res* 1994; **54:** 1634–7.

66. Chelly J, Concordet JP, Kaplan JC, Kahn A, Illegitimate transcription: transcription of any gene in any cell. *Proc Natl Acad Sci USA* 1989; **86:** 2617–21.

2

Adjuvant therapy for colorectal cancers

Scott Wadler

INTRODUCTION

Carcinomas of the colon and rectum are the second leading cause of cancer mortality in the USA, and will have accounted for over 56 000 deaths in 1999.[1] At the time of diagnosis, only one-third of colorectal tumors are localized, with 20% having distant metastases and the remainder regional involvement.[2] While 80% of patients are potential candidates for surgical resection, the majority of these patients will not be cured with surgery alone. Thus the appropriateness of adjuvant therapy in patients with colorectal carcinoma has important public health implications as well as implications for patient care.

Patterns of failure in colorectal cancer have been well described, with distant failure being most common. For colon cancer, the most common sites of failure are lymph nodes, liver, lung and abdominal cavity. For rectal cancer, distal failure at these sites is common; however, one-fourth of these patients will fail locally as well. Failure is predicted by Dukes stage at the time of surgery. Approximately 25% of patients with transmural involvement, Dukes B2–3, will be dead by five years, and 50–60% of patients with positive lymph nodes, Dukes C, will be dead by five years.[3] For patients who present de novo with advanced disease, Dukes D, five-year survival is less than 10%.

The conceptual basis for the adjuvant therapy of colorectal cancer can be summarized by five basic principles:[4]

1. Residual tumor cells remain viable following colorectal surgery.
2. Risk factors for recurrence can be identified.
3. Therapy is most effective immediately postoperatively, when the tumor burden is low.
4. Agents with proven efficacy are available, and these must be administered at doses and for durations sufficient to eradicate these tumor cells.
5. Risk–benefit ratios must be acceptable, because many patients receiving adjuvant therapy will not benefit (either they are destined not to suffer recurrences or they will relapse despite therapy).

Current recommendations for adjuvant therapy are based on careful surgical–pathological staging criteria. As the molecular biology of colorectal carcinoma becomes better defined, it is likely that molecular markers will also become important tools for defining patient prognosis in the future.[5]

Among the systemic agents that have been tested against colorectal carcinoma, cytotoxic drugs have been the most extensively studied. Among currently available agents, only the fluorinated pyrimidine 5-fluorouracil (5-FU) has demonstrated reproducible, albeit modest, anticancer activity. Even this agent, widely regarded as the mainstay of therapy for colon cancer, in a meta-analysis produced objective responses in only 11% of patients with advanced disease.[6] Thus single-agent 5-FU must be considered to have at best only marginal activity. Combinations of 5-FU with other agents or modalities have been studied in the adjuvant setting in patients with colorectal cancer. Four main approaches have been employed:

- combination chemotherapy;
- biochemical modulation;
- chemoimmunotherapy;
- combined-modality therapy (chemotherapy plus radiation therapy).

COMBINATION CHEMOTHERAPY

Although few single agents have reproducible activity in colorectal carcinoma, there were a number of reasons for the introduction of combination chemotherapy in the treatment of this disease. Early theoretical models suggested that multiple agents, even with marginal activity would be more effective than single-agent therapy.[7] Early studies in other refractory gastrointestinal (GI) malignancies appeared to support the use of combinations of drugs.[8] Finally, an early trial from the Mayo Clinic suggested that combinations of fluoropyrimidines and nitrosoureas might be synergistic in the treatment of refractory GI malignancies.[9] Specifically, methyl-CCNU was initially felt to have activity independent of 5-FU, and this led to a number of trials with combinations of these agents.

Later trials demonstrated little single-agent activity for nitrosoureas. Therefore combinations of marginally active drugs, such as 5-FU with a nitrosourea or mitomycin C, have predictably resulted in only marginal activity, with no improvement in overall survival and a significant increase in toxicity. Therefore nitrosoureas have been eliminated from more modern regimens, and alternative approaches have been studied. These include the use of not only classical modulators of 5-FU activity, but also nonclassical modulators acting by mechanisms that may not be clearly defined and that may result in enhanced immune function.

BIOCHEMICAL MODULATION OF 5-FLUOROURACIL

5-Fluorouracil

Detailed biochemical studies of 5-FU metabolism have demonstrated that 5-FU is a prodrug, which is anabolized to the false nucleotides fluorouridine triphosphate (FUTP) and fluorodeoxyuridylate (FdUMP). FUTP is incorporated into RNA, resulting in inhibition of protein synthesis. In the presence of reduced folate, FdUMP binds covalently but reversibly to inhibit the enzyme thymidylate synthase (TS), which is the source for de novo synthesis of thymidine nucleotides. TS inhibition results in unbalanced pools of deoxynucleotide triphosphates, the immediate precursors for DNA synthesis, which may result in an increase in DNA strand breaks. 5-FU is nevertheless a relatively weak cytotoxic drug. Multiple mechanisms of resistance have been identified, involving virtually every step in 5-FU metabolism.

The process by which 5-FU acts at the cellular level is complex, and there is still considerable debate over the relative importance of RNA versus DNA effects in murine and human systems, the mechanism by which FUTP affects RNA, and the mechanism by which depletion of dTTP results in cell death. Nevertheless, there is substantial evidence that the effects of 5-FU can be modulated by a variety of agents that affect the anabolism of 5-FU and the activity of cellular cofactors and target enzymes, and that this process can enhance the lethality of 5-FU, both in experimental tumor model systems and in the clinical setting.

5-FU + leucovorin (LV)

The best studied modulating agent is the reduced folate leucovorin (LV), which is converted intracellularly to the TS cofactor N^5,N^{10}-methylenetetrahydrofolate, the donor for the methyl group that converts deoxyuridylate to thymidylate. In a murine leukemia cell model, LV stabilized the complex formed between FdUMP and TS, substantially prolonging the half-life of the complex.[10] Combinations of 5-FU and LV were more inhibitory of TS activity than 5-FU alone. There are multiple mechanisms of resistance to the combination of 5-FU + LV, however. In addition to those for 5-FU, LV requires conversion to its polyglutamylated form; an additional mechanism of resistance is impairment of the polyglutamylation mechanism.

Combinations of 5-FU and LV have been extensively studied in clinical trials. Ten randomized trials comparing 5-FU alone with 5-FU + LV in advanced colorectal cancer have been conducted. While the doses and schedules of 5-FU and 5-FU + LV differ among these trials, the results have been compared by the statistical method of meta-analysis. A summary of this analysis has been published;[6] the results indicate that the combination of 5-FU + LV doubled the objective response rates achieved with 5-FU alone (23% versus 11%); however, there was no improvement in overall survival in patients with measurable disease. In patients with evaluable disease only, the combination of 5-FU + LV did result in significant prolongation of survival and improved quality of life.[11] The combination of 5-FU + LV has been tested in large adjuvant trials in patients with colorectal cancer. Recent results indicate that six months of therapy with 5-FU + LV is equivalent both in overall survival and progression-free survival to one year of therapy with 5-FU + levamisole (see below). Because the toxicity profiles are comparable, and the shorter therapy offers some benefits in terms of overall cost of care and patient quality of life, six months of adjuvant therapy with 5-FU + LV is the preferred therapy in the adjuvant setting of colon cancer.

5-FU + methotrexate (MTX)

One of the earliest known modulators of 5-FU activity was the dihydrofolate reductase inhibitor methotrexate (MTX). MTX and its polyglutamated forms were shown to enhance binding of FdUMP to TS in mice bearing murine sarcoma S180 tumors.[12] Furthermore, pretreatment with MTX resulted in a significant increase in levels of phosphoribosyl pyrophosphate (PRPP), a cofactor necessary for the metabolism of 5-FU to FUTP. PRPP levels increased as a result of inhibition of purine synthesis by MTX. The synergistic interaction was markedly dependent on the sequence and schedule in which MTX and 5-FU were employed.[13] Reversing the sequence could result in drug antagonism.[14] In clinical trials, combinations of MTX and 5-FU have demonstrated activity in patients with advanced colorectal carcinoma, and in one trial there was an improvement in overall survival.[11] In an innovative trial, the exquisite sensitivity to schedule of administration was demonstrated for the combination.[15] The role of MTX + 5-FU combinations has been inadequately tested in the adjuvant setting.

5-FU + N-(phosphonoacetyl)-L-aspartate (PALA)

One agent that has been extensively studied as a modulating agent is the aspartate transcarbamylase inhibitor N-(phosphonoacetyl)-L-aspartate (PALA).[16] Administration of PALA in vitro or in vivo resulted in decreases in pools of UTP, CTP, dCTP, dTTP and dGTP, but not ATP, GTP or dATP. Mechanisms of synergy between 5-FU and PALA include, among others:[16]

- depletion of UTP pools, favoring incorporation of FUTP into RNA,
- decreased dCTP pools, further augmenting 5FU-induced pool imbalances;
- decreased formation of dUMP, resulting in a favorable FdUMP/dUMP ratio at the level of TS.

Combinations of PALA and 5-FU, initially felt to be highly toxic, were improved with the discovery that low-dose PALA was as effective as higher doses, but significantly more tolerable.[17] Several phase II studies have demonstrated efficacy for the combination of 5-FU + PALA alone or with LV, and a phase III trial by the Eastern Cooperative Oncology Group to compare this regimen with other modulating regimens has been completed. The results of this trial (currently in preparation) will determine whether this combination will go into further adjuvant trials.

COMBINATIONS OF FLUOROPYRIMIDINES AND IMMUNOMODULATORY AGENTS

Nonspecific immunomodulators

Interest in nonspecific immunotherapy arose from a number of early reports of tumor regression in experimental animals treated with bacterial biologic response modifiers, such as attenuated BCG, methanol extraction residue (MER) of BCG, and attenuated *Corynebacterium parvum*. Several cooperative groups in the 1970s employed immunotherapy with BCG or MER either alone or in combination with cytotoxic agents in surgical adjuvant trials, where the tumor burden was presumably low and thus where immune stimulation was postulated to be most effective. For the most part, these trials produced negative results with no improvement in survival attributed to immune therapy. The most significant improvement in overall survival, however, was observed in the NCCTG trial of 5-FU + levamisole versus levamisole alone or no adjuvant therapy,[18] which was subsequently confirmed in a larger intergroup trial. This has resulted in further clinical trials using levamisole-based modulation of 5-FU (see Table 2.4).

5-FU + levamisole

Levamisole is an antihelminthic agent, which has been employed as an immunomodulating agent (for a review see reference 19). The precise mechanism of action has not been identified. Detailed biochemical studies in human colon cancer cell lines (HCT 116, SNU-C4 and NCI-H630) demonstrated that levamisole was cytotoxic, but only at concentrations that are two logs higher than that achievable clinically. Furthermore, levamisole additively enhanced the cytotoxic effects of 5-FU against these cell lines, but only at supraphysiologic doses.[20] Thus the mechanism by which levamisole potentiates the effects of 5-FU remains to be identified.

5-FU + interferon (IFN)

As recombinant molecular techniques have allowed the purification and pharmaceutical preparation of specific cytokines to be used for clinical trials, these recombinant molecules have preferentially replaced the older immunomodulatory preparations that were either crude mixtures, such as BCG, or immunomodulators with ill-defined mechanisms, such as levamisole. The best studied of these has been the biologic response modifier interferon (IFN). IFN augments the cytotoxic effects of a variety of unrelated chemotherapeutic agents.[21] The precise cellular mechanism of action of IFN remains unclear. IFN binds to specific cellular receptors, which appear to be unique either to IFN-α and -β or to IFN-γ. A second-messenger system preserves the integrity of the message delivered to the cell. The precise nature of the second message is unknown; however, there is evidence that the pathway is mediated by a staurosporine/K252a-sensitive protein kinase.[22] As a result of IFN binding, cytoplasmic polypeptides, termed IFN-stimulated gene factors (ISGF3α and -γ), are activated, translocate to the nucleus, assemble, and bind an IFN-stimulated response element (ISRE), a 15-nucleotide sequence, resulting in activation of multiple IFN-stimulated genes.

The combination of 5-FU and IFN-α or -β exhibited therapeutic synergism against two human colon cancer cell lines, HT-29 and SW480, in vitro.[23] In HL-60 cells and a murine adenocarcinoma cell line, these effects were reversed by exogenous thymidine,[24,25] suggesting that inhibition of TS was one important locus for the interaction. Further support for this view came from the observation in H630 human colon cancer cells that IFN inhibited translation of TS at the ribosomal level, suppressing a 5-FU-induced increase in levels of the enzyme.[26] One explanation for these effects is that IFN augments the activity of the 5-FU-anabolic enzyme thymidine phosphorylase, which results in higher intracellular levels of FdUMP,[27] and thus more thorough inhibition of TS. Potentially of greater importance, IFN induces thymidine phosphorylase (TP), which catalyzes the first step in the direct conversion of 5-FU to FdUMP. This results in higher levels of TP mRNA[28] and protein,[27] and higher levels of FdUMP, the active anabolite of 5-FU.

The level of TP expression mediates the sensitivity of human colon carcinoma cells to 5-FU.[29] The in vitro TP studies have been confirmed in vivo. TP is induced in patients receiving 5-FU + IFN, and maximal induction of activity may not occur for several hours after the administration of the IFN.[30] Induction of TP by IFN, with subsequent inhibition of TS and perturbation of nucleotide pools, is accompanied by a significant increase in DNA double-strand breaks, whether measured by neutral elution[31] or pulsed field gel electrophoresis,[32,33] as compared to treatment with 5-FU alone. Presumably, this contributes to the synergy between 5-FU and IFN. Thus it is likely that the specific time points at which IFN is administered relative to 5-FU in the clinic will be critical to the modulation of the antimetabolite.

Phase I/pharmacokinetic clinical trials have demonstrated a pharmacokinetic advantage for the addition of IFN-α to 5-FU.[34-38] Using a moderate-dose infusion of 5-FU in combination with IFN ± LV, catabolism of 5-FU has decreased and area-under-the-curve for 5-FU has increased. Questions remain about whether this is a dose-dependent phenomenon. Furthermore, it was not observed using a low-dose infusion of 5-FU, suggesting that the plasma concentration of 5-FU may be a critical factor.

Despite promising preclinical and pharmacokinetic data, the results of randomized clinical trials in patients with advanced colorectal cancer treated with 5-FU + IFN have been equivocal. The first comparative study, the Corfu trial,[39] demonstrated therapeutic equivalence for 5-FU + LV versus 5-FU + IFN, with equal response rates, response durations, survival and numbers of adverse events. In contrast, the Royal Marsden study[40] demonstrated that 5-FU + IFN was no better than 5-FU administered alone. These results are in further contrast to the Strasbourg study,[41] in which there was a significant improvement in response rates, event-free survival and overall survival for 5-FU + IFN versus 5-FU alone. Other comparative clinical trials have demonstrated either no benefit or a significant benefit for 5-FU + IFN versus 5-FU alone or 5-FU + LV in patients with advanced colorectal carcinoma. In retrospect, it is clear that the sequences employed in the Royal Marsden and Corfu trials may not have offered the optimal opportunity for modulation of 5-FU by IFN, at least with respect to the data cited above for TP induction and TS inhibition. Further studies of this combination with specific attention to the interval between IFN and 5-FU as well as other dosing and scheduling issues are warranted. Furthermore, an international trial of the combination of 5-FU and IFN-β is in progress to test the efficacy of this combination. Preliminary results do not suggest a benefit for IFN-β. A recent NSABP trial (C-05) failed to demonstrate a benefit for 5-FU + LV + IFN-α versus 5-FU + LV.[42]

NEW AGENTS IN COLORECTAL CANCER

Several new agents are currently being studied in the treatment of advanced colorectal cancer: CPT-11, oxaliplatin, doxifluridine and UFT.

CPT-11 (irinotecan)

CPT-11 (irinotecan) is a derivative of camptothecin, a natural product derived from the bark and wood of the Chinese tree *Camptotheca acuminata*. CPT-11 is unique among the camptothecins in the addition of a bulky piperidino side-chain at the C-10 position. In vivo, this side-chain is cleaved enzymatically by a carboxylesterase to the active metabolite SN-38. The camptothecins are inhibitors of the cellular enzyme topoisomerase I, which is necessary for the unwinding of DNA during synthesis. Inhibition of topoisomerase I results in DNA strand breaks and cell death. CPT-11 has been shown to have activity against a broad spectrum of human tumor xenografts, including colon cancer and ovarian cancer. The dose-limiting toxicity of CPT-11 is diarrhea, probably resulting from conversion of the inactive form of the drug excreted into the bile into an activated form within the colon by bacterial enzymes. CPT-11 has been approved for the treatment of colorectal carcinomas in Europe and the USA following two randomized trials from Europe that demonstrated a survival benefit versus best supportive care or versus additional fluoropyrimidine-based treatment.[43,44]

Oxaliplatin (1-OHP)

Oxaliplatin (1-OHP) is one of a family of derivatives of cisplatin containing the 1,2-diaminocyclohexane (DACH) ligand. Oxaliplatin is of interest because of the absence of complete cross-resistance with cisplatin and for the absence of renal and significant hematologic toxicities. In preclinical systems, oxaliplatin has demonstrated activity against ovarian, breast and colon carcinomas. In current clinical trials, it has been employed using an infusional schedule alone or with 5-FU and LV in a chronomodulated schedule. Early results suggest excellent clinical activity in combination with 5-FU + LV.[45] Further trials are in progress.

Doxifluridine

Doxifluridine (5'-deoxy-5-fluorouridine, 5'-dFUrd) is a fluoropyrimidine derivative that potentially has greater clinical advantages than its anabolite, 5-FU. First, it can be administered orally, because of its excellent absorption from the gastrointestinal tract. Second, because the 5'-carbon of the ribose group lacks a hydroxyl group, it cannot serve as a substrate for uridine kinase, but can be metabolized by uridine and thymidine phosphorylase to 5-FU, which can then undergo further metabolic activation. Because of differential tissue levels of these anabolic enzymes, doxifluridine may potentially have greater tissue specificity than 5-FU. In a transplantable colon carcinoma in the rat, treatment with doxifluridine resulted in a decrease of free TS to undetectable levels for 4 hours, with 70% inhibition persisting for 24 hours. In a randomized trial, doxifluridine has demonstrated greater clinical activity than 5-FU, with a different toxicity profile.

UFT

UFT is a fixed-ratio combination of the 5-FU prodrug ftorafur (Tegafur) with uracil, which has been added to inhibit the catabolism of 5-FU. Ftorafur, originally synthesized in the Soviet Union, is slowly metabolized to 5-FU by two different pathways: one mediated by the P450 microsomal enzyme pathway and the second mediated by soluble enzymes that cleave the N-1–C-2' bond to yield 5-FU. In randomized trials, ftorafur and 5-FU have demonstrated similar clinical activity, with different toxicity profiles. UFT has largely been developed in Japan, where it has demonstrated activity against a variety of transplanted tumors in rodents. In the USA, an oral regimen of UFT in combination with LV has been tested in a phase II clinical trial in patients with advanced colorectal cancer, with activity comparable to intravenous 5-FU and LV, and is currently in phase III trials in the adjuvant setting.

FLUOROPYRIMIDINES AS RADIATION SENSITIZERS

Combinations of fluoropyrimidines and radiation therapy are important in the adjuvant therapy of rectal cancer. Despite over 30 years of study, which has demonstrated radiosensitization properties for 5-FU, there is only limited information about the mechanism by which radiation therapy and fluoropyrimidines interact at the cellular level. 5-FU-induced perturbations in cellular pools of nucleotides, rather than direct incorporation of 5-FU metabolites into DNA, are likely to be the critical step in radiosensitization.[46] Schedule questions related to cell synchronization and duration of inhibition of TS are of critical importance for determining optimal treatment strategies.

CLINICAL TRIALS OF ADJUVANT THERAPY

Early clinical trials

In the 1950s and 1960s clinical trials were organized by the Veterans Administration Surgical Oncology Group (VASOG) and the Central Oncology Group (COG) to test the efficacy of chemotherapy in patients following curative surgery for colorectal cancer.[47] The earliest agents tested included the alkylating agent thiotepa, and the fluoropyrimidines floxuridine and 5-FU. Various schedules of 5-FU were employed in sequential trials, and it subsequently became the standard for future adjuvant trials because of its acceptable side-effect profile.

Several factors may have contributed to the negative outcome of these early clinical trials. Relatively small numbers of patients were enrolled. Patients with early stages (Dukes A and B1) disease were included in the trials, and, while adequate drug doses were employed, these were rapidly attenuated for even modest toxicity, thus reducing the overall dose intensity of treatment. An important finding derived from these studies was the benefit in overall survival for the small group of patients with rectal cancer studied by the Central Oncology Group.[48] This observation subsequently formed the basis for the separation of patients with rectal and colon cancer in future studies.

Combination chemotherapy and chemoimmunotherapy trials

Based on studies that suggested synergy for the combination of 5-FU and nitrosoureas and for emerging theories of combined chemotherapy and immunotherapy, a series of adjuvant clinical trials were conducted in the 1970s to test these concepts. Most combined 5-FU with the nitrosourea methyl-CCNU (MeCCNU, semustine) in the FUMe regimen, with or without vincristine (Oncovin) in the MOF regimen (Table 2.1). Unlike the earlier trials, these trials employed larger numbers of patients, with more rigorous eligibility requirements and dose modifications. While not definitive, there was a suggestion of a survival benefit for specific subsets of patients or of a disease-free survival benefit without an overall survival benefit in the four earlier trials.

In 1988, in the National Surgical Adjuvant Breast and Bowel Project adjuvant trial C-O1, there was a statistically significant increase in survival for patients treated with BCG as compared with those undergoing surgery alone; however, this was attributed exclusively to a decrease in noncancer deaths.[53] In subsequent analyses, this survival advantage failed to be maintained.

Rectal cancer trials

Possibly the most important results to emerge from this period were from a trial of FUMe, radiation therapy (RT) or the combination versus surgery alone in rectal cancer.[54] As shown in Table 2.2, this trial demonstrated a small survival benefit for either RT or FUMe and a larger, additive benefit for the combination. These results were statistically significant, and were confirmed at a later eight-year analysis with even further separation of the survival curves. A subsequent clinical trial by the NSABP (Table 2.2) confirmed the value of adjuvant chemotherapy for patients with rectal cancer; however, in this trial, the benefits of radiation therapy alone were equivocal, with the benefits for decreased local failure only reaching borderline statistical significance.[55]

Table 2.1 Second-generation adjuvant trials

Study	n	Regimen	Outcome[a]	Ref
VASOG 5	654	• 5-FU + MeCCNU (FUMe)	Survival benefit, Dukes C1 C1	49
ECOG 2276	866	• 5-FU • 5-FU + MeCCNU (FUMe)	No differences	50
GITSG 6175	621	• 5-FU + MeCCNU (FUMe) • BCG–MER • 5-FU + MeCCNU + BCG–MER	No differences	51
SWOG 7510	626	• 5-FU + MeCCNU (FUMe) • 5-FU + MeCCNU + BCG	Improved DFS with BCG	52
NSABP C-01	1166	• 5-FU + vincristine + MeCCNU (MOF) • BCG	Better survival for MOF	53

[a] DFS, disease-free survival.

As shown in Table 2.2, more recent clinical trials have confirmed a benefit for combined modality therapy in patients with rectal cancer. In a trial by the NCCTG, employing conventional RT alone versus a 'sandwich' approach (5-FU followed by RT followed by additional 5-FU), there was a survival benefit for the combination.[56] This prompted an NCI Clinical Announcement recommending adjuvant therapy with 5-FU + RT for patients with Dukes B2–3 and C rectal cancer ('Adjuvant therapy of rectal cancer', March 14, 1991). Subsequent trials have demonstrated that the addition of the nitrosourea MeCCNU resulted in no additional survival benefit, but did result in greater toxicity, including an increase in the incidence of acute leukemia among patients receiving this drug. A trial by the NCCTG has demonstrated the value of administering 5-FU as a prolonged, venous infusion (PVI) in combination with RT, rather than in the more conventional bolus fashion.[58]

Table 2.2 Adjuvant therapy of rectal carcinoma: combined-modality therapy

Institution	n	Chemotherapy[a]	Radiation therapy	Outcome[b]	Ref
NSABP R-01	184	• None	None	Improved DFS and OS for MOF	55
	184	• None	46 Gy, 2 Gy/fx		
	187	• MeCCNU + vincristine + 5-FU (MOF)	None		
GITSG 7175	48	• None	None	Improved OS for combined-modality therapy versus surgery alone	54
	50	• None	44–48 Gy, 2 Gy/fx		
	58	• 5-FU + MeCCNU (FUMe)	None		
	46	• 5-FU + MeCCNU (FUMe)	40–44 Gy, 2 Gy/fx		
NCCTG	204	• None	45 Gy, 1.8 Gy/fx	Improved OS for combined-modality therapy	56
		• 5-FU + MeCCNU (FUMe)	45 Gy, 1.8 Gy/fx		
GITSG	199	• 5-FU	41 Gy, 1.8 Gy/fx	No benefit for MeCCNU	57
		• 5-FU + MeCCNU (FUMe)	41 Gy, 1.8 Gy/fx		
NCCTG	660	• 5-FU + MeCCNU + bolus 5-FU	54 Gy, 1.8 Gy/fx	Improved RFS and OS with PVI 5-FU; no benefit for MeCCNU	58
		• 5-FU + MeCCNU + PVI 5-FU	54 Gy, 1.8 Gy/fx		

[a] PVI, prolonged venous infusion.
[b] DFS, disease-free survival; OS, overall survival; RFS, relapse-free survival.

Radiation therapy alone as adjuvant therapy for rectal cancer

As shown in Table 2.3, a series of trials, primarily from Europe, have investigated the optimal scheduling of RT in relation to definitive surgery for rectal cancer. The advantage of preoperative radiation was that it potentially allowed a smaller operation for 'downsized' tumors. The advantages of postoperative RT were that it did not delay definitive surgical therapy; surgeons did not have to operate in a previously irradiated field, and staging could be performed more accurately. Preoperative RT resulted in a decrease in local failure as compared with surgery alone, with a small survival benefit. Trials comparing preoperative versus postoperative RT failed to demonstrate a definitive benefit for either approach in the absence of concurrent chemotherapy.

Recent clinical trials in colon cancer

One of the nonspecific immunoaugmenting agents incorporated into clinical trials in colorectal cancer in the 1980s was the antihelminthic drug levamisole. As shown in

Institution	n	Pre/postoperative	Local failure (%)	Survival	Ref
Stockholm Rectal Cancer Study Group	849	• None	25	$p = 0.02$	59
		• Preop 25 Gy	11		
EORTC	459	• None	30	No difference	60
		• Preop 34.5 Gy	15		
Danish Multicenter	494	• None	No difference	No difference	61
		• Postop 50 Gy			
Netherlands Multicenter Study	172	• None	29	No difference	62
		• Postop 50 Gy	18		
RTOG/ECOG	304	• Preop + postop	21	No difference	63
		• Postop 45 Gy	31		
Stockholm Rectal Cancer Study Group	471	• Preop 25.5 Gy	12	No difference	64
		• Postop 60 Gy	21		

Table 2.3 Adjuvant therapy of rectal carcinoma: preoperative versus postoperative radiation therapy

Table 2.4 FU/levamisole or FU/leucovorin-based adjuvant trials

Institution	n	Regimen[a]	Outcome	Ref
Windle	131	• 5-FU + Lev • 5-FU • None	5-year survival advantage for 5-FU + Lev	65
Mayo	401	• 5-FU + Lev • Lev • None	5-year survival advantage for adjuvant therapy	18
NCCTG	929	• 5-FU + Lev • Lev • None	8-year survival advantage for 5-FU + Lev	3
INT-0089	3759	• 5-FU/Lev • 5-FU/LDLV • 5-FU/HDLV • 5-FU/LDLV/Lev	6 months therapy with 5-FU/LV = 12 months with 5-FU/Lev	66

[a] Lev, levamisole; LV, leucovorin; LD, low-dose; HD, high-dose.

Table 2.4, an early British trial demonstrated an advantage for the combination of 5-FU + levamisole versus 5-FU alone or no adjuvant therapy in patients with colon cancer.[65] A subsequent, larger randomized trial was conducted by the Mayo Clinic to test 5-FU + levamisole versus levamisole alone or versus no adjuvant therapy.[18] The positive effects on overall survival for the combination therapy prompted a large intergroup trial, which demonstrated a conclusive survival advantage for patients with Dukes C colon cancer who received adjuvant therapy with this combination.[3] This intergroup trial demonstrated a 41% decrease in recurrence and a 33% decrease in the death rate, and these results have been substantiated with longer follow-up. At an update, the survival benefit was 40%.[67] The benefit for patients with Dukes B2 disease is suggestive, but questionable. Levamisole alone did not result in a survival benefit. Earlier recommendations for the adjuvant treatment of Dukes C colon cancer included the combination of 5-FU with levamisole administered as per the intergroup trial for one year. These have now been supplanted by recommendations to use 5-FU + leucovorin

Institution	Study	Projected accrual	Regimens[a]
ECOG	1292, INT-0136	2000	• Perioperative 5-FU + postoperative 5-FU/LV • Postoperative 5-FU/LV
NCCTG	914653, INT-0135	1402	• 5-FU/LV + high-dose Lev • 5-FU/LV + standard-dose Lev
EORTC	40911	1982	• 5-FU + Lev versus 5-FU + LV • Early post-operative regional 5-FU versus no early treatment
SWOG	SWOG, 9415, INT-0153	1800	• Bolus 5-FU/LV/Lev • CIVI 5-FU + Lev
NSABP	C-06	1500	• UFT + LV • 5-FU + LV

Table 2.5 Ongoing adjuvant trials in colon cancer

[a] LV, leucovorin; Lev, levamisole; CIVI, continuous intravenous infusion.

(see below) for six months, which appear to offer an equivalent benefit. In a recent trial from the Mayo Clinic,[68] six months of 5-FU-based therapy was compared with one year. There was no significant improvement in patient survival when chemotherapy was given for one year compared with six months. When chemotherapy was given for six months, standard 5-FU + levamisole was associated with inferior patient survival compared with intensive-course 5-FU + leucovorin + levamisole. These data suggest that 5-FU + levamisole for six months should not be used in clinical practice, whereas six months of treatment with 5-FU + leucovorin + levamisole is effective.

Adjuvant treatment of colon cancer with combinations of 5-FU and leucovorin

As the combination of 5-FU and the reduced folate leucovorin (LV) has been considered the standard of care for patients with advanced colorectal carcinoma, the therapeutic efficacy of the combination in the adjuvant setting is of great interest. In a trial with 1081 patients conducted by the NSABP, 5-FU + LV was found to be more effective than MOF.[69] Furthermore, the NSABP has found 5-FU + LV to be as effective as 5-FU + levamisole.[70] As shown in Table 2.5, further trials are in progress to evaluate the worth of this combination as compared to standard therapy with 5-FU + levamisole.

Adjuvant treatment of Dukes B colon cancer

Patients with tumor involvement of the bowel wall but without lymph node involvement constitute about one-third of regionally advanced disease; nevertheless, the optimal therapy for these patients is undetermined. Because these patients have a relatively good prognosis with an 80% five-year survival, subset analyses of prior adjuvant trials have failed to demonstrate a survival benefit for this subset of patients. An intergroup trial (INT-0035) was conducted from 1984 to 1987 to answer this question.[71] The results of this trial demonstrated an improvement in disease-free survival among patients receiving adjuvant chemotherapy, but no improvement in overall survival for these patients. Thus current recommendations are for adjuvant therapy only among those patients with Dukes B disease at high risk for recurrence in virtue of poor prognostic factors, such as obstruction, perforation or local invasion of adjacent organs. A recent overview from the NSABP, presented in preliminary form only,[72] has suggested, to the contrary, that all patients with Dukes B disease benefit from adjuvant therapy to the same extent as those with Dukes C disease.

Adjuvant treatment of 'D$_0$' colon cancer

A small proportion of patients with metastatic disease to the liver or lung are candidates for combined resection of all disease, including the metastases (stage D$_0$). Usually, such operations are restricted to patients who have a single focus of metastatic disease and are good surgical candidates. Approximately 25% of such patients will be long-term survivors following such an operation.[73,74] The optimal treatment, regional versus systemic, for such patients remains to be defined, as does a definitive demonstration of a survival benefit for this cohort. In a small trial from Germany, patients with isolated liver metastases underwent resection of tumor followed by intraarterial/intravenous fluorodeoxyuridine (FUdR). The preliminary report from this trial suggested a

disease-free interval of 15–31 months.[75] The North Central Cancer Treatment Group is currently conducting a randomized trial of systemic 5-FU + levamisole + LV versus 5-FU + levamisole in patients with surgical resection of total gross disease, including distant metastases (NCCTG 90-46-52). There is no conclusive evidence at this time that adjuvant therapy in this group of patients prolongs survival.

NOVEL IMMUNOLOGIC STRATEGIES IN THE ADJUVANT TREATMENT OF COLORECTAL CANCER

Immunologic strategies are of conceptual interest in the adjuvant therapy of colorectal cancer because of their greater anticancer specificity as compared with chemotherapy. Various strategies have been employed in recent years based on intriguing preclinical leads that indicate clinical activity against experimental colon cancer tumor models. One of the earliest therapies, active specific immunotherapy (ASI) using tumor-associated antigens (TAAs) as targets, dates from the 1960s, when data from animal models demonstrated that specific immunostimulation with killed tumor cells could delay the growth of isogeneic tumors in animal models.[76] The rationale for ASI was based on the premise that immunization with unique proteins on the tumor cell surface will, under appropriate conditions, elicit a host immune response that results in lethality for the tumor cell but spares normal host tissue. The major obstacle to development of these therapies was the inability to define the optimal conditions for eliciting this response.

Interest in ASI was revived in the late 1970s when it was demonstrated in an experimental guinea pig tumor model that vaccination with an admixture of irradiated syngeneic tumor cells and BCG could induce a systemic immunity capable of curing established micrometastases of line-10 hepatocellular carcinoma.[77] BCG was employed as an adjuvant because of the weak immunogenicity of the tumor cells. Induction of effective ASI depended on using large numbers of tumor cells, carefully controlling the ratio of viable BCG organisms to killed tumor cells, and using the appropriate vaccination regimen.[78] While the vaccine was effective only in animals with a limited tumor burden, this approach clearly had relevance for the treatment of patients in the adjuvant setting.

Based on these early preclinical studies, the methodology for autologous ASI was adapted to a randomized, controlled clinical trial for patients with surgically resectable but poor-prognosis colorectal carcinoma.[79,80] In this, a cryopreserved vaccine was prepared from enzymatically dissociated autologous tumor cells admixed with BCG. The results of this trial suggested a benefit in patients with colon cancer, but not rectal cancer;[81] however, this study was not definitive. The Eastern Cooperative Oncology Group has conducted a phase III trial of 5-FU + levamisole versus 5-FU + levamisole + ASI in patients with surgically resected colon cancer. Finally, a trial from the Netherlands has compared ASI alone versus no adjuvant therapy in patients with Dukes B and C disease. This trial demonstrated a recurrence-free survival benefit – especially for patients with stage II (Dukes B) disease, with a 44% risk reduction.[82]

Allogeneic ASI and generic vaccines

A far broader potential is envisioned for ASI using potent allogeneic or generic vaccines to TAAs common to most colorectal tumors. The current challenge is to identify these common TAAs and to prepare potent vaccines that recognize them. This approach, while beset with problems of antigenic heterogeneity, offers the benefits of standardization of therapy and does not require individual preparation of autologous vaccines.

In one early trial, an allogeneic vaccine was prepared from pooled, purified tumor cell membranes. In this trial, 28 patients with advanced colon cancer, Dukes B through D, were treated with a colon TAA preparation (300 µg administered monthly for three months), and antibody levels were measured.[83]

A preliminary report demonstrated antibody responses in all survivors, which correlated with long-lasting cell-mediated immunity. The median survival in this group of patients was encouraging, with 5/9 Dukes D patients surviving for more than five years.[84]

Monoclonal antibodies (MoAbs)

The use of monoclonal antibodies (MoAbs) in cancer therapy derives from the work of Pressman and Korngald, who employed radio-labelled antibodies to detect osteogenic sarcoma in vivo,[85] and from the development of the hybridoma technique,[86] which allowed the large-scale production of highly purified protein. MoAbs hold a great deal of promise in the treatment of colorectal carcinoma because of their high degree of specificity as compared with chemotherapy.

While MoAbs are currently approved for use in the radiodetection of recurrent colon cancers following definitive surgical resection, their clinical utility as therapy for colorectal carcinoma remains to be determined. A number of technical and conceptual problems remain to be overcome:

- complete identification of the broadest range of tumor-specific antigens;
- development of high-affinity antibodies;
- identification of the mechanism of cytolysis by an MoAb or MoAb conjugate;
- neutralizing antibodies against the MoAb;
- tumor cell heterogeneity and antigenic modulation.

Early clinical trials initiated against specific colon cancer antigens have failed to demonstrate a reproducible clinical benefit.

The most widely studied MoAb in colorectal carcinoma is the murine MoAb 17-1A, an IgG_{2A} molecule that recognizes a TAA (CO17-1A) expressed by virtually all colorectal carcinoma cells. In early clinical trials in patients with advanced disease, objective tumor regression has been noted; however, response rates were relatively low. Furthermore, almost all patients developed human antibodies against 17-1A.[87–89]

Table 2.6 Controlled trials of adjuvant immunotherapy in colorectal cancer

Institution	Immunotherapy[a]	Chemotherapy	Outcome[b]	Ref
Munich	• 17-1A MoAb	None	Improved RFS and OS with Ab	90
	• None	None		
Kanagawa	• None	Oral 5-FU + mitomycin C	Improved RFS and OS with combined therapy	91
	• PSK	Oral 5-FU + mitomycin C		
Harvard	• ASI	None	Improved RFS and OS with ASI in colon, but not rectal cancer	81
	• None	None		

[a] MoAb, monoclonal antibody; ASI, active specific immunotherapy.
[b] RFS, relapse-free survival; OS, overall survival.

In the adjuvant setting, however, a European trial using the MoAb 17-1A has demonstrated a survival benefit for patients treated with the antibody versus those undergoing surgery without adjuvant therapy (Table 2.6).[90] These survival benefits were confirmed at seven years.[92] Confirmatory trials are in progress.

Many other MoAbs have been identified with specificity for gastrointestinal malignancies and normal gastrointestinal tissue.[93–106] These have been employed therapeutically in patients with advanced colorectal carcinoma, either alone or as conjugates with radiopharmaceuticals, cytotoxic drugs or immunotoxins, such as ricin A chain. Still other MoAbs have been identified and studied for tumor localization.

As the vast majority of MoAbs employed clinically are murine-derived, a limiting factor remains the development of human anti-mouse antibodies by the patient, a phenomenon observed in nearly all patients treated with the 17-1A antibody. Once these anti-mouse antibodies appear, they effectively neutralize the clinical effects of the MoAb. One strategy to circumvent this problem has been immunization of patients with anti-idiotypic antibodies that induce host production of a human antibody against a specific TAA. In a rabbit model, immunization with an anti-idiotypic antibody (Ab2) to the murine MoAb 17-1A (Ab1) not only inhibited binding of Ab1 to the tumor target, but also induced production of a rabbit anti-anti-idiotypic antibody (Ab3) with specificity for both Ab2 and for the target antigen, CO17-1A. Ab3 lysed colon carcinoma cells in vitro in the presence of rabbit complement. More importantly, since this was a rabbit protein, no anti-antibody response was produced.

In a clinical trial, 30 patients with advanced colorectal carcinoma were immunized with the goat anti-idiotypic antibodies (Ab2) to monoclonal anti-CO17-1A antibody at doses of 0.5–4.0 mg of protein.[107] All patients developed anti-anti-idiotypic antibodies (Ab3) with identical binding specificities to TAA CO17-1A as Ab1 (MoAb 17-1A). While strict criteria for response were not employed, six patients had clinical benefit from this treatment, defined as shrinkage of tumor or arrest of metastases. Thus this approach, which avoids the problems inherent in employing foreign proteins that provoke neutralizing antibodies, may have clinical utility.

Monoclonal antibody conjugates

Because of their high degree of specificity, MoAbs can be linked with potent toxins that either could not be employed systemically or have potent short-range activity. Examples include conjugates with radiopharmaceuticals, chemotherapeutic agents, immunotoxins such as *Pseudomonas* exotoxin or ricin A chain, or enzymes that are capable of metabolizing circulating benign molecules to potent toxins at the tumor cell surface.

A number of radiolabeled antibodies have been produced. The advantages of various α-, β- and γ-emitters remain controversial; β-emitters, for example, are less powerful than α-emitters, but penetrate further, allowing treatment of antigen-negative cells. Phase I and dosimetry studies have been initiated with a number of radioconjugates. In a phase I trial,[108] the β-emitter rhenium-186 was conjugated with the F(ab')$_2$ fragment of NR-CO-O2, an anti-CEA MoAb. Of 19 patients studied, 15 had advanced colorectal carcinoma. The major toxicity was myelosuppression. One patient achieved a partial response. In a dosimetry study using the anti-CEA MoAb T84.66, conjugated with indium-111,[109] wide variability in tumor uptake of the radioconjugate was observed among 11 patients, suggesting that such factors as vascularity of the tumor, interstitial pressure, and antigen exposure and modulation may play an important role in antibody–tumor cell binding.[110] Thus major questions remain concerning the use of these radioconjugates. Other approaches to augmenting the biological activity of MoAbs are reviewed in reference 111.

In summary, conjugated MoAbs are a promising strategy for the development of potent, but highly specific, and therefore less toxic, agents for use in an adjuvant setting.

CONCLUSIONS

Adjuvant therapy of patients following definitive surgical resection of the primary tumor is effective in prolonging disease-free survival and overall survival, and is well tolerated in the vast majority of patients. The development of such effective therapies has had important public health implications for thousands of patients. The current standard of care for patients with Dukes C colon cancer was defined by the results of several large intergroup trials, which have demonstrated survival benefits in the range of 40% among patients receiving either one year of therapy with 5-FU and levamisole or six months of therapy with 5-FU + leucovorin. The latter is probably preferable because of the shorter course of treatment. Adjuvant therapy for patients with Dukes B2 and D$_0$ disease is unproven, although patients with poor-prognosis Dukes B2 disease are likely to benefit. For patients with rectal cancer, six months of therapy with 5-FU and radiation therapy administered concurrently prolongs overall survival. Protracted-infusion therapy with 5-FU appears to be superior to bolus 5-FU, although this approach is more costly and requires prolonged intravenous access. Biologic response modifiers and other agents that augment immune function may have a role in the adjuvant therapy of colorectal cancer, although their utility remains to be clearly defined. Preliminary data are encouraging, however. Despite significant advances, adjuvant therapy is still expensive and relatively toxic; thus further studies for shorter, less-toxic and less-expensive therapies are warranted.

REFERENCES

1. Landis SH, Murray T, Bolden S, Wingo PA, Cancer statistics, 1999. *CA Cancer J Clin* 1999; **49:** 8–32.

2. Thomas RM, Sobin LH, Gastrointestinal cancer. *Cancer* 1995; **75**(Suppl): 154–71.

3. Moertel CG, Fleming TR, MacDonald JS et al, Levamisole and fluorouracil for adjuvant therapy of resected colon carcinoma. *N Engl J Med* 1990; **322:** 352–8.

4. Steele G, Augenlicht LH, Begg CB et al, National Institutes of Health Consensus Development Conference Statement – Adjuvant therapy for patients with colon and rectal cancer. *J Am Med Assoc* 1990; **264:** 1444–50.

5. O'Connell MJ, Schaid DJ, Ganju V et al, Current status of adjuvant chemotherapy for colorectal cancer: Can molecular markers play a role in predicting prognosis? *Cancer* 1992; **70:** 1732–9.

6. Advanced Colorectal Cancer Meta-analysis Project, *J Clin Oncol* 1992; **10:** 896–903.

7. Goldie JH, Coldman AJ, Gudauskas GA, Rationale for the use of alternating, non-cross-resistant chemotherapy. *Cancer Treat Rep* 1982; **66:** 439–49.

8. Macdonald JS, Woolley PV, Smythe T et al, 5-fluorouracil, Adriamycin and mitomycin C (FAM) combination chemotherapy in the treatment of advanced gastric cancer. *Cancer* 1979; **44:** 42–7.

9. Kovach JS, Moertel CG, Schutt A et al, A controlled study of combined 1,3-bis-(2-chloroethyl)-1-nitrosourea and 5-fluorouracil therapy for advanced gastric and pancreatic cancer. *Cancer* 1974; **33:** 563–7.

10. Keyomarsi K, Moran RG, Mechanism of the cytotoxic synergism of fluoropyrimidines and folinic acid in mouse leukemic cells. *J Biol Chem* 1988; **263:** 14402–9.

11. Poon MA, O'Connell MJ, Moertel CG et al, Biochemical modulation of 5-fluorouracil: evidence of significant improvement of survival and quality of life in patients with advanced colorectal cancer. *J Clin Oncol* 1989; **7:** 1407–18.

12. Bertino JR, Fernandes DJ, Sequential methotrexate and fluorouracil: mechanisms of synergy. *Semin Oncol* 1983; **10**(Suppl 2): 2–5.

13. Benz C, Schoenberg M, Choti M, Cadman E, Schedule-dependent cytotoxicity of methotrexate and 5-fluorouracil in human colon and breast tumor cell lines. *J Clin Invest* 1980; **66:** 1162–5.

14. Tattersall MHN, Jackson RG, Connors TA, Harrap KR, Combination chemotherapy: the interaction of methotrexate and 5-fluorouracil. *Eur J Cancer* 1973; **9:** 733–41.

15. Marsh JC, Bertino JR, Katz KH et al, The influence of drug interval on the effect of methotrexate and fluorouracil in the treatment of advanced colorectal cancer. *J Clin Oncol* 1991; **9:** 371–9.

16. Grem JL, King SA, O'Dwyer PJ, Leyland-Jones B, Biochemistry and clinical activity of N-(phosphonacetyl)-L-aspartate: a review. *Cancer Res* 1988; **48:** 4441–54.

17. Martin DS, Stolfi RL, Sawyer RC et al, Therapeutic utility of utilizing low doses of N-(phosphonoacetyl)-L-aspartic acid in combination with 5-fluorouracil: a murine study with clinical relevance. *Cancer Res* 1983; **43:** 2317–21.

18. Laurie JA, Moertel CG, Fleming TR et al, Surgical adjuvant therapy of large bowel carcinoma: an evaluation of levamisole and the combination of levamisole and fluorouracil: the North Central Cancer Treatment Group and the Mayo Clinic. *J Clin Oncol* 1989; **7:** 1447–56.

19. Grem JL, Levamisole as a therapeutic agent for colorectal carcinoma. *Cancer Cells* 1990; **2:** 131–7.

20. Grem JL, Allegra CJ, Toxicity of levamisole and 5-fluorouracil in human colon carcinoma cells. *J Natl Cancer Inst* 1989; **81:** 1413–17.

21. Wadler S, Schwartz EL, Antineoplastic activity of the combination of interferon and cytotoxic agents against experimental and human malignancies: a review. *Cancer Res* 1990; **50:** 3473–86.

22. Kessler DS, Levy DE, Protein kinase activity required for an early step in interferon-α signaling. *J Biol Chem* 1991; **266:** 23471–6.

23. Wadler S, Wersto R, Weinberg V et al, Interaction of fluorouracil and interferon in human colon cancer cell lines: cytotoxic and cytokinetic effects. *Cancer Res* 1990; **50:** 5735–9.

24. Elias L, Crissman HA, Interferon effects upon the adenocarcinoma 38 and HL-60 cell lines: antiproliferative responses and synergistic interactions with halogenated pyrimidine antimetabolites. *Cancer Res* 1988; **48:** 4868–73.

25. Elias L, Sandoval JM, Interferon effects upon fluorouracil metabolism by HL-60 cells. *Biochem Biophys Res Commun* 1989; **163:** 867–74.

26. Chu E, Zinn S, Boarman D, Allegra C, Interaction of gamma-interferon and 5-fluorouracil in the H630 human colon carcinoma

cell line. *Cancer Res* 1990; **50:** 5834–40.

27. Schwartz EL, Hoffman M, O'Connor CJ, Wadler S, Stimulation of 5-fluorouracil metabolic activation by interferon-α in human colon carcinoma cells. *Biochem Biophys Res Commun* 1992; **182:** 1232–9.

28. Schwartz EL, Baptiste N, O'Connor CJ et al, Potentiation of the antitumor activity of 5-fluorouracil in colon carcinoma cells by the combination of interferon and deoxyribonucleosides results from complementary results on thymidine phosphorylase. *Cancer Res* 1994; **54:** 1472–8.

29. Schwartz EL, Baptiste N, Wadler S, Makower D, Thymidine phosphorylase mediates the sensitivity of human colon carcinoma cells to 5-fluorouracil. *J Biol Chem* 1995; **270:** 19073–7.

30. Makower D, Wadler S, Haynes H, Schwartz EL, Interferon induces thymidine phosphorylase/platelet-derived endothelial cell growth factor expression in vivo. *Clin Cancer Res* 1997; **3:** 923–32.

31. Houghton JA, Morton CL, Adkins DA, Rahman A, Locus of interaction among 5-fluorouracil, leucovorin and interferon-α2a in colon carcinoma cells. *Cancer Res* 1993; **53:** 4243–50.

32. Horowitz R, Heerdt BG, Hu X et al, Combination therapy with 5-fluorouracil and interferon-α2a induces a non-random increase in <3 mb DNA fragments in HT29 colon carcinoma cells. *Clin Cancer Res* 1997; **3:** 1317–22.

33. Horowitz RW, Zhang H-Y, Schwartz EL, Wadler, S, Measurement of deoxyuridine triphosphate and thymidine triphosphate in the extracts of thymidylate synthase-inhibited cells using a modified DNA polymerase assay. *Biochem Pharmacol* 1997; **54:** 635–8.

34. Grem JL, McAtee N, Murphy RF, Balis FM et al, A pilot study of interferon alfa-2a in combination with fluorouracil plus high-dose leucovorin in metastatic gastrointestinal carcinoma. *J Clin Oncol* 1991; **9:** 1811–21.

35. Lindley C, Bernard S, Gavigan M et al, Interferon-alpha increases 5-fluorouracil (5FU) plasma levels 64-fold within one hour: results of a phase I study. *J Interferon Res* 1990; **10:** S132.

36. Danhauser L, Gilchrist T, Friemann J et al, Effect of recombinant interferon-α 2b on the plasma pharmacokinetics of fluorouracil in patients with advanced cancer. *Proc Am Assoc Cancer Res* 1991; **32:** 176.

37. Schuller J, Czejka M, Miksche M et al, Influence of interferon α2b (IFN) ± leucovorin (LV) on pharmacokinetics (PK) of 5-fluorouracil. *Proc*

Am Soc Clin Oncol 1991; **10:** 98.

38. Sparano J, Wadler S, Einzig A et al, Phase I trial of prolonged, continuous infusion (PCI) 5-fluorouracil (5FU) and alpha-2a interferon (IFN): greater FU dose-intensity and responses in refractory cancer. *Proc Am Soc Clin Oncol* 1991; **10:** 160.

39. Corfu-A Study Group, Phase III randomized study of two fluorouracil combinations with either interferon alfa-2a or leucovorin for advanced colorectal cancer. *J Clin Oncol* 1995; **13:** 921–8.

40. Hill M, Norman A, Cunningham D et al, Royal Marsden phase III trial of fluorouracil with or without interferon alfa-2b in advanced colorectal cancer. *J Clin Oncol* 1995; **13:** 1297–302.

41. DuFour R, Husseini F, Dreyfus B, Randomized study of 5-fluorouracil (5FU) versus 5FU + alpha 2A interferon (IFN) as treatment for metastatic colorectal carcinoma (MCRC). *Ann Oncol* 1994; **5**(Suppl 8): 44.

42. Wolmark N, Bryant J, Smith R et al, Adjuvant 5-fluorouracil and leucovorin with or without interferon alfa-2a in colon carcinoma: National Surgical Adjuvant Breast and Bowel Project Protocol C-05. *J Natl Cancer Inst* 1998; **90:** 1810–16.

43. Cunningham D, Pyrhonen S, James RD et al, Randomised trial of irinotecan plus supportive care versus supportive care alone after fluorouracil failure for patients with metastatic colorectal cancer. *Lancet* 1998; **352:** 1413–18.

44. Rougier P, Van Cutsem E, Bajetta E et al, Randomised trial of irinotecan versus fluorouracil by continuous infusion after fluorouracil failure in patients with metastatic colorectal cancer. *Lancet* 1998; **352:** 1407–12.

45. Levi F, Zidani R, Misset JL, Randomised multi-centre trial of chronotherapy with oxaliplatin, fluorouracil, and folinic acid in metastatic colorectal cancer. International Organization for Cancer Chronotherapy. *Lancet* 1997; **350:** 681–6.

46. Miller EM, Kinsella TJ, Radiosensitization by fluorodeoxyuridine: effects of thymidylate synthase inhibition and cell synchronization. *Cancer Res* 1992; **52:** 1687–94.

47. Higgins GA, Donaldson RC, Humphrey EW et al, Adjuvant therapy for large bowel cancer: update of Veterans Administration Surgical Oncology Group trials. *Surg Clin North Am* 1981; **61:** 1311–20.

48. Grage TB, Moss SE, Adjuvant chemotherapy in cancer of the colon and rectum: demonstration

of effectiveness of prolonged 5-FU chemotherapy in a prospective controlled randomized trial. *Surg Clin North Am* 1981; **61**: 1321–9.

49. Higgins GA, Amadeo JH, McElhinney J et al, Efficacy of prolonged intermittent therapy with combined 5-fluorouracil and Me-CCNU following resection for carcinomas of the large bowel. *Cancer* 1984; **53**: 1–9.

50. Mansour EG, MacIntyre JW, Johnson R et al, Adjuvant studies in colorectal carcinoma: experience of the Eastern Cooperative Oncology Group (ECOG) – preliminary report. In: *Progress and Perspective in the Treatment of Gastrointestinal Tumors* (Gerard A, ed). Pergamon Press: New York, 1981: 68–75.

51. Gastrointestinal Tumor Study Group (GITSG), Adjuvant therapy of colon cancer: results of a prospectively randomized trial. *N Engl J Med* 1984; **310**: 737–41.

52. Panettiere FJ, Goodman PJ, Costanzi JJ et al, Adjuvant therapy in large bowel adenocarcinoma: long-term results of a Southwest Oncology Group study. *J Clin Oncol* 1988; **6**: 947–53.

53. Wolmark N, Fisher B, Rockette H et al, Postoperative adjuvant chemotherapy or BCG for colon cancer: results from NSABP protocol C-01. *J Natl Cancer Inst* 1988; **80**: 30–6.

54. Gastrointestinal Tumor Study Group (GITSG), Prolongation of the disease-free interval in surgically treated rectal carcinoma. *N Engl J Med* 1985; **312**: 1465–72.

55. Fisher B, Wolmark N, Rockette H et al, Postoperative adjuvant chemotherapy or radiation therapy for rectal cancer: results from NSABP R-01. *J Natl Cancer Inst* 1988; **80**: 21–9.

56. Krook JE, Moertel CG, Gunderson LL et al, Effective surgical adjuvant therapy for high-risk rectal carcinoma. *N Engl J Med* 1991; **324**: 709–15.

57. Gastrointestinal Tumor Study Group (GITSG), Radiation therapy and 5-fluorouracil (5-FU) with or without MeCCNU for the treatment of patients with surgically adjuvant adenocarcinoma of the rectum. *Proc Am Soc Clin Oncol* 1990; **9**: 106.

58. O'Connell MJ, Martensen JA, Weiand HS et al, Improving adjuvant therapy for rectal cancer by combining protracted-infusion fluorouracil with radiation therapy after curative surgery. *N Engl J Med* 1994; **331**: 502–7.

59. Stockholm Colorectal Cancer Study Group, Randomized study on preoperative radiother-apy in rectal carcinoma. *Ann Surg Oncol* 1996; **3**: 423–30.

60. Gerard A, Buyse M, Nordlinger B et al, Preoperative radiotherapy as adjuvant treatment in rectal cancer. *Ann Surg* 1988; **208**: 606–12.

61. Balslev JB, Pedersen M, Tegobuaerg PS et al, Postoperative radiotherapy in Dukes' B and C carcinoma of the rectum and rectosigmoid. A randomized multicenter study. *Cancer* 1986; **58**: 22–31.

62. Treurneit-Donker AD, van Putten WLJ, Wereldsma JCJ et al, Postoperative radiation therapy for rectal cancer. An interim analysis of a prospective randomized multicenter trial in the Netherlands. *Cancer* 1991; **67**: 2042–53.

63. Sause WT, Martz KL, Noyes D et al, RTOG-81-15 ECOG 83-23 evaluation of preoperative radiation therapy in operable rectal carcinoma. *Int J Radiat Oncol Biol Phys* 1990; **19**: 179–84.

64. Pahlman L, Glimelius B, Pre- or postoperative radiotherapy in rectal and rectosigmoid carcinoma. Report from a randomized multicenter trial. *Ann Surg* 1990; **211**: 187–95.

65. Windle R, Bell PR, Shaw D, Five year results of a randomized trial of adjuvant 5-fluorouracil and levamisole in colorectal cancer. *Br J Surg* 1987; **74**: 569–72.

66. Haller DG, Catalano PJ, Macdonald JS, Mayer RJ, Fluorouracil (FU), leucovorin (LV), and levamisole (Lev) adjuvant therapy for colon cancer: four year results of INT-0089. *Proc Am Soc Clin Oncol* 1997; **16**: 265a.

67. Moertel CG, Fleming TR, Macdonald JS et al, Fluorouracil plus levamisole as effective adjuvant therapy after resection of stage III colon carcinoma: a final report. *Ann Int Med* 1995; **122**: 321–6.

68. O'Connell MJ, Laurie JA, Kahn M et al, Prospectively randomized trial of postoperative adjuvant chemotherapy in patients with high-risk colon cancer. *J Clin Oncol* 1998; **16**: 295–300.

69. Wolmark N, Rockette H, Fisher B et al, The benefit of leucovorin-modulated fluorouracil as postoperative adjuvant therapy for primary colon cancer: results from National Surgical Adjuvant Breast and Bowel Project C-03. *J Clin Oncol* 1993; **11**: 1879–87.

70. Wolmark N, Rockette H, Mamounas EP et al, The relative efficacy of 5-FU + leucovorin (FU-LV), 5-FU + levamisole (FU-Lev), and 5-FU + leucovorin + levamisole (FU-LV-Lev)

in patients with Dukes B and C carcinoma of the colon: first report of NSABP C-04. *Proc Am Soc Clin Oncol* 1996; **15**: 205.

71. Moertel CG, Fleming TR, Macdonald JS et al, Intergroup study of fluorouracil plus levamisole as adjuvant therapy for stage II/Dukes' B2 colon cancer. *J Clin Oncol* 1995; **13**: 2936–43.

72. Mamounas EP, Rockette H, Jones et al, Comparative efficacy of adjuvant chemotherapy in patients with Duke's B vs Duke's C colon cancer: results from four NSABP adjuvant studies (C-01, C-02, C-03, C-04). *Proc Am Soc Clin Oncol* 1996; **15**: 205.

73. Adson MA, Van Heerden JA, Major hepatic resections for metastatic colorectal cancer. *Ann Surg* 1980; **191**: 576–80.

74. Mountain CF, Khalil KG, Hermes KE et al, The contribution of surgery to the management of carcinomatous pulmonary metastases. *Cancer* 1978; **41**: 833–40.

75. Safi F, Hepp G, Link KH, Beger HG, Simultaneous adjuvant regional and systemic chemotherapy after resection of liver metastases of colorectal cancer. *Proc Am Soc Clin Oncol* 1995; **14**: A544.

76. Hanna MG Jr, Hoover HC Jr, Peters LC et al, Fundamental applied aspects of successful active specific immunotherapy of cancer. In: *Principles of Cancer Biotherapy* (Oldham RK, ed). Raven Press: New York, 1987: 195–221.

77. Hanna MG Jr, Peters LC, Specific immunotherapy of established visceral micrometastases by BCG–tumor cell vaccine alone or an adjuvant to surgery. *Cancer* 1978; **42**: 2613–25.

78. Hanna MG Jr, Brandhorst JS, Peters LC, Active specific immunotherapy of residual micrometastasis: an evaluation of sources, doses and ratios of BCG with tumor cells. *Cancer Immunol Immunother* 1979; **7**: 165–73.

79. Hoover HC Jr, Surdyke MG, Dangel RB et al, Prospectively randomized trial of adjuvant active-specific immunotherapy for human colorectal cancer. *Cancer* 1985; **55**: 1236–43.

80. Hoover HC Jr, Hanna MG Jr, Active immunotherapy in colorectal cancer. *Semin Surg Oncol* 1989; **5**: 436–40.

81. Hoover HC, Brandhorst JS, Peters LC et al, Adjuvant active specific immunotherapy for human colorectal cancer: 6.5 year median follow-up of a phase III prospectively randomized trial. *J Clin Oncol* 1993; **11**: 390–9.

82. Vermorken JB, Claessen AM, van Tinteren H et al, Active specific immunotherapy for stage II

and stage III human colon cancer: a randomised trial. *Lancet* 1999; **353**: 345–50.

83. Hollinshead A, Elias EG, Arlen M et al, Specific active immunotherapy in patients with adenocarcinoma of the colon utilizing tumor-associated antigens (TAA). *Cancer* 1985; **56**: 480–9.

84. Hollinshead A, Stewart T, Elias G, Arlen M, Update on phase I specific active immunotherapy colon cancer trial: humoral/cellular specific immunity studies. *Proc Am Soc Clin Oncol* 1990; **9**: 120.

85. Adams DO, Hall T, Steplewski Z et al, Tumors undergoing rejection induced by monoclonal antibodies of the IgG_{2A} isotype contain increased numbers of macrophages activated for a distinctive form of antibody-dependent cytolysis. *Proc Natl Acad Sci USA* 1984; **81**: 3506–10.

86. Herlyn D, Steplewski Z, Herlyn M et al, Inhibition of growth of colorectal carcinoma in nude mice by monoclonal antibody. *Cancer Res* 1980; **40**: 717–21.

87. LoBuglio A, Saleh M, Lee J et al, Phase I trial of multiple large doses of murine monoclonal antibody CO-17A. I. Clinical aspects. *J Natl Cancer Inst* 1988; **80**: 932–6.

88. Sears HF, Herlyn D, Steplewski Z et al, Initial trial use of murine monoclonal antibodies as immunotherapeutic agents for gastrointestinal adenocarcinoma. *Hybridoma* 1986; **5**: S109.

89. Sears HF, Herlyn D, Steplewski Z et al, Phase II clinical trial of a murine monoclonal antibody cytotoxic for gastrointestinal carcinoma. *Cancer Res* 1990; **45**: 5910–13.

90. Riethmuller G, Schneider-Gadicke E, Schlimok G et al, Randomised trial of monoclonal antibody for adjuvant therapy of Dukes' C colorectal carcinoma. German Cancer Aid 17-1A Study Group. *Lancet* 1994; **343**: 1177–83.

91. Cooperative Study Group of Surgical Adjuvant Immunochemotherapy for Cancer of Colon and Rectum (Kanagawa), Randomized, controlled study on adjuvant immunochemotherapy with PSK in curatively resected colorectal cancer. *Dis Colon Rectum* 1992; **35**: 123–30.

92. Riethmuller G, Holz E, Schlimok G et al, Monoclonal antibody (MAB) adjuvant therapy of Dukes C colorectal carcinoma: 7-year update of a prospective randomized trial. *Proc Am Soc Clin Oncol* 1996; **15**: 444.

93. Weiner LM, Steplewski Z, Koprowski H et al, Biologic effects of gamma interferon pre-

treatment followed by monoclonal antibody 17-1A administration in patients with gastrointestinal carcinoma. *Hybridoma* 1986; **5**: S65–71.

94. Frodin J-E, Harmenberg U, Biberfeld P et al, Clinical effects of monoclonal antibodies (MAb 17-1A) in patients with metastatic colorectal carcinomas. *Hybridoma* 1988; **7**: 309–21.

95. Douillard JY, Lehur PA, Vignoud J et al, Monoclonal antibodies specific immunotherapy of gastrointestinal tumors. *Hybridoma* 1986; **5**: S139–49.

96. Verrill H, Goldberg M, Rosenbaum R et al, Clinical trial of Wistar Institute 17-1A monoclonal antibody in patients with advanced gastrointestinal adenocarcinoma: a preliminary report. *Hybridoma* 1986; **5**: S175–83.

97. Weiner LM, Moldofsky PJ, Gatenby RA et al, Antibody delivery and effector cell activation in a phase II trial of recombinant gamma-interferon and the murine monoclonal antibody CO17-1A in advanced colorectal carcinoma. *Cancer Res* 1988; **48**: 2568–73.

98. Herlyn D, Herlyn M, Ross AH et al, Efficient selection of human tumor growth-inhibitory monoclonal antibodies. *J Immunol Meth* 1984; **73**: 156–67.

99. Koprowski H, Steplewski Z, Mitchall K et al, Colorectal carcinoma antigens detected by hybridoma antibodies. *Somat Cell Genet* 1979; **5**: 957–61.

100. Blaszczyk-Thurin M, Thurin J, Hindsgaul O et al, Y and blood group B type 2 glycolipid antigens accumulate in a human gastric carcinoma cell line as detected by monoclonal antibody. Isolation and characterization by mass spectrometry and NMR spectroscopy. *J Biol Chem* 1987; **262**: 372–9.

101. Hellstrom J, Horn D, Linsley P et al, Monoclonal mouse antibodies raised against human lung carcinoma. *Cancer Res* 1986; **46**: 3917–23.

102. Epenetos AA, Courtenay-Luck N, Dhokia B et al, Antibody-guided irradiation of hepatic metastases using intrahepatically administered radiolabelled anti-CEA antibodies with simulta-neous and reversible hepatic blood flow stasis using biodegradable starch microspheres. *Nucl Med Commun* 1987; **8**: 1047–58.

103. Takahashi Y, Yamaguchi T, Kitamura K et al, Clinical application of monoclonal antibody–drug conjugates for immunotargeting chemotherapy of colorectal carcinoma. *Cancer* 1988; **61**: 881–8.

104. Drew SI, Terasaki PI, Johnson C et al, Phase I study of high dose serotherapy with cytotoxic monoclonal antibodies in patients with gastrointestinal malignancies. In: *Monoclonal Antibodies* (Chatterjee SN, ed). PSG: Littleton, 1985: 127–36.

105. Rodvien R, Grant K, Darrant L et al, Phase I study of monoclonal antibody–ricin A chain immunotoxin in metastatic colon cancer. *Proc Am Soc Clin Oncol* 1988; **7**: 427.

106. Steis R, Smith J, Bookman M et al, Evaluation of a human anti-colorectal carcinoma monoclonal antibody in patients with metastatic colorectal cancer. In: *Proceedings of Second International Conference on Monoclonal Antibody Immunoconjugates for Cancer, San Diego, CA, March 12–14, 1987*: 42.

107. Herlyn D, Wettendorff M, Schmoll E et al, Anti-idiotypic immunization of cancer patients: modulation of the immune response. *Proc Natl Acad Sci USA* 1987; **84**: 8055–9.

108. Weiden P, Fer M, Schroff R et al, RE-186 anti-CEA monoclonal antibody (mAb) therapy: phase I dose escalation study. *Proc Am Soc Clin Oncol* 1990; **9**: 185.

109. Williams LE, Beatty BG, Beatty JD et al, Estimation of monoclonal antibody-associated ^{90}Y activity needed to achieve certain tumor radiation doses in colorectal cancer patients. *Cancer Res* 1990; **50**: 1029s–30s.

110. Order SE, Sleeper AM, Stillwagon GB et al, Radiolabeled antibodies: results and potential in cancer therapy. *Cancer Res* 1990; **50**: 1011s–13s.

111. Pullyblank AM, Monson JR, Monoclonal antibody treatment of colorectal cancer. *Br J Surg* 1997; **84**: 1511–17.

3

Malignant lymphoma

Timothy M Kuzel, Ann E Traynor, Steven T Rosen

INTRODUCTION

The study of molecular mechanisms of neoplasia has provided insight into the rational development of new therapeutics for the treatment of cancer. The study of hematologic neoplasms has led to the identification and clinical exploitation of a number of novel approaches that have activity against non-Hodgkin's lymphomas (NHL). Much of the work described in this chapter represents early preclinical or clinical findings, so the precise role these agents will play in the treatment of these disorders is not clear. Drugs, such as the purine analogs, the targeted therapies or the interferons, are further along in development and have displayed activity as single agents in relapsed disease. However, they are actively being studied with other standard treatments in adjuvant approaches. A number of compounds are also described, such as the glucocorticoids, retinoids, and protein kinase A and protein kinase C modulators, which are less likely to have significant single-agent activity. These therapies, however, may lend themselves to adjuvant strategies, since toxicity with these agents will be non-overlapping with conventional chemotherapeutics.

PURINE ANTIMETABOLITE THERAPY

A newer family of drugs, the purine antimetabolites, has been developed and shown to be active in the treatment of both B- and T-lymphocyte NHL. These compounds do not have a single mechanism of action, but all ultimately interfere with intracellular regulation of deoxyribonucleotide pools, and this imbalance partially explains their cytotoxicity. This family of drugs includes 2-deoxycoformycin (DCF), fludarabine phosphate and 2-chlorodeoxyadenosine (2-CdA).[1]

DCF was the first drug to be developed. It is a transition-state inhibitor of adenosine deaminase. Inhibition of this enzyme, necessary for the conversion of adenosine to inosine, results in accumulation of 2-deoxy-ATP and subsequent inhibition of the enzyme ribonucleotide diphosphate reductase, which is necessary for DNA synthesis in dividing cells. However, DCF is also effective against cells in the resting state, where ribonucleotide diphosphate reductase levels are barely detectable. It has now been shown that deoxy-ATP accumulation in resting lymphocytes results in increased DNA strand breaks over time; this results in the activation of

Table 3.1 Response rates (%) with purine antimetabolite treatment of lymphoma

Author[ref]/drug[a]	B-cell lymphoma		T-cell lymphoma	
	Low grade	Intermediate/ high grade	MF/SS[b]	Others
ECOG[2]/DCF	29	14	66	—
ECOG[4]/fludarabine	52	14	—	—
Whelan[5]/fludarabine	48	<20	—	—
Kay[6]/2-CDA	43	—	—	—
Hickish[7]/2-CDA	31	—	—	—
Hoffman[8]/2-CDA	43	—	—	—
Betticher[9]/2-CDA	75	36	100	—
Emanuele[10]/2-CDA[c]	88	—	—	—
Canfield[11]/2-CDA[c]	50	—	—	—
Liliemark[12]/2-CDA[c]	60	—	—	—
CALGB[13]/2-CDA[c]	100	—	—	—
Grever[16]/DCF	—	—	100	—
Dearden[17]/DCF	—	—	54	15
von Hoff[18]/fludarabine	—	—	18	—
Saven[19]/2-CDA	—	—	38	57
Kuzel[20]/2-CDA	—	—	28	—
O'Brien[21]/2-CDA	—	—	18	—

[a] DCF, 2-deoxycoformycin; 2-CDA, 2-chlorodeoxyadenosine.
[b] MF, mycosis fungoides; SS, Sézary syndrome.
[c] Previously untreated patients.

a Ca^{2+}/Mg^{2+}-dependent endonuclease that produces double-stranded DNA strand breaks at internucleosomal regions, and also activation of a poly-ADP-ribose polymerase that consumes both NAD and ATP. These perturbations lead to apoptotic cell death.

Fludarabine phosphate is a fluorinated derivative of ara-A (vidarabine). This compound was known to retain cytotoxic action against leukemias, and was resistant to degradation by adenosine deaminase. Solubility was poor, however, unless the 5'-monophosphate derivative was utilized; hence fludarabine monophosphate is the 5'-monophosphate form of F-ara-A. Similarly to the mechanism of action of cytarabine (ara-C) or ara-A, fludarabine phosphate requires phosphorylation by deoxycytidine kinase to the active triphosphate metabolite F-ara-ATP. Again, this triphosphate derivative inhibits ribonucleotide reductase, resulting in nucleotide pool imbalances that prevent DNA repair, and ultimately cause apoptosis.

2-CdA represents another chemical modification of deoxyadenosine that renders the drug resistant to adenosine deaminase. After activation via deoxycytidine kinase, the triphosphate derivative similarly inhibits ribonucleotide reductase, and accumulates intracellularly, perturbing the deoxyribonucleotide pool balance, resulting in DNA damage and cell death.

Certain enzymes such as cytoplasmic 5'-nucleotidease catalyze the degradation of the active triphosphate derivatives noted above. Cells with relatively greater levels of the enzyme for activation versus that for degradation were identified as likely clinical targets. Lymphocytic disorders make good targets for these agents for these reasons, including high levels of deoxycytidine kinase, low levels of 5'-nucleotidase, and their dependence on polymerase alpha for DNA repair. It was known that T-lymphoblastoid cell lines are most sensitive to these drugs, and thus it was thought that T-lymphocyte disorders would be most sensitive in vivo.[2] However, B-lymphocyte neoplasms have also been shown to be quite responsive to these agents. See Table 3.1 for a listing of studies utilizing the purine antimetabolites for therapy of lymphoma.

B-cell lymphomas

DCF was tested in an early study conducted by the Eastern Cooperative Oncology Group (ECOG).[3] They administered the DCF at 5 mg/m²/day for three consecutive days every 21 days. There were 31 eligible patients, with a variety of histologies, all of whom had failed multiple prior therapies. Of these, 21 patients with B-lymphocytic NHL were included, and 4 (19%) achieved partial responses. Twenty-nine percent of patients with low-grade follicular lymphomas responded, while only 14% of patients with intermediate- or high-grade lym-

phomas responded. The median duration of response was 16 months among eligible patients. This study suggested that DCF has some activity in the treatment of low-grade NHL.

Subsequently, fludarabine was studied by ECOG in 62 previously treated patients with NHL.[4] Patients received 18 mg/m² of drug by intravenous bolus daily for five days every 28 days. Of 60 patients evaluable for response, 9 achieved a complete response and 9 a partial response (overall response rate 30%). Again, histologic subtype was associated with the likelihood of achieving a response. Approximately 52% of low-grade patients but only 14% of patients with intermediate- or high-grade histologies responded. The high rate of response observed for low-grade histologies confirmed the findings of Whelan et al.[5] In this study, 48% of 23 patients with low-grade histologies achieved an objective response. Less than 20% of patients with more aggressive histologies responded.

Given the responses observed in the early trials with purine antimetabolites, it was reasonable to test 2-CdA for these disorders when it became available. The group at Scripps Clinic reported the results in 40 patients with relapsed or refractory indolent NHL in 1992. Patients received 2-CdA at 0.1 mg/kg/day for seven days as a continuous infusion. In this phase II trial, eight patients achieved a complete remission, and nine a partial remission (an overall response rate of 43%).[6] The median duration of response was only five months, but responses in excess of 33 months were noted. Several smaller studies have confirmed this activity in previously treated patients. Hickish et al[7] treated 21 patients with a variety of NHLs (eight low-grade). Thirty-one percent of the patients having low-grade lymphomas responded. In collaboration with investigators at Long Island Jewish Medical Center, we treated 21 patients with a variety of relapsed low-grade lymphomas, and observed an overall response rate of 43%.[8] Longer remissions were noted, with a median duration of response of 10 months. Finally, Betticher et al[9] reported their experience with 2-CdA for the treatment of a variety of hematologic neoplasms, including 16 patients with low-grade NHL. Seventy-five percent of the patients with low-grade lymphomas responded to therapy, compared with only 36% with intermediate- or high-grade NHL ($p = 0.06$).

This demonstration of activity in relapsed patients has led to a number of trials of 2-CdA in previously untreated patients. Emanuele et al[10] administered 2-CdA to 28 patients at a dose of 0.1 mg/kg/day for seven days by continuous infusion. They observed 9 complete remissions and 14 partial remissions for an overall response rate of 88%. The median response duration was nine months. Canfield et al[11] reported results in 14 patients treated with a similar dose. The overall response rate was 50%, with two complete remissions and five partial remissions. Finally, Liliemark et al[12] treated 20 patients with a two-hour infusion schedule (5 mg/m^2) each day for five days every four weeks. They observed four complete remissions and eight partial remissions, for an overall response rate of 60%. The Cancer and Leukemia Group B (CALGB) has reported results of a two-hour infusion schedule, administering 0.14 mg/kg/day for five days[13] every 28 days for a maximum of six cycles. They have observed a 100% response rate, with 31% complete remissions. Although these results are impressive, ultimately decisions regarding choice of initial therapy for these indolent lymphomas will require randomized trials of standard alkylator therapy versus 2-CdA, comparing survival as well as response outcomes.

Finally, the encouraging results with fludarabine and 2-CdA in patients with relapsed lymphomas and as initial therapy have led to a number of trials utilizing these agents in combination with other chemotherapeutics or biologic response modifiers. Results of a phase I trial with fixed doses of fludarabine (20 mg/m^2/day $\times$ 5) and escalating doses of interferon-α (3 or 6 million IU three times a week subcutaneously) for patients with relapsed low-grade NHL established that only low doses of interferon on this schedule would be tolerated by patients (3 million IU three times a week).[14] However, of nine evaluable patients, eight achieved a partial response. Phase II studies are needed to confirm this high rate of activity for the combination. Another phase I study combined 2-CdA (escalating doses) with chlorambucil (30 mg/m^2 every two weeks) for the treatment of patients with relapsed chronic lymphocytic leukemia and low-grade NHL.[15] Only two cycles of 2-CdA at 2 mg/m^2/day for seven days by continuous infusion were tolerable. Efficacy data are pending.

T-cell lymphomas

Because of the preclinical data suggesting that the purine antimetabolites would possess significant activity against T-lymphocytic disorders, several clinical trials were performed to test this hypothesis. Unfortunately, most of the study results are difficult to interpret because of the relatively small patient populations. Two small studies utilizing DCF as a single agent at doses ranging from 4 to 10 mg/m^2 daily for three doses every 28 days included patients with mycosis fungoides (MF) or Sézary syndrome (SS).[3,16] Combining the study findings, 12 patients were treated, with 2 complete responses (16.6%) and 6 partial responses (50%). A larger study of a variety of hematologic disorders treated with DCF also included patients with MF or SS, and human T-lymphotropic virus I (HTLV I)-related adult T-cell leukemia/lymphoma (ATLL).[17] With the 4 mg/m^2 dosage for three days every 28 days, a similarly impressive response rate of 54% (1 complete response and 6 partial responses in 13 patients with MF/SS) was seen, but, interestingly, all responses were in patients with the SS; there were none in the MF patients. In the aggressive variant cutaneous T-cell lymphoma ATLL, only 3 responses in 20 patients (15%) were observed. Patients only responded if they had recently been pretreated to reduce large tumor burdens, prior to the DCF administration.

The use of fludarabine for the treatment of MF/SS has been more thoroughly tested by von Hoff et al.[18] They treated 33 patients with MF categorized as good risk (patients with no prior systemic therapy) or poor risk (patients with prior systemic therapy) with fludarabine alone at doses of 25 mg/m²/day (good risk) or 18 mg/m²/day (poor risk) for five consecutive days. One complete response and five partial responses were observed for an overall response rate of 18%.

Finally, 2-CdA has also been evaluated as a single agent for the treatment of MF/SS. Investigators at the Scripps Clinic treated eight patients with a variety of doses of the drug.[19] They observed an overall response rate of 38%, with a median duration of response of three months. A number of patients with non-MF cutaneous T-cell lymphomas were also treated in this study; these patients experienced a 57% response rate. At Northwestern University, we have treated 21 patients with MF/SS.[20] All patients had failed at least one prior therapy. There were three complete responses and three partial responses (overall response rate 28%). However, the median duration of response in this heavily pretreated population was only four months. No patient with a large-cell variant histology (three patients) responded. Two other trials included small numbers of patients with MF/SS, and have been published.[9,21] Betticher et al[9] summarized their experience with 2-CdA for a number of malignancies; two patients with MF were included in this group. Both patients achieved responses persisting at three and six months at the time of the report. O'Brien et al[21] treated 11 patients with MF/SS as part of a larger trial of T-cell malignancies. They witnessed two responses, for a response rate of 18%.

Given the single-agent activity of this class of drugs cited above, several groups have combined these compounds with interferon-α (IFN-α). Investigators at the National Cancer Institute (NCI) conducted a phase II trial alternating cycles of DCF at a dose of 4 mg/m²/day for three days with intermittent high-dose IFN-α.[22] They observed a response rate of 41%, with a median time to progression of 13.1 months, not dramatically different from might be expected with either agent used singly. Of note, however, two SS patients achieved complete responses – one lasting in excess of five

years. Another NCI trial combined fludarabine (25 mg/m²/day for five days) with concurrent low-dose IFN-α2a (5 million IU/m² three times a week).[23] A response rate of 51% was reported, with four (11%) complete responses and 14 partial responses in a group of heavily pretreated patients. Three of the complete responders had SS and one had tumor-stage MF. The median time to progression was 5.8 months, which is shorter than that reported for the combination of DCF and IFN-α, but three of the four complete responders had unmaintained remissions for 18+, 20+ and 35+ months.

Toxicity

The similarity in the mechanisms of action of these compounds would suggest that toxicities associated with the various compounds would be similar. However, this has definitely not been the case. There are distinct differences in the spectrum of both acute and chronic toxicities with these compounds. The trials with DCF and fludarabine have revealed a much higher incidence of nausea and vomiting, and alopecia than is commonly associated with 2-CdA. The most significant toxicities seen with DCF and fludarabine, however, are neurotoxicity and immunosuppression. In reviewing the two studies combining IFN-α with either DCF or fludarabine, a 15–17% incidence of sepsis and a 5–14% incidence of opportunistic infections, including disseminated toxoplasmosis, cytomegaloviral infection, *Pneumocystis carinii* pneumonia, atypical mycobacterial infection and fungemia, was observed. This was likely due to both immunosuppression related to purine analog therapy and intrinsically impaired immune function.[14,22] In addition, 14–17% of patients developed severe neurotoxicity in the form of confusion, motor weakness, parasthesias and central nervous system demyelination. A review by Cheson et al[24] documents the spectrum of neurotoxicities associated with purine analog therapy.

2-CdA therapy is extremely well tolerated acutely, but may result in somewhat greater myelosuppression than the earlier-developed agents. This myelosuppression may be even more significant when the agent is used to treat T-lymphocyte disorders compared with B-lymphocyte diseases.[25] In the study by Betticher et al,[9] significant decrements in neutrophils and lymphocyte populations occurred in 46% and 41% respectively. Interestingly, the degree of lymphopenia correlated with the likelihood of response to therapy for patients with NHL, with lower lymphocyte counts on day 14 for responders versus non-responders. A number of the studies detailed above suggest that myelosuppression is worse in patients having pretreatment with alkylator agents, with involvement of bone marrow by lymphoma, or undergoing a greater number of cycles of 2-CdA therapy. In our study of 2-CdA for MF/SS, we reduced the days of therapy delivered by continuous infusion to five, from the usual seven, because of a perception that the toxicity (primarily prolonged thrombocytopenia) was unacceptable.[20]

These results suggest that patients treated with these agents should be carefully evaluated for infectious complications, especially opportunistic infections, and that prophylactic therapy should be considered during and following therapy if significant immunosuppression is documented. Additionally, one should carefully consider the value of continuing to administer cycles of therapy if there is no evidence of further improvement in clinical response, because of the risk of sudden development of prolonged cytopenias that may limit further therapeutic approaches.

TARGETED THERAPY OF HEMATOLOGIC NEOPLASMS

Antibody-based therapies have now been utilized in an attempt to treat human disease for nearly 50 years. The initial trials involved unconjugated polyclonal antibodies or radiolabeled polyclonal antibodies developed by immunization of an intermediate species of animal with the target antigen. Since the late 1970s, however, the trials have taken advantage of a technique to raise monoclonal antibodies with desired specificity.[26] Despite some recent notable breakthroughs with the use of unconjugated 'naked' monoclonal antibodies, the overall benefit observed in cancer patients has been quite limited (overall response rates of 5%) when taken in aggregate.[27,28] The major benefit from these trials was the identification of the limitations of monoclonal antibody-based therapy. These included poor tumor penetration in terms of percentage of administered dose, poor interactions with antibody Fc receptors and human effector cells, and the recognition of the presence of tumor antigen-expression heterogeneity. Additionally, since many of the early trials were conducted with murine-derived monoclonal antibodies, development of human anti-mouse antibodies resulting in altered pharmacokinetics of the infused antibody was identified as the major obstacle to successful therapy of human malignancies. Still, lymphoma represents the most sensitive neoplasm to therapy with these agents. Therefore this chapter will broadly discuss some of the notable trial results, outline limitations of this treatment approach, and alert the reader to newer strategies being developed. A detailed discussion of all the clinical trials reviewed to date is, however, beyond the scope of this chapter. The interested reader should consult several thorough overviews of this approach.[29–32]

Unconjugated monoclonal antibody therapy

Theoretically, unconjugated monoclonal antibodies could be utilized to eradicate human neoplastic cells by several different mechanisms.[33] These include antibody-dependent cellular cytotoxicity, through complement activation, or by aiding in the phagocytosis of tumor cells. They may be able to regulate cellular proliferation by binding to growth factor receptors, to the growth factor directly, or to tumor antigens that trigger apoptosis. Finally, strategies utilizing the immunogenicity of these molecules to generate vaccine-type responses are being explored.

T-cell lymphomas

Mycosis fungoides was chosen as an early tumor type for study because of the ability to study tumor lesions for the presence of the target antigen prior to therapy, and to assess antibody penetration into lesions during and after treatment. The monoclonal antibody T-101, a 65 kDa protein, recognizes CD5, an antigen present on mature T-lymphocytes, the malignant cell in MF and the neoplastic B-lymphocyte in chronic lymphocytic leukemia. In several studies using a variety of dosage schemes, 6 of 14 patients with MF manifested significant but short responses (several months).[34,35] A decrease in circulating neoplastic cells was observed in all patients. Binding to tumor cells was demonstrated in vivo in skin, bone marrow, blood and lymph nodes. Toxicity consisted of fevers and chills; up to 30% of patients manifested allergic-type reactions, with pruritus and urticaria. There were anaphylactoid-type reactions when rapid infusion schedules were utilized, manifested as wheezing and hypotension. Pretreatment with steroids or diphenhydramine hydrochloride controlled or prevented many of these side-effects.

These early studies first identified the problem of human anti-mouse antibodies complicating this form of treatment. Approximately 50% of the MF patients developed these antibodies. High levels of the anti-mouse antibodies were associated with lower peak T-101 serum levels and a lack of clinical response. The investigators, recognizing the limitations of this approach, recommended further trials with radiolabeled antibody in order to attain greater cytotoxicity in a shorter period of therapy.

B-cell lymphomas

As the development of clearing or neutralizing anti-mouse antibodies was identified, strategies to circumvent this problem were devised. Attempts at plasmapheresis prior to retreatment have had modest success.[36] A 40–60% reduction in human anti-mouse antibodies can be demonstrated after each plasma exchange.[37] Treating patients with large doses of unconjugated monoclonal antibodies may serve to saturate the human anti-mouse antibody (or as a pre-treatment prior to infusion of an immunoconjugate). A single dose of unlabeled antibody (equal to the total calculated human anti-mouse antibody binding capacity based on in vitro high-performance liquid chromatography analysis) will bind approximately 99% of circulating neutralizing antibody.[37] Immunosuppression with low doses of cytotoxic agents, such as cyclophosphamide, azothioprine or cyclosporine (cyclosporin A), has also been utilized in an attempt to reduce the human anti-mouse immune response.[38,39] Treatment with cyclosporine for six days during a monoclonal antibody infusion (anti-CEA) reduced the mean levels of the human anti-mouse antibody response to 3.5 µg/ml (three patients) versus 1988 µg/ml (three control patients). A combination of azothioprine and prednisone afforded patients a greater likelihood of retreatment (based on anti-mouse antibody levels and skin tests) than patients who received either no immunosuppression or moderate-dose cyclophosphamide and prednisone.

Ultimately, however, the simplest strategy involved shifting cellular targets. B-cell lymphomas provide an ideal system for studying the repeated administration of a therapeutic monoclonal antibody, because patients with these lymphomas are often inherently immunocompromised owing to the underlying lymphoma, and thus manifest a lesser human anti-mouse antibody response. B-cell lymphomas also express a variety of pan-B-cell antigens against which therapy could be targeted. Finally, they also may express on their surface a true tumor-associated antigen, the surface immunoglobulin molecule, whose idiotype is unique to the neoplastic clone of lymphocytes.

Press et al[40] utilized a monoclonal antibody directed against CD20, a 35 kDa B-cell antigen. They administered to four patients 50–2380 mg of the antibody as a continuous infusion over several days. Even low doses (5–10 mg/m²/day) could clear circulating neoplastic lymphocytes, but much larger doses (100–800 mg/m²/day) were required to coat target lymphocytes in nodes or the bone marrow. One patient achieved a partial response, but again the duration was short-lived, lasting six weeks. Minimal toxicity was recognized.

Meeker et al[41] chose to treat 14 patients with refractory B-cell lymphomas with anti-idiotype antibodies. Patients were treated in a dose-escalation fashion with cumulative doses ranging from 500 mg to 15 000 mg. In this sentinel approach to lymphoma therapy with anti-idiotype antibodies, one complete response (duration six years) and seven partial responses were observed. Interestingly, free circulating antigen was noted to be present in many patients, and clearing of such material had to be achieved prior to the development of antitumor responses. Immunogenicity in this group of heavily pretreated B-cell lymphomas was minimal. Ultimately, however, this form of therapy was limited by the slow process of developing a monoclonal antibody specific for each patient's tumor. There was some hope that patients would have cross-reactivity to antibodies (shared idiotypes) developed for other patient tumors, but the cumbersome procedures required to evaluate this for a prospective patient limited the direct routine application of such therapy.

The striking efficacy noted in these early trials led to further trials with unconjugated antibodies, however, utilizing new technologies that may finally lead to therapeutic products available to practicing oncologists. These latest-generation monoclonal antibodies are 'chimeric' human–murine antibodies. The constant region of monoclonal antibodies proved to be the most immunogenic portion (probably because of relative size) compared with the binding site variable region. Using molecular biological techniques developed in the last decade, it has become possible to express the gene for a murine variable region and the gene for a human constant region in the same hybridoma. This has allowed for optimization of isotype selection for interaction with host effector cells, while retaining the specificity of the murine antibody. Most importantly, this approach greatly reduces the immunogenicity of the chimeric monoclonal antibody.

The best results to date have been obtained with a chimeric anti-CD20 monoclonal anti-

body (IDEC-C2B8; Rituxan). This molecule is an IgG1 κ antibody that recognizes the CD20 pan-B-cell antigen expressed on both normal and malignant B lymphocytes.[42] The antibody binds complement, and effects both cell-dependent cytotoxicity and antibody-dependent cellular cytotoxicity, but perhaps most importantly, induces tumor cell apoptosis in vitro after binding to the receptor.[43] A number of phase I trials in patients with low-grade relapsed NHL have been reported.[44-46] The antibody appeared to be well tolerated, with treatment-related symptoms correlating with the number of circulating $CD20^+$ cells in the blood. Common adverse events included fever, fatigue, rigors, rash, hypotension and thrombocytopenia. Side-effects were worst during the initial infusions in the multiple-dose trials, and rare during later infusions. No quantifiable human anti-chimeric antibody response was noted. The maximum tolerated dose of antibody was 375 mg/m². Despite being dose-escalation phase I trials, 9 partial responses in 33 evaluable patients were observed. Subsequently, these investigators performed a phase II trial administering 375 mg/m² once weekly for four consecutive weeks to 37 patients with advanced, low-grade NHL.[47] The toxicity noted did not differ markedly from that observed in phase I trials. Of 34 evaluable patients, 17 achieved a complete or partial response (50%), with a median duration of response of 10.3 months. Several patients treated on the phase I trials were allowed to be retreated in the phase II portion; 80% responded to rechallenge with the drug.

The results in a larger confirmatory pivotal trial involving 166 patients with relapsed low-grade NHL led to the molecule being approved by the Food and Drug Administration for this indication. Using the four-dose schedule described above, an overall response rate of 48% was achieved, including 6% complete responses.[48]

Investigators assessing bcl-2 status prospectively have noted that 12 of 19 patients with peripheral blood positivity by polymerase chain reaction prior to treatment have become negative by the fourth infusion, and 4/5 patients with three-month follow-up remain negative.[49] It remains to be shown that these results are a reliable surrogate marker of efficacy, or that this is dramatically different than the experience with other standard chemotherapeutics.

In addition to the mechanisms of action noted above, there is in vitro evidence of synergy with chemotherapeutic agents, suggesting that combination approaches to the treatment of lymphoma would be worthwhile.[50] Therefore Czuczman et al undertook a combination trial of IDEC-C2B8 with cyclophosphamide, doxorubicin, vincristine and prednisone for initial therapy of low-grade NHL. In this trial, the antibody was administered twice in week 1, and then once in weeks 7, 13, 20 and 21. In the preliminary report,[50] 100% of 14 evaluable patients responded to therapy. The biologic endpoint of bcl-2 positivity was again studied; 4/4 patients who had completed therapy and who were positive for bcl-2 by polymerase chain reaction pretreatment had converted to bcl-2-negative status.

Future directions

Some investigators have chosen to exploit the immunogenicity of murine monoclonal antibodies with therapeutic intent. Foon and his colleagues administered a murine monoclonal antibody (4DC6), an anti-idiotype antibody raised against a monoclonal antibody that targets a highly restricted T-lymphocyte antigen expressed on neoplastic T cells in a variety of neoplastic T-cell processes, to four patients with MF/SS.[51] A host antibody response to this murine monoclonal antibody should cross-react with the tumor antigen, and theoretically enhance the host antitumor response. One of four patients experienced a major reduction in tumor masses persisting for 11 months. Humoral and cell-mediated response to the antibody were noted in all patients but proof of antitumor effect due to this response has not been conclusively demonstrated.

Another group chose to administer murine anti-idiotype monoclonal antibodies generated from individual patient lymph node specimens obtained at the time of enrollment.[52] Thirty-eight patients with advanced-stage follicular lymphomas have completed therapy. Patients initially received cytoreductive chemotherapy (20 complete and 18 partial responders). They then received a series of at least five immunizations with antibody admixed with a carrier protein (plus or minus an immunologic adjuvant). Twenty patients developed some sort of specific humoral anti-idiotype response. All patients developed an immune response to the carrier protein (confirming immunocompetence). Time to progression was 4.7 years for patients who developed an immune response, versus 0.7 years for those who did not ($p < 0.001$). The presence of measurable lymphoma at the time of immunization correlated with ability to respond to the anti-idiotype response. These studies suggest that generation of a specific humoral response against patient lymphomas may have a therapeutic role in the future. Obviously these studies need to control for the possible prognostic importance of being able to mount an immune response as a marker of patients destined for prolonged survival.

Immunoconjugate targeted therapy

Although occasional dramatic successes are now being seen in trials utilizing unconjugated monoclonal antibodies, new approaches are still being explored. To enhance the cytotoxicity of monoclonal antibodies, agents such as chemotherapeutic drugs, radionuclides or toxins may be conjugated to the antibody (Table 3.2). The monoclonal antibody acts as a carrier for the delivery of these toxic agents to neoplastic cells, ideally sparing normal tissues. Attempts using antibodies to carry various chemotherapeutic agents have been the least studied in humans. At doses of drug adequate to achieve the desired clinical response, problems with precipitation of the complex, polymerization or loss of immunoreactivity (specificity of binding) were noted.[53] Therefore most clinical trials have focused on conjugates of monoclonal antibodies and radioisotopes or plant and bacterial protein toxins.

Table 3.2 Isotopes and toxins for monoclonal antibody therapy

Isotope	Decay type	Half-life	Path length (mm)	Advantages
^{131}I	β/γ	8 days	0.8	Inexpensive, standard labeling technique
^{125}I	Auger-electron low-energy γ	60 days	0.001–0.02	Minimal external radiation for healthcare personnel (isotope must be internalized for cell killing)
^{90}Y	β	2.6 days	5.3	High-energy emission; radiolabeling using bifunctional chelating agents
^{186}Re	β/γ	3.75 days	1.8	Therapeutic analog of technetium; γ emission ideal for imaging
^{188}Re	β/γ	18 h	4.4	See ^{186}Re; generator product
^{212}Bi	α	1 h	0.04–0.08	High energy/short range
^{211}At	α	7.2 h	0.04–0.08	High energy/short range

Toxin	Mechanism of action
Ricin (plant)	Blocks assembly of 60S ribosomal subunit via inhibition of EF-2
Saporin (plant)	Blocks assembly of 60S ribosomal subunit via modification of one of several nucleoside residues
Trichothecenes (fungus)	Family of toxins that inhibit synthesis of proteins by interfering with ribosomal initiation or peptide elongation
Diphtheria (bacterium)	Blocks assembly of 60S ribosomal subunit via inhibition of EF-2

Radioimmunoconjugates

The most extensively studied class of immuno-conjugate is the radioimmunoconjugate. In spite of the multitude of trials to date, no single isotope has been identified as optimal. Table 3.2 lists a number of commonly utilized radioisotopes and their physical characteristics. Early trials primarily were conducted with iodine-131 (^{131}I) for several reasons: it is an inexpensive isotope, the labeling techniques available were ideal for this isotope, and both imaging (γ emission) and therapeutic benefit (β emission) were achievable with the same isotope. The long range of penetration associated with γ rays, however, has limited the use of agents with significant γ emission. These agents give rise to radiation safety concerns when utilized in high doses. Patients require strict isolation to prevent harm to family members, other patients and allied health care professionals. In addition, dehalogenation (breakage of the linkage of the antibody to the isotope) occurs despite the standard conjugating methods, and elimination in urine or feces is seen.

With advances in radiochemical methodology, other isotopes have been evaluated for use as immunoconjugates. α-emitting radionuclides, which have a high linear energy transfer but a short range (astatine-211, ^{211}At, or bismuth-212, ^{212}Bi) are being investigated, but their γ radiation may have disadvantages similar to those arising with ^{131}I. ^{125}I produces low-energy γ radiation from its Auger-electron decay. These Auger electrons have very short ranges (10 μm) and may best be utilized in conjunction with antibodies that are internalized into cells.[54] Finally, isotopes with β emissions are increasingly utilized for radioimmunotherapy. These isotopes can have cytotoxic effects over a longer range without the bothersome γ decay. An example of a β-emitting isotope is yttrium-90 (^{90}Y), which has a half-life of 64 hours and an effective path length of 5.4 mm (the radius of a sphere in which 90% of the radiation is deposited). This allows effective tumor irradiation, even if substantial numbers of neoplastic cells are antigen-negative. Uptake into small tumor deposits may result in undesirable irradiation of normal tissue, and the avidity of ^{90}Y for bone also contributes to its toxicity. Improved radiochemical techniques to conjugate antibodies to ^{90}Y may reduce in vivo separation and resultant myelosuppression.

Immunotoxins

To avoid toxicity to normal organs (especially the bone marrow) associated with radio-immunoconjugates, plant or bacterial toxins are increasingly being used as the toxic moiety conjugated to an antibody (see Table 3.2). These molecules share a number of common features:

- they are heterodimers with two chains;
- one chain (the A chain) usually imparts cytotoxicity via inhibition of protein synthesis;
- the other chain (the B chain) is responsible for binding to mammalian cells and possesses a membrane-translocating ability.

The toxins most commonly chosen include the plant toxin ricin (either the A chain alone or with chemical modifications to 'block' non-specific cellular binding), the diphtheria toxin or *Pseudomonas* exotoxin. A variety of early-phase trials have demonstrated the ability of these constructs to induce tumor responses. However, these immunoconjugates have very short half-lives, and thus require continuous infusions or very high doses of therapy to achieve satisfactory tumor cell exposure times. Immune responses against these constructs can be brisk, directed against not only the antibody but also the toxin moiety. Antibodies can be either neutralizing or non-neutralizing (which can increase circulating half-life). Toxicity is related to hepatic scavenging of the immunoconjugate with non-specific injury (elevated liver function tests, hypoalbuminemia and a poorly understood capillary leak-like syndrome).

Radioimmunoconjugate therapy of T-cell lymphomas

Since much of the early work with unconjugated monoclonal antibodies utilized the antibody T-101 for therapy of T-cell lymphomas, this antibody was used in an early radioimmunotherapy trial conjugated to ^{131}I for the treatment of cutaneous T-cell lymphoma. Rosen et al[55] administered 5.6–13.1 mCi of ^{131}I conjugated to 9.6–10.5 mg of antibody to six patients to assess the biodistribution of the radiolabeled monoclonal antibody, and to predict radiation doses absorbed by specific tumor or organ sites. Inguinal and axillary adenopathy could be detected by γ scintigraphy during the imaging phase. Five patients subsequently received therapeutic doses of 100.5–150 mCi of ^{131}I conjugated to 9.9–16.9 mg of antibody. Two partial remissions of two months duration were observed. Regression of skin lesions and enlarged lymph nodes were observed, and all patients reported diminished pruritus after treatment. These responses were observed despite dosimetry calculations that suggested that responding skin lesions received only modest doses of radiation (40–510 cGy). Additionally, whole-body radiation exposures ranged from 28 to 89 cGy. Thus this study illustrated a finding common in many subsequent radiolabeled monoclonal antibody studies: microdosimetry calculations of radiation doses absorbed at the cellular level need to be developed, and the possible relation of exposure time, as well as total radiation dose, to tumor response needs to be explored. External planar imaging via a γ camera may not be the ideal way to define the dosimetry; there are now preliminary data suggesting that single-photon-emission computed tomography[56] or positron-emission tomography[57] may be preferable. The interested reader should seek out an excellent review[32] on radioimmunoconjugates for speculation on mechanisms whereby radioimmunotherapy exerts its cytotoxic effects despite lower theoretical radiation effectiveness. Mild reversible myelosuppression was the only toxicity witnessed in this trial.

Only a few other trials of radioimmunotherapy for T-cell diseases are underway, notably trials of radiolabeled anti-Tac (directed against the α chain of the human interleukin-2 receptor). Waldmann and his colleagues at the National Cancer Institute have treated patients with retrovirus-related acute T-cell lymphoma/leukemia, and have observed some partial and complete remissions.[58]

Radioimmunoconjugate therapy of B-cell lymphomas

DeNardo and co-workers[32,59] have performed many of the studies of radioimmunotherapy for B-cell lymphomas. They have used Lym-1, an IgG2a monoclonal antibody with specificity for malignant B cells, which binds to a polymorphic variant of the HLA-Dr antigen.[60] This antibody has been shown to be inactive as a single agent in unconjugated fashion.[61] In their initial phase I/II trials, 25 patients with relapsed low-grade NHL that expressed Lym-1 received 10–100 mCi ^{131}I-labeled antibody after a preload of unconjugated Lym-1. Twelve of the patients achieved a response to therapy; interestingly, 94% of patients who received cumulative radiation doses in excess of 180 mCi achieved remissions. In a subsequent trial, 21 patients were treated with escalating infusions of ^{131}I-labeled Lym-1 (40–100 mCi/m²) to determine the maximum tolerated dose; 75% of patients had intermediate- or high-grade lymphoma. Toxicity noted included myelosuppression, hypotension in one patient, and occasional vomiting. There were 7 complete and 4 partial responses (52%), with a mean duration and response of 10 months. It was found that 100 mCi/m² was a safe dose for multi-institution studies in patients selected to exclude more than 20% marrow involvement, or 80 mCi/m² if marrow status was not known.[62]

Another multicenter trial was attempted to determine the maximum tolerated dose of ^{131}I-labeled Lym-1 in single-dose escalating fashion in intermediate- and high-grade lymphomas.[63] Thirteen patients were treated, many with refractory disease. Four partial responses were observed, with a median duration of response of 4.5 months. Myelosuppression was established as the dose-limiting toxicity, with the maximum tolerated dose established at 65 mCi/m². The limited number and short duration of the responses suggested that this agent was no better than standard multi-agent chemotherapy for this population of patients.

Subsequently, DeNardo et al[64] have reported preliminary results with copper-67 ([67]Cu)-labeled Lym-1 in patients with low-grade NHL. Two of three patients achieved a response warranting further exploration. Thus the precise role for this antibody has not been established. The ideal dosing schedule has not been defined, nor has the isotope of choice been settled. Studies are underway in an attempt to clarify these issues.

Several other pan-B-cell monoclonal antibodies have been utilized in clinical trials. Goldenberg et al[65] studied the biodistribution, toxicity and efficacy of ^{131}I-labeled LL2, an antibody that targets the pan-B-cell antigen, CD22. In this combined radioimmunodiagnostic and radioimmunotherapy protocol, 16 patients were initially accrued. All patients had a history of B-cell NHL. Based on the results of imaging studies, seven patients were enrolled in the therapeutic portion of the study. Patients were to receive cycles of 30 and 20 mCi of radiation, one week apart. Two achieved partial responses after one cycle, with a median duration of response of approximately three months. Interestingly, one patient developed a partial response after a diagnostic dose of only 6.2 mCi, and, with subsequent doses of 8.0 and 9.9 mCi of ^{131}I, this evolved into a complete response. Total-body radiation exposure ranged from 2.4 to 61.4 cGy. Severe myelotoxicity was seen in three of the seven patients given therapeutic doses (the total radiation dose administered was approximately 50 mCi in all cases). Chimeric versions of LL2 have been developed, and may enter clinical testing.

Kaminski et al[66,67] investigated the efficacy of ^{131}I-labeled monoclonal antibody MB-1, directed against the pan-B-cell antigen CD37, and also explored radioimmunotherapy with ^{131}I-labeled B1, directed against CD20. In the first trial,[66] 40 mg of MB-1 antibody trace-labeled with 3–7 mCi of ^{131}I were administered to 12 patients. Ten patients had satisfactory tumor imaging on serial γ scans. The patients then received a minimum of one therapy dose with 40 mg of antibody labeled with 25–161 mCi of [131]I. Tumor to normal tissue radiation ratios of 1.1–3.1 were observed. At the highest doses, prolonged thrombocytopenia was observed, which precluded retreatment. Objective responses in two patients were noted, lasting two and six months.

More recently, the group studied ^{131}I-labeled monoclonal antibody B1, directed against CD20.[67] Forty-seven patients with low-grade (31) or intermediate-grade lymphomas (16) who had failed prior therapy were initially treated with 15–20 mg of antibody with 5 mCi of radiation. In a series of dose-escalating or phase II treatments at the maximum tolerated dose, 34 of the 47 patients (72%) experienced a response. Low-grade patients were more likely to respond than patients with intermediate-grade lymphomas ($p = 0.01$). The responses noted with unconjugated anti-CD20 antibodies (see above) raises the issue of ascribing benefit to radiation versus simple binding of antibody to antigen with consequent induction of apoptosis.

The above results were all obtained with ^{131}I-labeled antibodies. Another group has reported results of therapy with ^{90}Y-labeled anti-CD20 antibodies (4 patients with B1 and 14 with IDEC-Y2B8).[68] Relapsed low- or intermediate-grade B-cell lymphomas were eligible. The maximum tolerated dose was established as 50 mCi/m². Pretreatment with unlabeled antibody prior to the infusion of the immunoconjugate again improved biodistribution. An overall response rate of 72% was noted, with six complete responses and seven partial responses, with freedom from progression ranging from 3 to 29 months (median 8 months) for responders. Again, the benefit attributed to the radiolabel is difficult to discern, given the activity of the unconjugated anti-CD20 antibodies.

An alternative approach has been to utilize high-dose radioimmunoconjugates as a preparative regimen prior to autologous bone marrow transplantation. Press et al[69] have treated 21 patients with relapsed NHL with 345–785 mCi ^{131}I-labeled anti-CD20 (B1) followed by autologous stem cell rescue. Nineteen of the patients were evaluable for response. Complete responses were observed in 84% of the patients, a partial response in 10% and stable disease in the last case. A 62% progression-free survival rate, with a median two year follow-up, has been reported.

Immunotoxin therapy of T-cell lymphomas
Fewer clinical studies of immunotoxins have been reported, with results that have been less spectacular than with radioimmunoconjugates. An early trial utilized an antibody against CD5 conjugated to the A chain of ricin for therapy of MF.[70] Toxicity in this trial consisted of dyspnea at rest with higher doses, fatigue, fever and chills. A particular syndrome of toxicity seen with immunotoxins was noted here – a vascular leak syndrome with mild hypoalbuminemia, weight gain and pedal edema. The exact etiology of this side-effect is not understood. Patients received 10 daily infusions. Of 12 patients evaluated, 10 had anti-immunotoxin antibodies (either to the antibody itself or to the toxin component). Of the 10, 7 had blocking

antibodies, which interfere with binding. There were four partial responses, with a median duration of response of 3.5 months.

Immunotoxin therapy of B-cell lymphomas

Owing to the significantly reduced risks of anti-immunoconjugate antibody formation in relapsed B-cell NHL, more studies are available to be reviewed. A series of phase I/II trials have been conducted with a deglycosylated ricin A chain conjugated to RFB4, an anti-CD22 antibody.[71–72] Whole antibody and fragments have been tested. Although the clearance from the circulation was more rapid with the fragments and the maximum tolerated dose (as an intravenous bolus) was greater, dose-limiting toxicities were similar, consisting of the vascular leak-like syndrome and myalgias. Additionally, the response rates in these phase I trials were similar, leading the authors to suggest development of the less expensive full antibody.

The most recent study administered the immunotoxin over 192 hours as a continuous infusion.[73] Interestingly, the maximum tolerated dose was virtually identical to that observed in the bolus trials, as were the dose-limiting toxicities (vascular leak syndrome). This study also found a correlation between toxicity and the presence or lack of circulating malignant cells. In these early-phase small trials, responses have been observed. Antigen heterogeneity and poor tumor penetration are clearly major obstacles to successful therapy with these agents, because of the requirement for cell binding and internalization in order for cytotoxicity to result. For this reason, some investigators have reasoned that these agents with unique non-overlapping mechanisms of antineoplastic action may be most usefully administered in the setting of minimum residual disease.

That strategy is being evaluated with an anti-CD19 (anti-B4-blocked ricin). Blocked ricin contains the intact ricin modified only by blocking B-chain galactose-binding sites to prevent non-specific, indiscriminate mammalian cell binding. Early work with this agent suggested that either bolus injections or seven-day continuous

infusions were associated with the same maximum tolerated dose (50 µg/kg/day).[74,75] The typical toxicities of fever, chills, hypoalbuminemia, elevated liver function tests, and thrombocytopenia were observed. Response rates of 10–20% were observed. Since those trials, more recent work has focused on administration after autologous bone marrow transplantation for relapsed NHL. The initial work identified two seven-day continuous infusions of 40 µg/kg every 28 days as the maximum tolerated dose.[76] Administration commenced after engraftment occurred. Reversible thrombocytopenia determined the optimal dose. According to a preliminary report of a phase II study,[77] 41 patients (39 evaluable) in complete remission post autologous bone marrow transplantation were treated with 30 µg/kg/day every 14 days as a seven-day continuous infusion. Toxicity was modest and expected. Interestingly, 21 patients developed human anti-mouse or anti-ricin antibodies. Median disease-free survival was reported as 15 months. A phase III multi-institution trial has been launched to attempt to verify the potential benefits of this therapy administered in this fashion.

Ligand fusion toxin therapy of hematologic neoplasms

Because of the relatively low efficacy noted against established tumors with immunotoxins, and the high rate of host immune responses against the constructs, investigators began to experiment with alternative targeting systems. With the development of molecular biological techniques to fuse genes in plasmids, with expression in bacterial systems, ligands covalently linked to toxins, or replacing the toxin-binding domain, became feasible. The first such toxins to enter clinical trials were $DAB_{486}IL-2$ and $DAB_{389}IL-2$. These fusion toxins bind to the interleukin-2 (IL-2) receptor (IL-2R), and consist of nucleotide sequences of the enzymatically active and membrane-translocating domains of diphtheria toxin and the sequence for human IL-2.[78] $DAB_{389}IL-2$ is a second-generation molecule characterized by a deletion of 97 amino acids from the diphtheria toxin translocating domain of $DAB_{486}IL-2$, thus creating a fusion toxin with a more favorable pharmacokinetic profile.[79] Both fusion toxins bind to high-affinity IL-2 receptors, are internalized by receptor-mediated endocytosis, and subsequently inhibit protein synthesis by translocation of the active portion of diphtheria toxin into the cytosol, where it inhibits ADP-ribosylation of elongation factor 2.[78,80,81] Activity of both $DAB_{486}IL-2$ and $DAB_{389}IL-2$ has been limited to neoplastic lymphocytes or cell lines bearing the high-affinity (p55, p75, p64) IL-2 receptor complex, while those cells expressing only a partial form of the receptor (p55, p64, or p75, p64) are insensitive to these toxins.

Although initial phase I/II studies with these fusion toxins included patients with Hodgkin's disease, NHL and MF, the activity of the agents appeared to be greatest against MF. Twenty percent of patients with MF or SS treated in various phase I studies with $DAB_{486}IL2$ responded, including one patient with tumor-stage disease who has had a complete response of 36+ months duration.[82–85] A phase II study of $DAB_{486}IL2$ was conducted at the National Cancer Institute, which accrued 14 patients with advanced or refractory MF and SS.[86] One patient with extensive plaque-stage disease had a partial response, and two patients with SS had responses that fell just short of the required overall improvement to be considered a partial response. IL-2R expression was measured in skin and on circulating Sézary cells in the treated patients, and no patient who lacked expression of the high-affinity IL-2R responded to therapy.

A phase I clinical trial with $DAB_{389}IL-2$, the second-generation IL-2 fusion toxin, has been completed for patients with IL-2R-expressing lymphomas, including MF, Hodgkin's disease, and relapsed NHL.[87] Immunohistochemical analysis of tumor tissue for IL-2R expression was a prerequisite for entry into this study. IL-2R positivity was associated with the type of lymphoma: 45% of B-cell lymphomas, 60% of cutaneous T-cell lymphomas and 81% of Hodgkin's disease biopsy specimens were positive for p55 expression. In this large trial, 22% of patients achieved a response. Again, histological type was an important predictor for response. No patient with Hodgkin's disease

responded, 17% of patients with B-cell lymphomas responded and 34% of patients with cutaneous T-cell lymphomas responded. The median duration of response in this heavily pretreated population was approximately nine months. Toxicities have included mild and reversible elevations of hepatic transaminases, mild hypoalbuminemia, fever and also hypersensitivity reactions. Immunologic assessment of the non-Sézary patients demonstrated no change in total numbers of peripheral $CD4^+$, $CD8^+$ or $CD4^+/CD25^+$ lymphocyte populations, suggesting that there should be no secondary immunosuppressive effects associated with this therapy.

Future directions for targeted therapy of lymphoma

The development of the ligand fusion toxins appears to be an improvement compared with murine monoclonal antibody-targeted immunotoxins. Although immunogenicity is observed with the fusion toxins, it does not appear to interfere dramatically with efficacy.[82] Molecular size, however, remains a consideration. Monoclonal antibody fragments appear to penetrate tumors better than the whole antibodies, and, similarly, the fusion toxins function better with reduction in size ($DAB_{389}IL-2$ versus $DAB_{486}IL-2$). Therefore finding small substances that can target neoplastic cells may be an effective therapeutic enhancement.

Renschler and co-workers have been exploring these concepts. They have synthesized peptide ligands specific for the surface immunoglobulin receptor of a human Burkitt's lymphoma cell line.[88] Previously, they had demonstrated that the efficacy of anti-idiotypic antibodies against lymphomas was related to induction of crosslinking of surface immunoglobulin receptors after binding, leading to protein tyrosine phosphorylation by several tyrosine kinases, then phosphoinositol hydrolysis, leading to protein kinase C activation, and ultimately to increased intracellular calcium concentrations. They have been able to reproduce this cascade of events, as measured by extracellular acidification, using small multimeric peptides, presumably complementary to the portion of the antibody that binds to the receptor on this neoplastic cell line. Monomers were ineffective, further supporting the concept that crosslinking of the surface receptor is important. It is hoped that the synthesis and screening of such small peptide ligands would be more feasible for individual patients than anti-idiotype antibodies proved to be, and may be more favorably utilized in vivo.

Another approach to making targeted therapies specific but less immunogenic to enhance pharmacokinetics has been to develop recombinant toxins linked covalently to Fv fragments (the smallest functional portions of antibodies required to maintain binding and specificity of the whole antibody).[89] These Fv immunotoxins can be single-chain species if the variable heavy chain and variable light chains are linked by a peptide linker to allow the chains to fold back on themselves to form the antigen-binding site. These molecules have not been uniformly effective, because of poor affinity for antigen or problems with aggregation of the protein in the preparation.[90] Now, using protein engineering techniques, the Fv fragments have been stabilized with an interchain disulfide bond, creating double-stranded recombinant Fv immunotoxins.

Ultimately, the use of these recombinant strategies or patient-specific approaches, combined with protein engineering, may make the use of targeted therapies for lymphoma part of the practicing oncologist's armamentarium. Many of these new molecules are in advanced-phase testing, and the newer products described are being evaluated rigorously in preclinical trials. Increasingly, rational drug design is paying dividends for cancer patients.

Vaccination of patients with follicular lymphoma, using idiotypic determinants from their cell surface immunoglobulin, may be a future patient-specific approach to treatment. Twenty-one patients in complete remission after aggressive chemotherapy received five monthly injections of the immunoglobulin protein conjugated to a carrier. Autologous lymphoma-specific CD8+ cells were induced in the majority of patients. Eleven of the 21 patients were still positive for *bcl-2* by polymerase chain reaction prior to vaccination. Eight of the 11 reverted to negative after vaccination. The authors acknowledge that the long-term significance of molecular remission remains to be determined.[91]

INTERFERONS

The interferons (IFNs) represent a family of glycoproteins that have antiviral, antiproliferative and immunomodulatory activities. Several excellent reviews detail the mechanism of action of these pleiotropic cytokines (Figure 3.1).[92–94] IFNs mediate their biological effects by activating signal transduction pathways leading to transcriptional activation of genes involved in cell cycle regulation and differentiation. There are two major classes of human IFNs. Type I IFNs comprise the IFN-α family (subdivided into the IFN-α1 and IFN-α2 (as well as IFN-ω) families) together with IFN-β, while type II IFN is IFN-γ. Type I IFNs have significant homology and bind to the same cell surface receptor.[95] IFN-γ has a distinct amino acid sequence, and binds to a separate cell surface receptor.[96] IFNs were among the first recombinant DNA products to be used in the treatment of NHL.

IFN signaling is initiated through the tyrosine phosphorylation of their receptors.[97] The cascade of phosphorylation that follows appears to be regulated by Janus kinases (i.e. Tyk and Jak). The subsequent phosphorylation of cytoplasmic transcription factors called signal transducers and activators of transcription (STATs) leads to the formation of a peptide complex that translocates to the nucleus and recognizes a *cis*-acting DNA sequence present in the promoters of IFN-responsive genes.[98] Regulation of malignant cell growth may be mediated by the induction of select genes (for example of the *p68* protein kinase[99] or 2′,5′-oligoadenylate synthetase[100]) or by decreased expression (for example of c-*myc*,[101] c-*fos*[102] or *IL-6R*[103]). Induction of alternative pathways, including the insulin receptor substrate signaling system, may contribute to the cytotoxic effects of IFNs.[104] Resistance to IFNs may theoretically result from modification of receptor

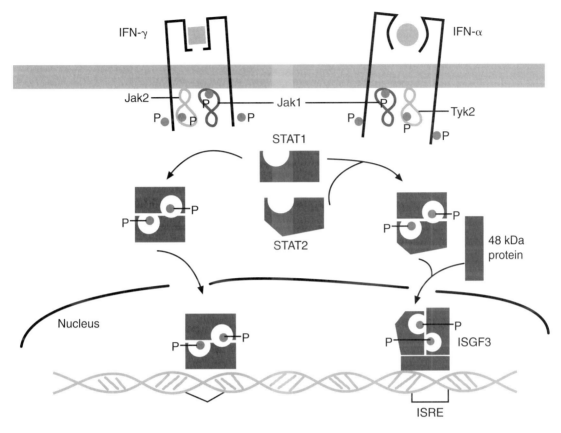

Figure 3.1 Interferon signal transduction pathway: IFN is interferon; Jak1 and Tyk2 are tyrosine kinases; STATs are signal transducers and activators of transcription; ISGF3 is an interferon-stimulated gene factor; ISRE is an interferon-specific response element (P = phosphate). (Reproduced with kind permission of RG Landes Company from Grunicke HH, *Signal Transduction Mechanism in Cancer*, 1995.)

expression or function or alterations in downstream signaling events.

T-cell lymphomas

IFNs are among the most active agents for the treatment of MF and SS. Bunn and colleagues conducted the first large phase II trial using IFN-α2a in 20 patients with advanced stages of these cutaneous T-cell lymphomas.[105] The IFN was administered intramuscularly at a dose of 50×10^6 U/m² three times weekly. All patients were heavily pretreated and had failed standard therapies. Two patients achieved a complete remission and seven had a partial remission. The median duration of response was 5.5 months, with a range from 3 months to more than 3 years.

A review of ten additional studies[106–115] involving 164 patients showed approximately 20% with complete remission and 40% with partial remission after treatment with either IFN-α2a or IFN-α2b. Objective responses in the range of 75% for previously untreated and 40% for previously treated patients have been seen. The optimal dose and frequency of IFN has not been defined. However, most patients tolerate between 3 and 9×10^6 IU given subcutaneously daily up to three times per week. The mean time to a complete remission is five to six months. Some patients on low-dose IFN who do not achieve a complete remission will have remission induced with dose escalation. The optimal duration of maintenance therapy has not been determined. Predictors of response include stage (early > late), morphology (small cell > large cell) and immunophenotype (CD7$^+$, CD5$^+$ > CD7$^-$, CD5$^-$).[116,117] Common side-effects include flu-like symptoms, anorexia and weight loss, depression, leukopenia, and liver function abnormalities, which are usually bearable and reversible. Cardiac toxicity, nephrotic syndrome and thyroid dysfunction have been noted. Approximately 20–30% of patients develop an antibody response against IFN, which on occasion may neutralize its therapeutic activity.

IFN-α has been combined with other agents for the treatment of T-cell lymphomas. The largest number of patients have received interferon with oral 13-*cis*-retinoic acid (isotretinoin) or with etretinate.[110,115,118,119] Although this combination regimen is well tolerated, it is not clear that response rate or duration is improved. Scheulen and colleagues[195] treated six patients with IFN-α2a at $10 \times 10^6/m^2$ daily plus vinblastine at 0.05–0.15 mg/kg every three weeks. There was one short-lived complete remission and three partial responses ranging from 5 to 49 weeks. Three studies have evaluated the combination of IFN with the purine analogs fludarabine monophosphate and deoxycoformycin (DCF).[120–122] Toxicity, including myelosuppression and opportunistic infections, was significant, and response rates and duration were similar to that seen with either agent used alone. Hermine et al[123] have described five patients with adult T-cell leukemia/lymphoma treated with zidovudine and IFN-α. There were two complete and three partial responses witnessed.

IFN-α has also been combined with photochemotherapy (PUVA or photophoresis). Kuzel et al[124] reported on 39 patients who were treated in phase I/II studies with IFN-α2a ($(6–24) \times 10^6$ IU three times per week for two years) and PUVA (three times a week until complete remission, and then tapered to a monthly maintenance dose). Patients with stage IB to IVB were enrolled, and the majority of patients had been previously treated. Overall,

36–39 patients achieved a complete response (62%) or partial response (28%) to therapy. The median response duration was 28 months (range 1–64+). IFN treatment resulted in increased photosensitivity. Notably, patients on this combined regimen did not develop antibodies against IFN.[125] There are several reports of the combination of extracorporeal photophoresis plus IFN.[126,127] Response rates and durations were similar to those seen with IFN used alone.

More-limited investigations have been performed with IFN-γ. Kaplan and colleagues administered recombinant human IFN-γ to 16 patients with refractory cutaneous T-cell lymphomas.[128] No complete responses were seen, but 31% of the patients achieved a partial remission, with a median response duration of 10 months. Toxicity was similar to that seen with IFN-α, with the exception of more frequent and severe headaches. One of the patients who responded to IFN-γ was resistant to IFN-α therapy.

B-cell lymphomas

IFN-α has activity against indolent B-cell lymphomas. Trials using both crude and recombinant forms of IFN-α have demonstrated antitumor response rates between 30% and 50%. Studies evaluating patients with intermediate-grade B-cell lymphomas suggest more modest activity. High-grade lymphomas rarely respond to IFN as a single agent.

Smalley and co-investigators randomized 291 patients with diffuse well-differentiated lymphocytic lymphoma, nodular poorly differentiated lymphocytic lymphoma, diffuse poorly differentiated lymphocytic lymphoma, nodular mixed lymphoma, or nodular histiocytic lymphoma to chemotherapy with or without IFN-α.[129] The chemotherapy regimen included cyclophosphamide, vincristine, prednisone and doxorubicin given every four weeks, for 8–10 cycles. IFN-α2a was administered at a dose of 6×10^6 IU/m^2 intramuscularly on days 22–26 of each cycle. Although the two regimens produced comparable objective remissions, the regimen including IFN had a greater effect in prolonging the time to treatment failure and the duration of complete response. When the results were adjusted for important covariates, the IFN arm had a greater effect on overall survival.

Molica and co-workers investigated the efficacy and toxicity of the combination of IFN-α2a, chlorambucil and prednisone in nine patients with low-grade NHL.[130] Monthly cycles of subcutaneous IFN (3×10^6 IU three times a week for three weeks), chlorambucil (5 mg/day for 21 days) and prednisone (30 mg three times a week for three weeks) were administered. There were four complete remissions and two partial remissions, with a median duration of 18.5 months (range 4–29 months). Notably, three of the four complete remissions were achieved in patients with histologically proven bone marrow involvement. Myelosuppression was common, and two patients experienced grade 3 hematologic toxicity, which did not preclude continuation of therapy.

The CALGB conducted a phase II pilot study of the combination of IFN-α2b (2×10^6 IU/m^2 subcutaneously, three times a week) and cyclophosphamide (100 mg/m^2/day orally).[131] The trial included 105 patients with stage III or stage IV International Working Formulation B or C histology. Both previously chemotherapy-treated patients (32) and patients without prior chemotherapy (73) were entered in the study. For individuals without prior chemotherapy, the overall response rate to the combination regimen was 86%, with 58% achieving a complete remission. For individuals who had previously been treated with chemotherapy, a 62% response rate was seen, and 25% of patients had achieved a complete remission. Myelosuppression was a consistent dose-limiting side-effect.

INTERLEUKIN-2

Interleukin 2 (IL-2) is a pleiotropic cytokine produced primarily by activated CD4$^+$ T cells and, under select conditions, by CD8$^+$ lymphocytes.[132–134] It is a 130-amino-acid polypeptide,

with a molecular weight of 14–17 kDa, depending on the degree of glycosylation. IL-2 is capable of activating killer T cells, natural killer (NK) cells and NK-derived cells known as lymphokine-activated killer (LAK) cells. IL-2 is also a growth factor for B cells. Release of secondary cytokines (namely IL-2, tumor necrosis factor (TNF) and IFN-γ) from IL-2-activated cells augments the immune response. Reports have suggested activity of IL-2 in NHL.[135–138]

The most comprehensive report comes from Gisselbrecht et al.[139] They treated 61 patients with a spectrum of low-, intermediate- and high-grade B- and T-cell lymphomas with high-dose IL-2. The majority of patients had been heavily pretreated. IL-2 was administered by continuous infusion at 20×10^6 IU/m^2 for three cycles of five days, four days and three days, during the first week, third week and fifth week respectively. After evaluation, a monthly maintenance treatment of five days of IL-2 at 20×10^6 IU/m^2/day was optional. Fourteen patients had their treatment stopped as a result of toxicity (e.g. cardiac, hypotension, vascular leak syndrome, renal, gastrointestinal, thrombocytopenia and neurologic). Responses were seen in low-grade lymphoma ($n = 24$; 1 CR), aggressive lymphoma ($n = 23$; 3 complete, 2 partial) and MF ($n = 7$; 1 complete, 4 partial). Response durations ranged from 3 to 29+ months. None of the seven Hodgkin's disease patients responded.

The use of immunotherapy after autologous bone marrow transplantation for lymphoma was evaluated in a feasibility study at the Fred Hutchinson Cancer Research Center. Seventeen patients with NHL and five patients with Hodgkin's disease underwent autologous bone marrow or peripheral stem cell transplantation followed by IL-2 plus LAK cells (16 patients) or IL-2 alone (6 patients).[140] Patients received an induction course of IL-2 at 3.0×10^6 U/m^2/day by continuous intravenous infusion over five days initially. Because of toxicity, the induction was diminished to a four-day infusion. A maintenance low-dose infusion of 0.3×10^6 U IL-2/m^2/day was administered over 10 days, days 12–22. Sixteen patients underwent apheresis for LAK-cell generation on days 7–9. Cells obtained by apheresis were cultured in media supplemented with IL-2 (3000 IU/ml) for five days and then administered over one to two hours on days 12–14. Patients were hospitalized on a regular oncology floor and received the maintenance IL-2 as outpatients. A phase III trial evaluating consolidative IL-2 therapy alone versus observation after autologous bone marrow transplant for NHL is currently in progress.

GLUCOCORTICOIDS AS THERAPEUTIC AGENTS IN LYMPHOPROLIFERATIVE DISEASES

Steroid receptors, as a superfamily of transcription factors, are defined by the fact that each is activated by binding a particular steroid hormone. The major groups of steroids, and some ligands with related molecular activity, are shown in Figure 3.2.[141] A steroid hormone can enter the cell by simple diffusion. Once within the cell, it may bind to a steroid receptor. When the hormone binds to the receptor, the latter is converted to an activated form with a markedly increased affinity for non-specific DNA. Thus the hormone–receptor complex becomes localized within the nucleus. The activated receptor recognizes a specific DNA consensus sequence, which is typically located within an enhancer, as seen in Figure 3.3. When the steroid hormone binds to the enhancer, the nearby promoter becomes activated, and transcription is initiated.[141]

Receptors for the diverse group of steroid hormones, thyroid hormones and retinoic acids all share similar structural features. They possess domains accounting (1) for DNA binding and (2) for hormone binding in the same relative positions, as seen in Figure 3.4.[141] The C-terminal domain is the hormone-binding domain, which regulates the receptor's activity. Some hormones bind with multiple closely related receptors (such as the three retinoic acid receptors, RARα, -β and -γ, and the three receptors for 9-*cis*-retinoic acid, RXRα, -β and -γ). The central DNA-binding domains are closely related for the various steroid receptors. Any

alterations in the central DNA-binding domain that prevent DNA binding likewise prevent transcriptional activation by the receptor. The N-terminal regions of the receptors show the least conservation of sequence, and they include other regions that allow for transcriptional activation function.

Each receptor of the superfamily binds at response elements related by a consensus sequence. Each consensus consists of two short repeats (or half-sites). The receptors fall into two groups. The first group of receptors form *homodimers* with themselves. The glucocorticoid (GR), mineralocorticoid (MR), androgen (AR) and progesterone (PR) receptors are all in this group. They all recognize response elements whose half-sites have the consensus TGTTCT. The half-sites are arranged as palindromes, and the spacing between them determines to which particular ligand the receptor for the consensus sequence binds.

The second group of the superfamily form heterodimers. The retinoic acid (RAR) and 9-*cis*-retinoic acid (RXR) receptors, as well as the thyroid (T3R) and vitamin D (VDR) receptors, form heterodimers, which recognize half-sites with the sequence TGACCT. The half-sites are arranged as direct repeats, and receptor recognition is again influenced by their base pair (bp) spatial separation as follows:

- 1 bp: RXR;
- 3 bp: VDR;
- 4 bp: T3R;
- 5 bp: RAR

This spacing applies only for the heterodimeric receptors constituting the second group. One subunit of the heterodimer is the receptor listed for the designated base-pair distance above, and the other is always RXR. (For a 1 bp distance, therefore, the dimer is actually a homodimer of RXR.)

The glucocorticoid receptor (GR) is a typical steroid receptor, consisting of three major domains. All of the functions of the C-terminal portion of the receptor are dependent on hormone binding for their activity. It appears that the activation of the receptor in some cases may result in cell death.

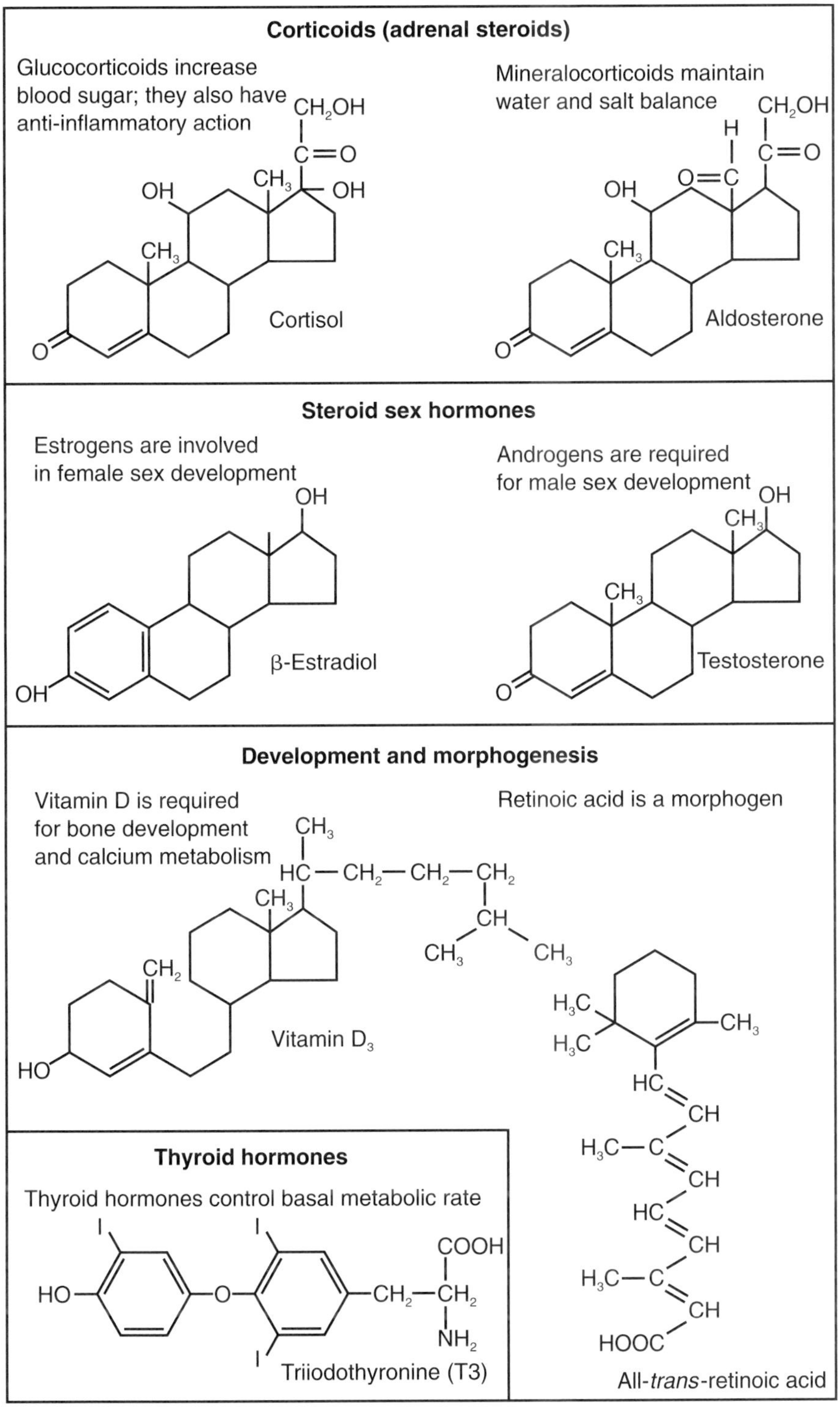

Figure 3.2 Several types of hydrophobic small molecules activate transcription factors. Corticoids and steroid sex hormones are synthesized from cholesterol, vitamin D is a steroid, thyroid hormones are synthesized from tyrosine, and retinoic acid is synthesized from isoprene (in fish liver). (Reproduced with permission of Oxford University Press from Lewin B, *Genes V*, 1994.)

Corticoids (adrenal steroids)

Glucocorticoids increase blood sugar; they also have anti-inflammatory action

Cortisol

Mineralocorticoids maintain water and salt balance

Aldosterone

Steroid sex hormones

Estrogens are involved in female sex development

β-Estradiol

Androgens are required for male sex development

Testosterone

Development and morphogenesis

Vitamin D is required for bone development and calcium metabolism

Vitamin D₃

Retinoic acid is a morphogen

All-*trans*-retinoic acid

Thyroid hormones

Thyroid hormones control basal metabolic rate

Triiodothyronine (T3)

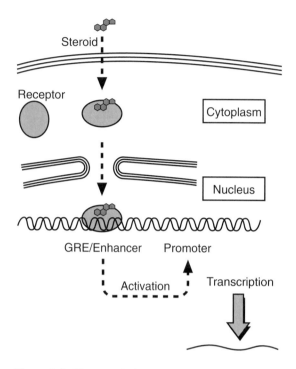

Figure 3.3 Glucocorticoids regulate gene transcription by causing their receptor to bind to an enhancer whose action is needed for promoter function (GRE = glucocorticoid response element). (Reproduced with permission of Oxford University Press from Lewin B, *Genes V*, 1994.)

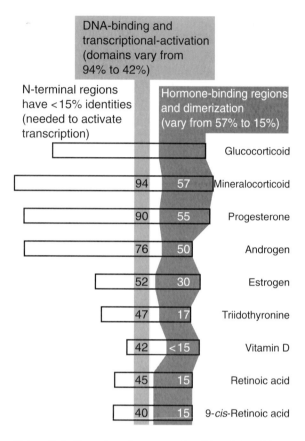

Figure 3.4 Receptors for many steroid and thyroid hormones have a similar organization, with an individual N-terminal region, conserved DNA-binding region and a C-terminal hormone-binding region. (Reproduced with permission of Oxford University Press from Lewin B, *Genes V*, 1994.)

In the specific cases of apoptosis induced by steroid hormones and similar ligands, there is a universal requirement for the intracellular hormone receptor, which suggests a role for transcriptional regulation in evoking cell death. Following exposure to glucocorticoid, proliferating cells undergo arrest at the G_0/G_1 transition of the cell cycle.[142-144] This is followed shortly by the activation of endonucleases, which ultimately cleave DNA. It has been proposed that the cell death induced by glucocorticoids may involve repression of a gene whose product is related to cell division and viability, the absence of which permits death to proceed by default.[145] One example of a gene thought to play such a crucial role is c-*myc*, constitutively upregulated in some B-cell lymphomas. Expression of c-*myc* is markedly decreased by glucocorticoid exposure in lymphoid cell lines.

Transfection of c-*myc* expression vectors has been shown to inhibit dexamethasone-induced apoptosis. Inversely, downregulation of c-*myc* by antisense oligonucleotides has produced cell death equivalent to that induced by glucocorticoid exposure.[146,147] Glucocorticoid-resistant cell lines do not suppress c-*myc* in response to glucocorticoid. Constitutive expression of c-*myc* may be one explanation of this phenomenon.

Other mechanisms have been noted in order to explain glucocorticoid insensitivity.[148,149] Glucocorticoid-resistant variants of leukemia and lymphoma cell lines are easily isolated by their ability to live in high concentrations of potent glucocorticoids. Following the examination of hundreds of such resistant variants in vitro, the majority have been found to express either low levels or a defective form of the GR protein.[148,149] Diminished or altered transcription[150,151] of the GR is therefore one well-described mechanism of this unresponsiveness. But resistant lymphoma can occur in patients expressing ample normal GR. Several investigators have measured the number of GRs in normal and neoplastic lymphoid tissue to see whether this correlates with glucocorticoid responsiveness in vitro or in vivo. No clear correlation could be established between the level of GR and the in vitro action of steroids in normal and neoplastic lymphoid tissue.[151] To add to the complexity, diminished GR activation function may not equate to resistance to glucocorticoid-induced cell death.[145] Recently an 'activation-deficient' glucocorticoid receptor mutant in leukemia cells was found to be as active as the wild-type receptor in repression of AP-1 activity, inhibition of IL-2 production, inhibition of c-*myc* expression, and the induction of apoptosis.[148] This reinforces the concept introduced above: that steroid-induced apoptosis can occur by repression of protective function rather than by induction of active apoptotic genes. There is nothing about this survival repression model that necessarily explains why it fails, leading to clonal survival. One could theorize that the protective or proliferative mechanisms become less repressible owing to a mutational event.

Withdrawal of growth or viability factors from dependent cells permits apoptosis, and, conversely, the presence of such growth factors may prevent the apoptosis induced by dexamethasone, by other anticancer drugs or by *p53*. Again this suggests a suppressive role for glucocorticoids in allowing cell death. As an example, dexamethasone was shown by Hardin et al to inhibit IL-6 gene expression in three of four B-cell myeloma lines studied, and to inhibit the transcription of the IL-6 receptor gene. Restoration of an exogenous source of IL-6 partially inhibited dexamethasone-mediated apoptosis, but not by suppressing GR-mediated transcription.[152] Thus GR activation may inhibit events associated with cell viability, such as those events stimulated by IL-6 or other growth factors. Recently, elucidation of the role of glucocorticoids in suppressing the NF-κB-mediated transcription of many cytokines, including IL-6, has suggested that this may be a more generalized phenomenon than was previously appreciated.[153,154] This inhibition of cytokine transcription would explain many glucocorticoid effects, and would also explain one aspect of glucocorticoid resistance, namely the ability of malignant cells to escape steroid efficacy given sufficient growth factor. Moreover, if the cell signaling and transcriptional regulation that is normally induced by the growth factor becomes constitutively upregulated, as it may by a mutation in the N-*ras* or c-*myc* pathway for example, then one would predict that growth factor dependence and much of the therapeutic efficacy of glucocorticoids could be lost. Cell death could become the exception rather than the default mode.

Bcl-2 is a protein whose oncogene was originally sequenced at the site of the t(14;18) chromosomal translocation common to follicular lymphomas and to some large cell lymphomas.[155] The protein associates with the mitochondrial membrane, nuclear envelope and parts of the endoplasmic reticulum, conferring resistance to apoptosis that is normally induced by either glucocorticoids or by growth factor withdrawal.[156] Bcl-2 has been shown to protect against the apoptosis evoked by glucocorticoid-induced downregulation of c-*myc*.[157] This Bcl-2 protection can be seen when glucocorticoid receptor expression remains normal.

Clinical trials

While glucocorticoids have been the most common component of combination regimens used in the treatment of lymphoma for the last 40 years, there are few publications that allow a comparison of regimens with and without glucocorticoids. Such studies have been performed in cohorts of small lymphocytic lymphoma (SLL)-like chronic lymphocytic leukemia (CLL) patients having lymphadenopathy and organomegaly, and in patients with multiple myeloma. High-dose glucocorticoid therapy has also been evaluated as the central component of a non-myelosuppressive regimen for heavily pretreated NHL.

Ezdinli et al[158] reviewed the outcome of 60 patients with CLL/SLL treated with prednisone alone, administered at a dose of 40–80 mg/day. Following a response, each patient was maintained on 10–30 mg of prednisone per day. Two-thirds of patients experienced a decrease in adenopathy and organomegaly. Anemia and thrombocytopenia also improved. There were no complete responses. The average duration of response was less than six months. The median survival was 30 months. Of 73 courses of prednisone, 20 were associated with major infections. Ezdinli et al found 20–30 mg doses to be nearly as effective as 40–80 mg doses. In 1973, Han et al[159] reported a double-blind study in which 15 patients treated with a combination of chlorambucil at a dose of 6 mg/day and prednisone at a dose of 30 mg/day were compared with 11 similar patients treated with chlorambucil therapy alone. The difference in response rate was statistically significant. Complete remissions were observed in 20% of the combination-treatment group, with another 67% of them achieving partial remissions. The partial remission rate in the chlorambucil group was 45%, with one patient achieving complete remission.[160] When the CALGB (Cancer and Leukemia Group B) randomized patients with CLL/SLL to receive prednisone alone or prednisone with one of two different schedules of chlorambucil, remissions were more durable for the patients receiving chlorambucil and prednisone together. The two-year survival was 93% for the chlorambucil/prednisone group and 54% for the chlorambucil group, not statistically significant in this small study, but suggestive of survival advantage. The two schedules of chlorambucil administration achieved equivalent results.[160] Japanese authors treated 12 patients with advanced NHL, including 8 T-cell lymphoma patients, with a combination regimen including vincristine at 0.25 mg/day, prednisolone at 1 g/m²/day and pepleomycin (a bleomycin analog) at 5 mg/day with no myelo-

suppressive agent for four days every two to three weeks until an improvement in cytopenia occurred. All patients responded to this therapy with at least 50% tumor regression. Toxicity included glycosuria, thrush, moniliasis and reactivation of herpes zoster.[161] The Southwest Oncology Group evaluated steroid intensity in myeloma. They randomized 522 previously untreated myeloma patients to each of three (VMCP/ VBAP-based) chemotherapy regimens distinguished by different glucocorticoid intensities.[162] Patients who achieved remission were then randomized to receive IFN or observation until relapse. Chemotherapy with higher-dose-intensity glucocorticoids yielded higher response rates and improved survival ($p = 0.02$ for the three-group comparison). One-hundred and ninety-three patients who achieved remission were randomized to receive IFN-α 3 MU three times weekly or observation. IFN was not superior to observation for relapse-free or overall survival from start of maintenance.

RETINOIDS: DIFFERENTIATION AND THE INDUCTION OF CELL DEATH

Retinoids modulate growth and differentiation in many malignant cells, including hematologic neoplasms such as promyelocytic leukemia. Liposomal all-*trans*-retinoic acid (L-ATRA) has been evaluated for its effect on different lymphoma cell lines.[163] It inhibited the growth of NHL B-cell lines by as much as 90%, and significant induction of apoptotic death was verified by propidium iodide flow-cytometric evaluation. After L-ATRA exposure, the expression of Bcl-2 protein was diminished by 50%. Bax protein, which has the capacity to heterodimerize with Bcl-2 or to homodimerize, enhancing cell death, was upregulated in the L-ATRA-exposed cells. Sundaresan et al[159] tested different analogs, and concluded that, of the retinoic acid receptors, the RARα, but not the RARβ or RARγ, were involved in this Bcl-2 modulation associated with lymphoma cell death. This suggests that ATRA may have a role in the treatment or suppression of NHL. It is a logical choice for an adjuvant therapy trial, but has never been evaluated in this way.

ATRA has been shown to downregulate the expression of the IL-6 receptor in myeloma cell lines and in purified B cells of patients with IgM monoclonal gammopathy who have not yet developed Waldenström's macroglobulinemia.[164] This change is associated with decreased IgM production in these patients, which may be a reflection of decreased plasmacytoid differentiation, and might theoretically be used to prevent hyperviscosity. Hyperviscosity is not generally a problem in the pre-Waldenström patient, however, and ATRA was of less impact on IL-6 expression, IL-6R expression and IgM production when Levy et al[164] applied it to the purified B cells of patients with established Waldenström's macroglobulinemia. This may suggest that in Waldenström's macroglobulinemia, additional clonal evolution has occurred, placing the B-cell population beyond effective ATRA modification of differentiation.

There may be a role for retinoic acid (RA) in immunotherapy trials. Transplantable syngeneic Moloney lymphoma tumors are immunogenic. In normal mice fed varied concentrations of RA and given injections of Moloney leukemia cells, RA caused a dose-dependent increase in the number of survivors. Athymic mice were not protected by the dietary RA, suggesting that the retinoid-induced antitumor effect was thymus-dependent.[165] This suggests a role for RA in conjunction with adaptive immunotherapy trials and vaccine trials.

Recently retinoids have been evaluated in combination with agonists of known signal transduction pathways for synergy against lymphoma cell lines. The neoplastic Hodgkin's Reed–Sternberg (RS) cell in culture has been shown to be cytokine-independent. Phorbol esters inhibit the growth of RS cells, and RA markedly potentiates the growth inhibition of RS cells that occurs in response to phorbol ester alone.[166] Phorbol esters influence the protein kinase C (PK-C) pathway, and this synergy suggests that lymphomas that have become growth-factor-independent may respond to manipulations of signal transduction pathways.

Retinoid therapy may be synergistic with PK-C manipulations in this way. When the human lymphoma cell line U937 is incubated with a combination of IFN-α or IFN-γ and RA, strong synergistic killing is witnessed.[167] Confirmation of this observation would suggest a trial of IFN with RA as adjuvant therapy for lymphoma.

Clinical trials

There have been few clinical trials of retinoids for the treatment of lymphomas. Most of the studies have been for the treatment of T-cell lymphomas. German investigators treated 16 patients (12 with cutanous T-cell lymphoma, 1 with SS, 1 with actinic reticuloid and 2 with parapsoriasis variegata) with either a potent arotinoid (a retinoid derivative) or a combination of the retinoid etretinate and PUVA therapy.[168] Ninety-two percent of patients responded, and more than 50% of the skin lesions cleared in 67% of patients. There was no difference between the efficacy of the arotinoid and the retinoid/PUVA combination, but the latter was less toxic.

A phase II trial of 13-*cis*-retinoic acid (isotretinoin, 1–2 mg/kg/day) for patients with MF demonstrated objective responses in 44% of 25 patients, including three clinical complete remissions.[169] In a smaller study, the combination of the retinoid etretinate with IFN-α produced objective responses in 4/7 patients with cutaneous T-cell lymphoma (CTCL).[170]

PROTEIN KINASE A (PK-A) ANALOGS AND PROTEIN KINASE C (PK-C) MODULATORS

Cyclic AMP (cAMP) is generated by adenylate cyclase, which is coupled to cellular receptors through G proteins. Most of the effects of cAMP are mediated through the cAMP-dependent protein kinase (PK-A). Two major types of cAMP-dependent protein kinases have been described: PK-A I and PK-A II. They differ in their regulatory subunits, RI and RII respectively. In some cells an enhanced expression of

PK-A I correlates with cell proliferation and transformation, while a decrease in PK-A I or an increase in PK-A II correlates with growth inhibition and differentiation. The regulatory subunits of PK-A contain cAMP-binding sites, and binding of the cAMP to the regulatory sub-unit results in a release of the activated catalytic subunit, permitting it to interact with its corre-sponding protein substrate. Site-selective cAMP analogs have been tested for their ability to alter the ratio of PK-A II to PK-A I activity, and the potency of the site-selective cAMP analogs in growth inhibition seems to correlate with downregulation of PK-A I and upregulation of PK-A II.[171]

In germinal centers, as the majority of B cells undergo apoptosis, their intracellular cAMP levels increase. Transforming growth factor β (TGF-β), isoproterenol and forskolin, all of which induce increases in intracellular cAMP, cause apoptotic death in resting human B lym-phocytes.[172] Agonists of PK-A have been shown to induce apoptotic cell death in lymphoma cell lines, including cells that have acquired resis-tance to the effects of glucocorticoids. These PK-A agonists, like glucocorticoids, induce an arrest in the G_1 phase of the cell cycle in B lym-phocytes prior to DNA fragmentation. It is interesting that after subculturing sensitive lymphoma cell lines, one can select a daughter cell line that is resistant to the cell death induced by glucocorticoids or PK-A and yet the cells express intact GRs and intact PK-A mol-ecules. This suggests that, while steroids and PK-A agonists may elicit cell death by mechan-isms unique proximally, more distally their mechanisms converge, allowing a single muta-tion to confer resistance to both agents.[173] In striking contrast, PK-C activators completely suppressed spontaneous death and the inhib-ited induction of apoptotic death by PK-A ago-nists in B lymphocytes.

PK-A agonists may serve as regulators of PK-C-induced stimulation, and may be used to induce lymphocytes to undergo apoptosis. This system may interact through the regulation of intercellular signaling with regard to growth factor activation of the Ras proteins that regu-late the mitogen-activated protein (MAP)

kinases (MAPKs) ERK1 and ERK2.[174–179] ERK1 and ERK2 (extracellular signal-related kinases 1 and 2) are serine–threonine kinases that require phosphorylation at both tyrosine and threonine sites for their activation (see Figure 3.5). These phosphorylations are catalyzed by the same upstream enzyme, MEK (MAPK/ERK kinase), which in turn is activated by the c-Raf-1 proto-oncogene product or by MEP kinase. Stimulation of quiescent cells with various growth factors or the introduction of oncogenic Ras proteins leads to the activation of ERKs within minutes, and Ras is required for growth factors to fully activate the Raf–MEK–ERK pathway. The Raf–MEK–ERK pathway is acti-vated by agonists of PK-C. Isoproterenol and agonists of PK-A were shown to inhibit signal transduction from Ras by uncoupling Ras-dependent activation of Raf-1. PK-A may phosphorylate Raf-1 at a PK-A consensus phos-phorylation site, preventing activation of the mitogenic pathway, arresting the cell cycle and allowing cell death. PK-A inhibition of MAP kinase signaling could affect transcriptional events brought about through the regulation of c-Myc, c-Jun, c-Fos and NF-IL-6, events associ-ated with proliferation and cell viability.[180–183] Finding a target-cell-specific mechanism of upregulating cAMP has to be a priority in maxi-mizing the efficacy and minimizing the toxicity of this manipulation. Phase I trials with cAMP analogs and their metabolites have begun.

In many cell lines, PK-C activation and signal transduction are associated with proliferation. In lymphocytes, this intracellular signal is asso-ciated with survival of germinal center B lym-phocytes. Ligation of CD40, a member of the TNF/NGF receptor family, prevents apoptosis of germinal center B lymphocytes, as well as a variety of lymphoma cell lines. Signaling through this receptor induces the activation and translocation of PK-C. PK-C signaling through this receptor was shown to markedly upregu-late *bcl-2* transcription.[184] Upon withdrawal of the growth factor IL-3 from a leukemia cell line, *bcl-2* mRNA and protein levels decreased, but this decrease was potentiated by downregula-tion of PK-C with phorbol ester. Even in the continued presence of growth factor, the PK-C

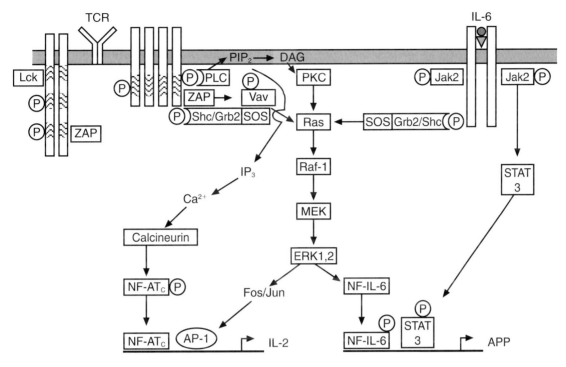

Figure 3.5 Signaling following T-cell and IL-6 receptor stimulation. The scheme is intended to show similarities in the signal transduction pathways employed by the two receptor types, but should not be interpreted as a model for a cooperative kind of action. TCR is the T-cell receptor, consisting of the extracellular α/β heterodimer, the associated ζ chain dimer and the CD3 complex. The darker blocks within the ζ chains and the CD3 complex symbolize the antigen recognition activation motifs (ARAM). Lck and ZAP are non-receptor tyrosine kinases. The proto-oncogene *vav* encodes a protein Vav with a putative Ras-specific guanine nucleotide exchange activity. NF-AT, NF-IL-6 and AP-1 are transcription factors. The activated IL-6 receptor is shown schematically on the right. The dark circle represents IL-6, the triangle the IL-6α receptor, and the two bars the gp130 signal transduction elements. Jak2 is Janus-type kinase 2; STAT3 is signal transducer and activator of transcription 3; APP is the acute-phase protein coding sequence.

inhibitors calphostin and H-7 substantially reduced *bcl-2* mRNA and protein expression.[185] Spontaneously apoptosing myelomonocytic cells showed increased PK-Cb and reduced PK-Cz, confirming prior observations of change in PK-C isoenzyme distribution in association with cell death.[186,187] PK-C agonists cause resistance to apoptosis in some lymphoma and leukemia cell lines,[188] and redistribution of PK-C isoenzymes to the nucleus has been associated with the enhancement of Bcl-2 expression. These studies and others have identified PK-C transduction through the Raf–MEK–ERK

system as a major pathway in the prevention of cell death, and suggest that its antagonism through PK-A agonists or PK-C inhibitors has potential for the treatment of lymphoma.

The bryostatins are closely related macrocyclic polyacetones first identified in marine animals. They bind to and activate PK-C, and are described as partial agonists. Depending on the cell line tested and the conditions employed, bryostatins may block or may mimic the induction of cell differentiation and proliferation induced by phorbol esters.[189–191] Bryostatin 1 has been shown to augment inhibitory effects of vincristine in a human diffuse large cell lymphoma cell line, and exposure to bryostatin prior to vincristine enhanced apoptotic death.[192]

Lastly, since there is evidence to suggest that intersection of two major pathways, the Ras–MEK pathway and the IFN-induced Jak–STAT pathway, occurs at the enzyme ERK2,[193] it is possible that manipulation of PK-C transduction will be of synergistic efficacy when applied in conjunction with interferon administration. This is an area of current investigation in lymphoma and myeloma cell lines, which may provide additional agents for therapy of lymphoma and myeloma.

Clinical trials

The first phase I study of the cAMP analog 8-chloro-cAMP (8-Cl-cAMP) in humans has been conducted to define the maximum tolerated dose, toxicity, plasma drug levels and immunological effects of 8-Cl-cAMP in patients with cancers refractory to standard treatments.[194] The drug was administered as a continuous intravenous infusion. The maximum tolerated dose (200 µg/kg/h) caused a grade 1 increase in serum creatinine. No cardiac toxicity was seen. We are evaluating infusional 8-Cl-cAMP as a single agent for the treatment of myeloma. We are also bringing to clinical trial the 8-chloroadenosine metabolite, which may be more target-selective and may achieve higher intracellular concentrations. The 8-chloroadenosine analog is highly effective in resistant myeloma cell lines. Whether it acts as a PK-A agonist or as a traditional purine analog is currently under investigation.

REFERENCES

1. Saven A, Piro LW, The newer purine analogs. *Cancer* 1993; **72**: 3470–83.
2. Carson DA, Kaye J, Wasson DB et al, Deoxycytidine kinase mediated toxicity of deoxyadenosine analogs towards malignant human lymphoblasts in vivo. *Proc Natl Acad Sci USA* 1980; **77**: 6865–9.
3. Cummings FJ, Kim K, Neiman RS et al, Phase II trial of pentostatin in refractory lymphomas and cutaneous T-cell disease. *J Clin Oncol* 1991; **9**: 565–71.
4. Hochester HS, Kim K, Green MD et al, Activity of fludarabine in previously treated non-Hodgkin's low grade lymphoma: results of an Eastern Cooperative Oncology Group study. *J Clin Oncol* 1992; **10**: 28–32.
5. Whelan JS, Davis CL, Ruse S et al, Fludarabine monophosphate for the treatment of low-grade lymphoid malignancy. *Br J Cancer* 1991; **64**: 120–3.
6. Kay AC, Saven A, Carrera CJ et al, 2-Chlorodeoxyadenosine treatment of low-grade lymphomas. *J Clin Oncol* 1992; **10**: 371–7.
7. Hickish T, Serafinowski P, Cunningham D et al, 2-Chlorodeoxyadenosine: evaluation of a novel predominantly lymphocytic selective agent in lymphoid malignancies. *Br J Cancer* 1993; **67**: 139–43.
8. Hoffman M, Tallman MS, Hakimian D et al, 2-Chlorodeoxyadenosine is an active salvage therapy in advanced indolent non-Hodgkin's lymphoma. *J Clin Oncol* 1994; **12**: 788–92.
9. Betticher DC, Fey MF, von Rohr A et al, High incidence of infections after 2-chlorodeoxyadenosine (2-CDA) therapy in patients with malignant lymphomas and chronic and acute leukemias. *Ann Oncol* 1994; **5**: 57–64.
10. Emanuele S, Saven A, Kosty M et al, 2-Chlorodeoxyadenosine activity in patients with untreated low-grade lymphoma. *J Clin Oncol* 1994; **13**: 306 (abst).
11. Canfield V, Vose J, Nichols C, Phase II trial of 2-chlorodeoxyadenosine in patients with untreated low grade non-Hodgkin's lymphoma. *Blood* 1994; **84**(Suppl 1): 168a (abst).
12. Liliemark J, Hagberg H, Cavallin-Stahl E et al, Cladribine for early low-grade non-Hodgkin's lymphoma. *Blood* 1994; **84**(Suppl 1): 168a (abst).
13. Piro LD, Petroni G, Barcos M et al, Bolus infusion of 2-chlorodeoxyadenosine (2-CdA) as

first-line therapy of low-grade non-Hodgkin's lymphoma: CALGB 9153. *Blood* 1995; **86**(Suppl 1): 274a (abst).

14. Chun HG, Ahmed T, Mittelman A et al, Phase I trial of fludarabine monophosphate (FAMP) plus alpha-interferon in refractory low-grade non-Hodgkin's lymphoma. *Blood* 1995; **86**(Suppl 1): 810 (abst).

15. Tefferi A, Witzig TE, Reid JM et al, Phase I study of combined 2-CdA and chlorambucil in chronic lymphocytic leukemia and low-grade lymphoma. *J Clin Oncol* 1994; **12**: 569–74.

16. Grever MR, Bisaccia E, Scarborough DA et al, An investigation of 2'-deoxycoformycin in the treatment of cutaneous T-cell lymphoma. *Blood* 1983; **61**: 279–82.

17. Dearden C, Matutes E, Catovsky D, Deoxy-coformycin in the treatment of mature T-cell leukemias. *Br J Cancer* 1991; **64**: 903–6.

18. von Hoff D, Dahlberg S, Hartstock R, Eyre HJ, Activity of fludarabine monophosphate in patients with advanced mycosis fungoides/Sézary syndrome. *J Natl Cancer Inst* 1990; **82**: 1353–5.

19. Saven A, Carrera CJ, Carson DA et al, 2-Chlorodeoxyadenosine: an active agent in the treatment of cutaneous T-cell lymphoma. *Blood* 1992; **80**: 587–92.

20. Kuzel TM, Huria A, Samuelson E et al, Phase II trial of 2-chlorodeoxyadenosine for the treatment of cutaneous T-cell lymphoma. *Blood* 1996; **87**: 906–11.

21. O'Brien S, Kurzrock R, Duvic M et al, 2-Chlorodeoxyadenosine therapy in patients with T-cell lymphoproliferative disorders. *Blood* 1994; **84**: 733–7.

22. Foss F, Breneman D, Ihde D et al, Phase II study of pentostatin and intermittent high-dose recombinant interferon alfa-2a in advanced mycosis fungoides/Sézary syndrome. *J Clin Oncol* 1992; **10**: 1907–13.

23. Foss F, Ihde D, Linnoila I et al, Phase II trial of fludarabine phosphate and interferon alfa-2a in advanced mycosis fungoides/Sézary syndrome. *J Clin Oncol* 1994; **12**: 2051–9.

24. Cheson B, Sorenson J, Foss F, Vena DA, Neurotoxicity of purine analogs: a review. *J Clin Oncol* 1994; **12**: 2216–28.

25. Piro LD, Cladribine in the treatment of low-grade non-Hodgkin's lymphoma. *Semin Hematol* 1996; **33**(Suppl 1): 34–9.

26. Kohler G, Milstein C, Continuous cultures of fused cells secreting antibody of predefined specificity. *Nature* 1975; **256**: 495–7.

27. Grossbard ML, Press OW, Appelbaum FR et al, Monoclonal antibody-based therapies of leukemias and lymphomas. *Blood* 1992; **80**: 863–78.

28. Riethmuller G, Schneider GdE, Johnson JP, Monoclonal antibodies in cancer therapy. *Curr Opin Immunol* 1993; **5**: 732–9.

29. Kuzel TM, Winter JN, Rosen ST, Zimmer AM, Monoclonal antibody therapy of lymphoprolif-erative disorders. *Oncology* 1990; **4**: 77–84.

30. Kuzel TM, Rosen ST, Radioimmunotherapy of lymphomas and leukemias. In: *Nuclear Medicine* (Heinken RE, Boles MA, Dillehay GL et al, eds). Mosby-Year Book, St Louis, MO, 1996: 594–600.

31. Frankel AE, FitzGerald D, Siegall C, Press OW, Advances in immunotoxin biology and therapy: a summary of the Fourth International Symposium on Immunotoxins. *Cancer Res* 1996; **56**: 926–32.

32. Wilder RB, DeNardo GL, DeNardo SJ, Radio-immunotherapy: recent results and future directions. *J Clin Oncol* 1996; **14**: 1383–400.

33. Houghlin A, Scheinberg D, Monoclonal anti-bodies in the treatment of the hematopoietic malignancies. *Semin Hematol* 1988; **25**(Suppl): 23–9.

34. Dillman RO, Shawler DL, Dillman JB et al, Therapy of chronic lymphocytic leukemia and cutaneous T-cell lymphoma with T-101 monoclonal antibody. *J Clin Oncol* 1984; **2**: 881–91.

35. Dillman RO, Beauregard J, Shawler DL et al, Continuous infusion of T-101 monoclonal anti-body in chronic lymphocytic leukemia and cutaneous T-cell lymphoma. *J Biol Response Modifiers* 1986; **5**: 394–410.

36. Rosen ST, Zimmer AM, Goldman-Leiken RE et al, Radioimmunodetection and radioim-munotherapy of cutaneous T-cell lymphomas using an I-131 labeled monoclonal antibody: an Illinois Cancer Council study. *J Clin Oncol* 1987; **5**: 562–73.

37. Zimmer AM, Kazikiewicz JM, Spies WG et al, Analysis of human antimurine mediated immunoglobulin complex formation in patients receiving murine monoclonal antibodies. *Antibody Immunoconj Radiopharm* 1989; **2**: 71–82.

38. Ledermann JA, Begent RHJ, Riggs SR et al, Suppression of the human anti-mouse antibody response by cyclosporin A during therapy with a monoclonal antibody. In: *Proceedings of 3rd International Conference on Monoclonal Antibody*

Immunoconjugates for Cancer, San Diego, CA, 1988, Vol 3: 26 (abst).

39. LoBuglio AF, Khazaeli M, Wheeler R et al, The effects of immunosuppressive regimens on human immune response to murine monoclonal anti-melanoma antibody ricin-A chain. In: *Proceedings of 3rd International Conference on Monoclonal Antibody Immunoconjugates for Cancer, San Diego, CA, 1988,* Vol 3: 27 (abst).

40. Press OW, Appelbaum F, Ledbetter JA et al, Monoclonal antibody IF-5 (anti-CD-20) serotherapy of human B-cell lymphomas. *Blood* 1987; **69:** 584.

41. Meeker TC, Lowder J, Maloney DG et al, A clinical trial of anti-idiotype therapy for B-cell malignancy. *Blood* 1985; **65:** 1349–63.

42. Reff ME, Carner K, Chambers KS et al, Depletion of B cells in vivo by a chimeric mouse human monoclonal antibody to CD-20. *Blood* 1994; **83:** 435–45.

43. Maloney DG, Smith B, Appelbaum FR, The anti-tumor effect of monoclonal anti-CD20 antibody therapy includes direct anti-proliferative activity and induction of apoptosis in CD20 positive NHL cell lines. *Blood* 1996; **88**(Suppl 1): 637a (abst).

44. Maloney DG, Liles TM, Czerwinski DK et al, Phase I clinical trial using escalating single-dose infusion of chimeric anti-CD20 monoclonal antibody in patients with recurrent B-cell lymphoma. *Blood* 1994; **84:** 2457–66.

45. Maloney DG, White C, Bodkin D et al, Initial report on a phase I/II multiple dose clinical trial of IDEC-C2B8 in relapsed B-cell lymphoma. *Proc Am Soc Clin Oncol* 1994; **13:** 304 (abst).

46. Maloney DG, Liles TM, Czerwinski DK et al, Phase I/II clinical trials of IDEC-C2B8 in relapsed B-cell lymphoma. *Cancer Invest* 1995; **13**(Suppl 1): 31–2 (abst).

47. Maloney DG, Bodkin D, Grillo-Lopez AJ et al, IDEC-C2B8: final report on a phase II trial in relapsed non-Hodgkin's lymphoma. *Blood* 1995; **86**(Suppl 1): 54a (abst).

48. McLaughlin P, Grillo-Lopez AJ, Link BK et al, Rituximab chimeric anti-CD20 monoclonal antibody therapy for relapsed indolent lymphoma: Half of patients respond to a four-dose treatment program. *J Clin Oncol* 1998; **16:** 2825–33.

49. McLaughlin P, Grillo-Lopez AJ, Czucsman MS et al, Preliminary report on a phase III pivot trial of the anti-CD20 antibody IDEC-C2B8 in patients with relapsed low-grade or follicular lymphoma. *Proc Am Soc Clin Oncol* 1996; **15:** 417 (abst).

50. Czuczman MS, Grillo-Lopez AJ, Jonas C et al, IDEC-C2B8 and CHOP chemoimmunotherapy of low-grade lymphoma. *Blood* 1995; **86**(Suppl 1): 55a (abst).

51. Foon KA, Oseroff AR, Vaic Kus L et al, Immune responses in patients with T-cell lymphoma treated with an anti-idiotype antibody mimicking a highly restricted T-cell antigen. *Clin Cancer Res* 1995; **1:** 1285–94.

52. Hsu FJ, Caspar CB, Kwak LW et al, Results of a clinical trial of idiotype specific vaccine therapy for B-cell lymphoma. *Blood* 1995; **86**(Suppl 1): 273a (abst).

53. Dillman RO, Johnson DE, Shawler DL, Comparisons of drug and toxin immunoconjugates. *Antibody Immunoconj Radiopharm* 1988; **1:** 65–77.

54. Vriesendorp HM, Quadari SM, Williams JR, Radioimmunoglobulin therapy. In: *High-Dose Cancer Therapy: Pharmacology, Hematopoietins, Stem Cells* (Armitage JO, Antman KH, eds). Williams and Wilkins: Baltimore, 1992: 87–123.

55. Rosen ST, Zimmer AM, Goldman-Leiken R et al, Radioimmunodetection and radioimmunotherapy of cutaneous T-cell lymphomas using an ^{131}I-labeled monoclonal antibody: an Illinois Cancer Council study. *J Clin Oncol* 1987; **5:** 562–73.

56. DeNardo GL, Macey DJ, DeNardo SJ et al, Quantitative SPECT of uptake of monoclonal antibodies. *Semin Nucl Med* 1989; **19:** 22–32.

57. Daghighian F, Pentlow KS, Larson SM et al, Development of a method to measure kinetics of radiolabelled monoclonal antibody in human tumour with applications to microdosimetry: positron emission tomography studies of iodine-124 labelled 3F8 monoclonal antibody in glioma. *Eur J Nucl Med* 1993; **20:** 402–9.

58. Waldmann TA, The IL-2/IL-2 receptor system: a target for rational immune intervention. *Trends Pharmacol Sci* 1993; **14:** 159–64.

59. Lewis JP, DeNardo GL, DeNardo SJ, Radioimmunotherapy of lymphoma; a UC Davis experience. *Hybridoma* 1995; **14:** 115–20.

60. Epstein AL, Marder RJ, Winter JN, Two new monoclonal antibodies, Lym-1 and Lym-2, reactive with human B-lymphocytes and derived tumors, with immunodiagnostic and immunotherapeutic potential. *Cancer Res* 1987; **47:** 830–40.

61. Hu E, Epstein AL, Naeve GS et al, A phase Ia

clinical trial of Lym-1 monoclonal antibody serotherapy in patients with refractory B-cell malignancies. *Hematol Oncol* 1989; **7:** 155–66.

62. DeNardo GL, DeNardo SJ, Goldstein DS et al, Maximum-tolerated dose, toxicity, and efficacy of (131)I-Lym-1 antibody for fractionated radioimmunotherapy of non-Hodgkin's lymphoma. *J Clin Oncol* 1998; **16:** 3246–56.

63. Kuzel TM, Rosen ST, Zimmer AM et al, A phase I escalating-dose, safety, dosimetry, and efficacy study of radiolabeled monoclonal antibody Lym-1. *Cancer Biother* 1993; **8:** 3–16.

64. DeNardo GL, DeNardo SJ, Treatment of B-lymphocyte malignancies with iodine-131–Lym-1 and copper-67–2IT–BAT–Lym-1 and opportunities for improvement. In: *Cancer Therapy with Radiolabeled Antibodies* (Goldenberg DM, ed). CRC Press: Boca Raton, FL, 1995: 217–27.

65. Goldenberg DM, Horowitz JA, Sharkey RM et al, Targeting, dosimetry, and radioimmunotherapy of B-cell lymphomas with iodine-131 labeled LL2 monoclonal antibody. *J Clin Oncol* 1991; **9:** 548–64.

66. Kaminski MS, Fig LM, Aasadny KR et al, Imaging, dosimetry, and radioimmunotherapy with iodine-131 labeled anti-CD37 antibody in B-cell lymphoma. *J Clin Oncol* 1992; **10:** 1696–711.

67. Kaminski MS, Fenner MC, Estes J et al, Phase I/II trial results of 131-I–anti B1 (anti-CD20) non myeloablative radioimmunotherapy (9RIT) for refractory B-cell lymphoma. *Proc Am Soc Clin Oncol* 1996; **15:** 414 (abst 1266).

68. Knox SJ, Goris ML, Trisler K et al, Yttrium-90-labeled anti-CD20 monoclonal antibody therapy of recurrent B-cell lymphoma. *Clin Cancer Res* 1996; **2:** 457–70.

69. Press OW, Eary JF, Appelbaum FR et al, Phase II trial of iodine-131–B1 (anti-CD20) antibody therapy with autologous stem cell transplantation for relapsed B-cell lymphomas. *Lancet* 1995; **346:** 336–40.

70. LeMaistre CF, Rosen S, Frankel A et al, Phase I trial of H65–RTA immunoconjugate in patients with cutaneous T-cell lymphoma. *Blood* 1991; **78:** 1173–82.

71. Amlot PL, Stone MJ, Cunningham D et al, Phase I study of an anti-CD22 deglycosylated ricin A-chain immunotoxin in the treatment of B-cell lymphomas resistant to conventional treatment. *Blood* 1993; **82:** 2624–33.

72. Vitetta ES, Stone M, Amlot P et al, Phase I immunotoxin trial in patients with B-cell lymphoma. *Cancer Res* 1991; **51:** 4052–8.

73. Sausville EA, Headlee D, Stetler-Stevenson M et al, Continuous infusion of the anti-CD22 immunotoxin IgG–RFB4–SMPT–dgA in patients with B-cell lymphoma: a phase I study. *Blood* 1995; **85:** 3457–65.

74. Grossbard ML, Freedman AS, Ritz J et al, Serotherapy of B-cell neoplasms with anti-B4-blocked ricin: a phase I study. *Blood* 1992; **79:** 576–85.

75. Grossbard ML, Lambert JM, Goldmacher VS et al, Anti-B4-blocked ricin: a phase I trial of 7-day continuous infusion in patients with B-cell neoplasms. *J Clin Oncol* 1993; **11:** 726–37.

76. Grossbard ML, Gribben JG, Freeman AS et al, Adjuvant immunotoxin therapy with anti-B4-blocked ricin after autologous bone marrow transplantation for patients with B-cell non-Hodgkin's lymphoma. *Blood* 1993; **81:** 2263–71.

77. Grossbard ML, O'Day S, Gribben JG et al, A phase II study of anti-B4 blocked ricin (anti-B4-bR) therapy following autologous bone marrow transplantation for B-cell non-Hodgkin's lymphoma. *Proc Am Soc Clin Oncol* 1994; **13:** 293 (abst 951).

78. Williams D, Snyder C, Strom T et al, Structure/function analysis of interleukin-2 toxin (DAB$_{486}$IL2). *J Biol Chem* 1990; **285:** 11885–9.

79. Bacha PA, Forte SE, McCarthy DM et al, Impact of interleukin-2 receptor targeted cytotoxins on a unique model of murine interleukin-2 receptor expressing malignancy. *Int J Cancer* 1991; **49:** 96–101.

80. Bacha P, Williams D, Waters C et al, Interleukin-2 receptor mediated action of a diphtheria toxin related interleukin-2 fusion protein. *J Exp Med* 1988; **167:** 612–22.

81. Williams D, Parker K, Bacha P et al, Diphtheria toxin receptor binding domain substitution with interleukin-2: genetic reconstruction and properties of a diphtheria toxin-related interleukin-2 fusion protein. *Protein Eng* 1987; **1:** 493–8.

82. LeMaistre CF, Meneghetti C, Rosenblum M et al, Phase I trial of an interleukin-2 fusion toxin (DAB486IL2) in hematologic malignancies expressing the IL-2 receptor. *Blood* 1992; **79:** 2547–54.

83. LeMaistre CF, Craig F, Meneghetti C et al, Phase I trial of a 90-minute infusion of the fusion toxin DAB(486IL2) in hematologic cancers. *Cancer Res* 1993; **11:** 1682–90.

84. Kuzel TM, Rosen ST, Gordon LI et al, Phase I trial of the diphtheria toxin/interleukin-2 fusion protein DAB486IL-2: efficacy in mycosis fungoides and other non-Hodgkin's lymphomas. *Leuk Lymphoma* 1993; **11:** 369–77.

85. Hesketh P, Caguioa P, Koh H et al, Clinical activity of a cytotoxic fusion protein in the treatment of cutaneous T-cell lymphoma. *J Clin Oncol* 1993; **11:** 1682–90.

86. Foss F, Borkowski T, Gilliom M et al, Chimeric fusion protein toxin (DAB486IL-2) in refractory mycosis fungoides and the Sézary syndrome: correlation of activity and IL-2 receptor expression in a phase II study. *Blood* 1994; **84:** 1765–74.

87. LeMaistre CF, Saleh MN, Kuzel TM, et al, Phase I trial of a ligand fusion-protein (DAB389IL-2) in lymphomas expressing the receptor for interleukin-2. *Blood* 1998; **91:** 399–405.

88. Renschler MF, Wada G, Fok KS et al, B-lymphoma cells are activated by peptide ligands of the antigen binding receptor or by anti-idiotypic antibody to induced extracellulary acidification. *Cancer Res* 1995; **55:** 5642–7.

89. Reiter Y, Pastan I, Antibody engineering of recombinant Fv immunotoxins for improved targeting of cancer: disulfide-stabilized Fv immunotoxins. *Clin Cancer Res* 1996; **2:** 245–52.

90. Raag R, Whitlow M, Single-chain Fvs. *FASEB J* 1995; **9:** 73–80.

91. Bendandi M, Gocke C, Kubrin C et al, Molecular complete remissions induced by patient-specific vaccination in most patients with follicular lymphoma. *Blood* 1998; **92**(Suppl 1): 153a (abst).

92. Petska S, Langer JA, Zoon KC, Samuel CE, Interferons and their actions. *Annu Rev Biochem* 1987; **56:** 727–77.

93. Platanias L, Interferons: laboratory to clinic investigations. *Curr Opin Oncol* 1995; **7:** 560–5.

94. Uzej G, Lutfalla G, Mongensen K, α and β interferons and their receptor and their friends and relations. *J Interferon Cytokine Res* 1995; **15:** 3–26.

95. Dron M, Tovey MG, Interferon α/β gene structure and regulation. In: *Interferon: Principles and Medical Applications* (Baron S, Coppenhaver DH, Dianzani WR et al, eds). The University of Texas Medical Branch at Galveston, Department of Microbiology: Galveston, TX, 1992: 33–45.

96. Naylor SL, Sakaguchi AY, Shows TB et al, Human immune interferon gene is located on chromosome 12. *J Exp Med* 1983; **157:** 1020–7.

97. Platanias LC, Uddin S, Colamonici OR, Tyrosine phosphorylation of the α and β subunits of the type I interferon receptor: interferon β selectively induces tyrosine phosphorylation of an α subunit associated protein. *J Biol Chem* 1994; **27:** 17761–4.

98. Darnell JE Jr., Kerr IM, Stark GR, Jak–STAT pathways and transcriptional activation in response to IFNs and other extracellular signaling proteins. *Science* 1994; **264:** 1415–21.

99. Staeheli P, Interferon-induced proteins and the antiviral state. *Adv Virus Res* 1990; **38:** 147–99.

100. Samuel CE, Antiviral actions of interferon: interferon-regulated cellular proteins and their surprisingly selective antiviral activities. *Virology* 1991; **183:** 1–11.

101. Einat M, Resnitzky D, Kimchi A, Close link between reduction of c-myc expression by interferon and G_0/G_1 arrest. *Nature* 1985; **313:** 597–600.

102. Einat M, Resnitzky D, Kimchi A, Inhibitory effects of interferon on the expression of genes regulated by platelet-derived growth factor. *Proc Natl Acad Sci USA* 1985; **82:** 7608–12.

103. Schwabe M, Brini AT, Bosco MC et al, Disruption by interferon-α of an autocrine interleukin-6 loop in IL-6-dependent U266 myeloma cells by homologous and heterologous down-regulation of the IL-6 receptor α- and β-chains. *J Clin Invest* 1994; **94:** 2317–25.

104. Uddin S, Yenush L, Sun X-J et al, Interferon α engages the insulin receptor substrate-1 to associate with the phosphatidylinositol 3′-kinase. *J Biol Chem* 1995; **270:** 15938–41.

105. Bunn PA, Foon KA, Inde DC et al, Recombinant leukocyte A interferon: an active agent in advanced cutaneous T-cell lymphomas. *Ann Intern Med* 1984; **101:** 484–7.

106. Lang MH, Altmeyer P, Lodemann E et al, Therapy of cutaneous T-cell lymphoma with α-interferon. *Z Hautkr* 1986; **61:** 599–608.

107. Covelli A, Cavaliere R, Coppola G, Recombinant leukocyte A interferon (IFN-rA) as initial therapy in mycosis fungoides and Sézary syndrome. *Proc Am Soc Clin Oncol* 1987; **6:** 189 (abst).

108. Ihde DC, Stays R, Sausville EA, Phase II trial of intermittent high-dose recombinant interferon alpha-2a in mycosis fungoides and Sézary syndrome. *Proc Am Assoc Cancer Res* 1987: 208.

109. Tura S, Mazza P, Zinzani PL et al, Alpha recombinant interferon in the treatment of mycosis fungoides. *Haematologica* 1987; **72:** 337–40.

110. Thestrup-Pedersen K, Hammer R, Kaltoft K et

al, Treatment of mycosis fungoides with recombinant interferon-alpha-2a alone and in combination with etretinate. *Br J Dermatol* 1988; **118:** 811–18.

111. Hagberg H, Juhlin L, Scheynius A, Tjernlund U, Low dosage alpha-interferon treatment in patients with advanced cutaneous T-cell lymphoma. *Eur J Haematol* 1988; **40:** 31–4.

112. Olsen EA, Rosen ST, Vollmer RT et al, Interferon alfa-2a in the treatment of cutaneous T-cell lymphoma. *J Am Acad Dermatol* 1989; **20:** 395–407.

113. Estrach T, Vicente MA, Marti R et al, Tratamiento de linfomas cutanos de células T con dosis bajas de interferon alfa 2b recombinante: estudio de nueve casos. *Med Cut Iber Lat Am* 1990; **18:** 354–8.

114. Papa G, Tura S, Mandelli F et al, Is interferon alpha in cutaneous T-cell lymphoma a treatment of choice? *Br J Haematol* 1991; **79**(Suppl): 48–51.

115. Dreno B, Claudy A, Meynaier J et al, The treatment of 45 patients with cutaneous T-cell lymphoma with low doses of interferon-α2a and etretinate. *Br J Dermatol* 1991; **125:** 456–9.

116. Kohn EC, Steis RG, Sausville EA et al, Phase II trial of intermittent high-dose recombinant interferon alfa-2a in mycosis fungoides and the Sézary syndrome. *J Clin Oncol* 1990; **8:** 155–60.

117. Springer EA, Kuzel TM, Varakojis D et al, Correlation of clinical responses with immunologic and morphologic characteristics in patients with cutaneous T-cell lymphoma treated with interferon alfa-2a. *J Am Acad Dermatol* 1993; **29:** 42–6.

118. Braathen LS, McFadden N, Successful treatment of mycosis fungoides with the combination of etretinate and human recombinant interferon alfa-2a. *J Dermatol Treat* 1989; **1:** 29–32.

119. Knobler RM, Trautinger F, Radaszkiewicz T et al, Treatment of cutaneous T-cell lymphoma with a combination of low-dose interferon alfa-2b and retinoids. *J Am Acad Dermatol* 1991; **24:** 247–52.

120. Bernard S, Gill P, Rosen P et al, A phase I trial of α-interferon in combination with pentostatin in hematologic malignancies. *Med Pediatr Oncol* 1991; **19:** 276–82.

121. Foss F, Ihde D, Phelps R et al, Phase II study of fludarabine and interferon alfa 2A in advanced mycosis fungoides/Sézary syndrome. *Proc Am Soc Clin Oncol* 1992; **11:** A1065 (abst).

122. Foss FM, Ihde DC, Breneman DL et al, Phase II study of pentostatin and intermittent high-dose recombinant interferon alfa-2a in advanced mycosis fungoides/Sézary syndrome. *J Clin Oncol* 1992; **10:** 1907–13.

123. Hermine O, Bovscary D, Gessain A et al, Brief report: treatment of adult T-cell leukemia–lymphoma with zidovudine and interferon alfa. *N Engl J Med* 1995; **332:** 1749–51.

124. Kuzel TM, Roenigk HH, Samuelson E et al, Effectiveness of interferon alfa-2a combined with phototherapy for mycosis fungoides and the Sézary syndrome. *J Clin Oncol* 1995; **13:** 257–63.

125. Kuzel TM, Roenigk HH, Samuelson E et al, Suppression of anti-interferon alpha-2a antibody formation in patients with mycosis fungoides by exposure to long-wave UV radiation in the A range and methoxsalen ingestion. *J Natl Cancer Inst* 1992; **84:** 119–21.

126. Rook AH, Prystowsky MB, Cassin M et al, Combined therapy for Sézary syndrome with extracorporeal photochemotherapy and low-dose interferon alfa therapy. *Arch Dermatol* 1991; **127:** 1535–40.

127. Olsen EA, Bunn PA, Interferon in the treatment of cutaneous T-cell lymphoma. *Haematol Oncol Clin North Am* 1995; **9:** 1089–107.

128. Kaplan EH, Rosen ST, Norris DB et al, Phase II study of recombinant human interferon gamma for treatment of cutaneous T-cell lymphoma. *J Natl Cancer Inst* 1990; **82:** 208–12.

129. Smalley RV, Andersen JW, Hawkins MJ et al, Interferon alfa combined with cytotoxic chemotherapy for patients with non-Hodgkin's lymphoma. *N Engl J Med* 1992; **327:** 1336–41.

130. Molica S, Tucci L, Levato D et al, Combined use of interferon alpha-2, chlorambucil and prednisone in previously treated patients with low grade non-Hodgkin's lymphomas: results of a phase II study. *Tumori* 1993; **79:** 195–7.

131. Ozer H, Anderson JR, Peterson BA et al, Combination trial of subcutaneous recombinant α2b interferon and oral cyclophosphamide in follicular low grade non-Hodgkin's lymphoma. *Med Pediatr Oncol* 1994; **22:** 228–35.

132. Grimm EA, Mazumder A, Zhagn HZ, Rosenberg SA, Lymphokine-activated killer cell phenomenon: lysis of NK-resistant fresh solid tumor cells by interleukin 2-activated autologous human peripheral blood lymphocytes. *J Exp Med* 1982; **155:** 1823–41.

133. Ochoa AC, Hasz DE, Rezonzew R et al, Lymphokine-activated killer activity in long-

term cultures with anti-CD3 plus interleukin-2: identification and isolation of effector subsets. *Cancer Res* 1989; **49**: 963–8.

134. Bertagnolli M, *Cytokines and T Lymphocytes*. RG Landes: Austin, TX, 1993.

135. Margolin KA, Aronson FR, Sznol M et al, Phase II trial of high-dose interleukin-2 and lymphokine-activated killer cells in Hodgkin's disease and non-Hodgkin's lymphoma. *J Immunother* 1991; **10**: 214–20.

136. Allison MA, Jones SE, McGuffy P, Phase I trial of outpatient interleukin-2 in malignant lymphoma, chronic lymphocytic leukemia and selected solid tumors. *J Clin Oncol* 1989; **7**: 75.

137. Bernstein ZP, Vaickus L, Friedman N et al, Interleukin-2 lymphokine-activated killer cells therapy of non-Hodgkin's lymphoma and Hodgkin's disease. *J Immunother* 1991; **10**: 141.

138. Weber JS, Yang JC, Topalian SL et al, The use of interleukin-2 and lymphokine-activated killer cells for treatment of patients with non-Hodgkin's lymphoma. *J Clin Oncol* 1992; **10**: 33.

139. Gisselbrecht C, Maraninchi D, Pico JL et al, Interleukin-2 treatment in lymphoma: a phase II multicenter study. *Blood* 1994; **83**: 2081–5.

140. Benyunes MC, Higuchi C, York A et al, Immunotherapy with interleukin 2 with or without lymphokine activated killer cells after autologous bone marrow transplantation for malignant lymphoma: a feasibility trial. *Bone Marrow Transplant* 1995; **16**: 283–8.

141. Lewin B, *Genes V.* Oxford University Press: Oxford, 1994: 879–909.

142. Hard T, Kellenbach E, Boelens R et al, Solution structure of the GR DNA binding domain. *Science* 1990; **249**: 157–60.

143. Wyllie AH, Glucocorticoid induced thymocyte apoptosis is associated with endogenous endonuclease activation. *Nature* 1980; **284**: 555–6.

144. Harbour DV, Chambon P, Thompson EB, Steroid mediated lysis of lymphoblasts requires the DNA binding region of the steroid hormone receptor. *J Steroid Biochem* 1990; **35**: 1–9.

145. Helmberg A, Auphan N, Caelles C, Karin M, Glucocorticoid induced apoptosis of human leukemic cells is caused by the repressive function of the glucocorticoid receptor. *EMBO J* 1995; **14**: 452–60.

146. Thulasi R, Harbour DV, Thompson EB, Suppression of c-myc is a critical step in glucocorticoid induced human leukemic cell lysis. *J Biol Chem* 1993; **268**: 18306–12.

147. Pfal M, Kelleher RJ, Bougeois S, General fea-

tures of steroid resistance in lymphoid cell lines. *Mol Cell Endocrinol* 1978; **10**: 193–207.

148. Sibley CH, Tomkins GM, Isolation of lymphoma cell variants resistant to killing by glucocorticoids. *Cell* 1974; **2**: 213–20.

149. Homo-Delarch F, Glucocorticoid receptors and steroid sensitivity in normal and neoplastic human lymphoid tissue: a review. *Cancer Res* 1984; **44**: 431–7.

150. Moalli PA, Pillay S, Krett NL, Rosen ST, Alternatively spliced glucocorticoid receptor messenger RNAs in glucocorticoid resistant human multiple myeloma cells. *Cancer Res* 1993; **53**: 3877–9.

151. Strasser-Wozak EM, Hattmanstorfer R, Hala M et al, Splice site mutation in the glucocorticoid receptor gene causes resistance to glucocorticoid induced apoptosis in a human acute leukemic cell line. *Cancer Res* 1995; **55**: 348–53.

152. Hardin J, MacLeod S, Grigorieva I et al, Interleukin-6 prevents dexamethasone-induced myeloma cell death. *Blood* 1994; **84**: 3063–70.

153. Auphan A, DiDonato JA, Rosette C et al, Immunosuppression by glucocorticoids: inhibition of NF-kB activity through induction of IkB synthesis. *Science* 1996; **270**: 286–90.

154. Scheinman RI, Cogswell PC, Lofquist AK, Baldwin AS, Role of transcriptional activation of IkBa in mediation of immunosuppression by glucocorticoids. *Science* 1996; **270**: 283–6.

155. Korsmeyer SJ, Bcl-2: a repressor of lymphocyte death. *Immunol Today* 1992; **13**: 285–8.

156. Biussonnette RP, Echeverri F, Mahboubi A, Green DR, Apoptotic cell death induced by c-myc is inhibited by bcl-2. *Nature* 1992; **359**: 552–4.

157. Caron-Leslie LA, Evans RB, Cidlowski JA, Bcl-2 inhibits glucocorticoid induced apoptosis but only partially blocks calcium ionophore or cyclophosphamide-regulated apoptosis in S49 cells. *FASEB J* 1994; **8**: 639–45.

158. Ezdinli EZ, Stutzman L, William Aungst C, Firat D, Corticosteroid therapy for lymphomas and chronic lymphocytic leukemia. *Cancer* 1969; **23**: 900.

159. Han T, Ezdinli EZ, Shimaoka K, Desai DV, Chlorambucil vs. combined chlorambucil–corticosteroid therapy in chronic lymphocytic leukemia. *Cancer* 1973; **31**: 502.

160. Sawitsky A, Rai KR, Glidewell O, Silver RT and participating members of the CALGB, Comparison of daily vs. intermittent chlorambucil and prednisone therapy in the treatment

of patients with chronic lymphocytic leukemia. *Blood* 1997; **50**: 1049–55.

161. Tamura K, Araki Y, Seita M, Treatment for advanced malignant lymphoma in patients with compromised bone marrow – a combination therapy using pepleomycin, vincristine and high-dose adrenocorticoids (POP regimen). *Jpn J Cancer Chemother* 1984; **11**: 2568–72.

162. Salmon S, Crowley J, Impact of glucocorticoids and interferon on outcome in multiple myeloma. *Proc Am Soc Clin Oncol* 1992; **11**: 316 (abst).

163. Sundaresan A, Claypool CK, Lopez-Berestein G et al, Inhibition of cell growth and bcl-2 expression in aggressive B-cell lymphomas in retinoic acid. *Blood* 1995; **86**(10 Suppl 1): 603a.

164. Levy Y, Labaume S, Gendron MC, Brouet JC, Modulation of spontaneous B-cell differentiation in macroglobulinemia by retinoic acid. *Blood* 1994; **83**: 2206–10.

165. Dillehay DL, Shealy YF, Lamon EW, Inhibition of Moloney murine lymphoma and sarcoma growth in vivo by dietary retinoids. *Cancer Res* 1989; **49**: 44–50.

166. Hsu SM, Hsu PL, Lack of effect of colony-stimulating factors, interleukins, interferons and tumor necrosis factor on the growth and differentiation of cultured Reed–Sternberg cells. *Am J Pathol* 1990; **136**: 181–9.

167. Ho CK, Synergistic anticellular effect of a combination of beta-interferon and retinoic acid against U937 cells. *Cancer Res* 1985; **45**: 5348–51.

168. Mahrle G, Thiele B, Retinoids in cutaneous T cell lymphomas. *Dermatologica* 1987; **175**(Suppl 1): 145–50.

169. Kessler J, Levine N, Meyskens F et al, Treatment of cutaneous T-cell lymphoma (mycoses fungoides) with 13-*cis*-retinoic acid. *Lancet* 1983; **i**: 1345–7.

170. Zachariae H, Thestrup-Pederson H, Interferon alpha and etretinate combination treatment of cutaneous T-cell lymphoma. *J Invest Dermatol* 1990; **95**: 206S–8S.

171. Cho-Chung YS, Perspectives in cancer research: role of cAMP-receptor proteins in growth, differentiation and suppression of malignancy: new approaches to therapy. *Cancer Res* 1990; **50**: 7093–100.

172. Lomo J, Kiil Blomhoff H, Beiske K et al, TGF-b1 and cyclic AMP promote apoptosis in resting human B lymphocytes. *J Immunol* 1995; **154**: 1634–43.

173. Dowd D, Miesfeld R, Evidence that glucocorticoid- and cyclic AMP-induced apop-

totic pathways in lymphocytes share distal events. *Mol Cell Biol* 1992; **12**: 3600–8.

174. Bollag G, McCormick F, Regulators and effectors of ras proteins. *Annu Rev Cell Biol* 1991; **7**: 601–32.

175. Hall A, Ras-related proteins. *Curr Opin Cell Biol* 1993; **5**: 265–8.

176. Leevers SL, Marshall J, Activation of extracellular signal-regulated kinase, ERK2, by p21ras oncoprotein. *EMBO J* 1992; **11**: 569–74.

177. Thomas SM, DeMarco M, D'Arcangelo G et al, Ras is essential for nerve growth factor- and phorbol ester-induced tyrosine phosphorylation of MAP kinases. *Cell* 1992; **68**: 1031–40.

178. Wood KW, Sarnecki C, Roberts TM, Blenis J, Ras mediates nerve growth factor receptor modulation of three signal-transducing protein kinases: MAP kinase, Raf-1, and RSK. *Cell* 1992; **68**: 1041–50.

179. de Vries-Smits AM, Burgering BM, Leevers SJ et al, Involvement of p21ras in activation of extracellular signal-regulated kinase 2. *Nature* 1992; **357**: 602–4.

180. Sevetson BR, Kong X, Larwrence JC Jr, Increasing cAMP attenuates activation of mitogen-activated protein kinase. *Proc Natl Acad Sci USA* 1993; **90**: 10305–9.

181. Wu J, Dentt P, Jelinek T et al, Inhibition of the EGF-activated MAP kinase signaling pathway by adenosine 3'5' monophosphate. *Science* 1993; **262**: 1065–9.

182. Cook SJ, McCormick F, Inhibition by cAMP of Ras-dependent activation of Raf. *Science* 1993; **262**: 1069–72.

183. Graves LM, Bornfeldt KE, Raines EW et al, Protein kinase A antagonizes platelet derived growth factor induced signaling by mitogen activated protein kinase in human arterial smooth muscle cells. *Proc Natl Acad Sci USA* 1993; **90**: 10300–4.

184. Mochy-Rosen D, Khaner H, Lopez J, Identification of intracellular receptor proteins for activated protein kinase C. *Proc Natl Acad Sci USA* 1991; **88**: 3997–4000.

185. Rinaudo MS, Su K, Falk LA et al, Human interleukin-3 receptor modulates bcl-2 mRNA and protein levels through protein kinase C in TF-1 cells. *Blood* 1995; **86**: 80–8.

186. Pongracz J, Tuffley W, Johnson GD et al, Changes in protein kinase C isoenzyme expression associated with apoptosis in U937 myelomonocytic cells. *Exp Cell Res* 1995; **218**: 430–8.

187. Knox KA, Johnson GD, Gordon J, A study of protein kinase C isozyme distribution in relation to Bcl-2 expression during apoptosis of epithelial cells in vivo. *Exp Cell Res* 1993; **207:** 68–73.

188. Genestier L, Bonnefoy-Berard N, Roualt JP et al, Tumor necrosis factor, a PKC agonist, up-regulates Bcl-2 expression and decreases calcium-dependent apoptosis in human B cell lines. *Int Immunol* 1995; **7:** 533–40.

189. Hu ZB, Gignac SM, Uphoff GC et al, Induction of differentiation of B cell leukemia cell lines JVM-2 and EHEB by bryostatin 1. *Leuk Lymphoma* 1993; **10:** 135–42.

190. Szallasi Z, Smith CB, Pettit GR, Blumberg PM, Differential regulation of protein kinase C isozymes by bryostatin 1 and phorbol-12-myristate-13-acetate in NIH 3T3 fibroblasts. *J Biol Chem* 1994; **269:** 2118–24.

191. Isakove N, Galron D, Mustelin T et al, Inhibition of phorbol ester induced T-cell proliferation by bryostatin is associated with rapid degradation of protein kinase C. *J Immunol* 1993; **150:** 1195–204.

192. Mohammad RM, Diwakaran H, Maki A et al, Bryostatin 1 induces apoptosis and augments inhibitory effects of vincristine in human diffuse large cell lymphoma. *Leuk Res* 1995; **19:** 667–73.

193. David M, Petricoid E III, Benjamin C et al, Requirement for MAP kinase (ERK2) activity in interferon-a and interferon-b stimulated gene expression through STAT proteins. *Science* 1995; **269:** 1721–3.

194. Tortora G, Ciardiello F, Pepe S et al, Phase I clinical study with 8-chloro cAMP and evaluation of immunological effects in cancer patients. *Clin Cancer Res* 1995; **1:** 377–84.

195. Scheulen ME, Ohl S, Baumberg M et al, Treatment of mycosis fungoides by recombinant leukocyte alpha-A interferon and vinblastine. *J Cancer Res Clin Oncol* 1986; **111:** 540.

4

Low-dose IFN-α adjuvant therapy in intermediate- and high-risk melanoma

Jean-Jacques Grob

INTRODUCTION

The incidence of cutaneous melanoma has increased dramatically in many countries over the last four decades. The progress achieved in melanoma prognosis has mostly been due to an increase in early detection. Much attention has been devoted to adjuvant therapies, since, once distant metastases have developed, chemo- and immunotherapies are unable to modify the course of the disease.

Adjuvant therapies are based on the principle that micrometastatic disease persisting after the removal of the clinically evident disease can be treated more easily than the subsequent macrometastatic disease. However, in only a few malignancies has adjuvant treatment been demonstrated to improve survival in high-risk patients.

Efficacy of an agent in an adjuvant setting can only be established by randomized placebo-controlled studies in a large sample of patients carefully followed for years. This is why the number of trials is necessarily limited, and why the answers to questions posed in 1988–90 are being obtained now – when they are sometimes no longer relevant.

In melanoma patients, several adjuvant therapies have been evaluated, including elective node dissection, chemotherapy with dacarbazine (DTIC) or nitrosourea, radiotherapy, nonspecific immunotherapy with levamisole, BCG, or *Corynebacterium parvum*, and the first generation of vaccines.[1] Recently, two adjuvant regimens using interferon (IFN)-α have been demonstrated in a randomized control study to provide a benefit in high-risk melanoma patients.[2,3] The two trials were completely different with regard to the dose of IFN-α and to the status of tumours in the treated melanoma patients: low-dose IFN-α in early invasive intermediate-risk melanoma without clinical evidence of node metastases[3] versus high-dose IFN-α in node-invasive high-risk melanoma.[2] In this chapter, we shall focus on an analysis of results to date with the low-dose regimen.

RATIONALE FOR ADJUVANT THERAPY OF MELANOMA USING IFNs

The assessment of therapeutic value for an adjuvant regimen in melanoma requires long follow-up: more than five years after resection of primary melanoma, and at least three years after resection of tumour-involved nodes. All of the trials that have recently been published were designed before 1990. Little information was available at that date, and many questions were posed.

Reasons for use of IFNs

IFNs were initially proposed for adjuvant therapy of melanoma because of the results obtained in the metastatic setting. It is generally believed that a treatment proven to be effective for macrometastatic disease is a reasonable candidate for micrometastatic disease. However, IFNs were evaluated not only because of their specific properties but also because they were the first recombinant cytokines to become available for routine use. Fortunately, the first results of IFN therapy in a metastatic setting were optimistic. It is likely that if the original trials conducted with IFN-α2 had correctly estimated their true level of antitumour activity (15% response), many trials in an adjuvant setting would not have been started. This is the 'first paradox' of IFN adjuvant therapy in melanoma.

Choice of IFN

IFNs exert multiple effects upon tumours, which may be mediated indirectly by modifying gene expression or the effects of other cytokines or effectors.[4] These effects of IFNs are usually separated into two categories:[5] direct antitumour activity, and immunomodulation including modification of tumour antigens. IFN-γ is a more potent immunomodulator than IFN-α, particularly through its ability to regulate the expression of class II antigens of the major histocompatibility complex. However, IFN-α has been the most intensively tested in adjuvant trials, because most of the therapeutic results in metastatic melanoma have been obtained with IFN-α[6].

Selection of candidates for adjuvant therapy with IFN

Candidates can be selected on the basis of their expected disease-free or overall survival. In primary melanoma, thickness remains the best marker of poor prognosis. Other markers, such as sentinel lymph node involvement or expression of histochemistry markers, have not yet been validated, but sentinel node involvement may surpass the predictive value of Breslow thickness.[7] In melanoma patients with clinically involved lymph nodes, the number of nodes involved has proven to be the best prognostic indicator. However, while these markers are statistically correlated with prognosis, none can predict whether or not a given individual will develop recurrence. This inability to predict prognosis for individual patients is still a major limitation for adjuvant therapy in melanoma. When most of the first adjuvant trials were started, adjuvant therapy was proposed in populations that were designated as 'high risk'. The definition of 'high-risk' melanoma may be very subjective: a five-year recurrence rate over 20%? 40%? 60%? 80%? 'High-risk' patients included in adjuvant trials have been variously defined as primary melanoma with a Breslow thickness over 1.5 mm, or over 1.7 mm, or over 3 mm, or over 4 mm, or else melanoma with clinically and/or histologically involved regional nodes.

Candidates for adjuvant therapy can be selected on the basis of the tumour burden before surgery. It can be assumed that a patient is more likely to respond to adjuvant immunotherapy after removal of a small tumour burden (resection of a primary melanoma) than after removal of a high tumour burden (resection of multiple tumour-involved nodes). Therefore patients with clinically evident nodes were excluded from some trials.[3,8] Other investigators chose to enrol patients after removal of clinically evident nodal disease for two main reasons: the toxic regimen they used was more acceptable in patients with a higher risk of short-term death,[2] and this population permitted a more rapid analysis of efficacy, because of the higher probability of short-term recurrence. However, this approach might have led to the wrong conclusions. For instance, the low-dose IFN regimen would have been considered ineffective if tested only in patients with clinically evident nodal disease,[9] whereas it was shown to be effective in patients with intermediate-risk primary melanoma.[3]

Candidates for adjuvant therapy would ideally be selected on the basis of their chances to respond to the adjuvant therapy with IFNs. Unfortunately, the factors that are predictive of response to IFNs have not yet been identified.

Choice of regimen

When most IFN adjuvant trials in melanoma were originally designed, no biological data were available to decide the ideal dosage or duration of an adjuvant therapy using IFNs. We and others[3,8–10] considered that a long duration of treatment is probably more important to achieve immunomodulation and that this goal was to be desired over a cytostatic effect. Others[11] have tested the effect of a shorter course of therapy.

The dose of IFN was also a matter of debate. Experience in the treatment of disseminated metastatic melanoma showed that very high doses of IFN-α (>20 MU) do not provide a greater benefit than intermediate to high doses (3–9 MU).[12] Intravenous high doses were expected to provide high serum concentrations, but there are no clear data showing that these high levels are needed in adjuvant therapy. High doses of IFN-α were supposed to induce more intensive cytostatic effects, but the dose–effect relationship in the immune anticancer effect of IFNs is not clearly established. Furthermore, enhancement of natural killer (NK) activity is suspected to be optimal using low-dose IFNs with an intermittent schedule.[5] The search for a cytostatic effect was certainly an important argument for the groups who evaluated high doses in trials started before 1990. It is likely that if IFN trials had been started after 1995, high doses might not have been tested in an adjuvant setting, and the clinical effect would have been missed. This is the 'second paradox' of IFN adjuvant therapy in melanoma.

Definition of a good adjuvant therapy

The ideal adjuvant therapy is well tolerated, and improves survival in a large proportion of high-risk melanoma patients. The most suitable endpoints for IFN adjuvant trials are thus overall survival and toxicity. However, in order to have a rapid evaluation of IFN in the adjuvant setting, relapse-free survival was selected as an endpoint in several adjuvant trials. Although a benefit in relapse-free survival does not always convert to a prolonged overall survival, a benefit in relapse-free survival is also a reasonable target in a disease with no active treatment options once advanced stage has been diagnosed. As a patient, or as a public health decision-maker, there is no doubt that delaying recurrence and its complications (surgery, post-surgical lymphoedema, etc.) can be considered as a benefit, even without prolongation of survival.

Risk–benefit assessment for adjuvant therapy is different from that for metastatic disease. Many patients considered statistically to be at intermediate to high risk of relapse are actually free of disease, and thus will not relapse with or without adjuvant treatment. They will, however, be submitted to the treatment and its toxic effects. There are basically two solutions that allow a good risk–benefit ratio to be maintained for adjuvant trials: using a well-tolerated treatment, or restricting the treatment to populations with a 'very high risk', which limits the possibility that a surgically cured individual is treated. The first solution was chosen in the French and Austrian multicentre trials[3,8] and the second in the ECOG 1684 trial.[2]

Among the presently published adjuvant trials using IFNs, assessment of toxicity was a main endpoint, but none prospectively assessed quality of life. Retrospective evaluation is possible, and has been accomplished in two trials.[13–15] We should like to underline the particular importance of the impact of an adjuvant treatment on the quality of life. Benefit in a few cases must be weighed against the impact on the quality of life of all the treated individuals. In this regard, a prolongation of survival in a subgroup of patients is certainly a benefit when it is obtained with a well-tolerated adjuvant treatment, but the benefit is questionable when it is obtained with a poorly tolerated regimen. In other words, one can discuss the benefit of a particular survival gain after a very toxic therapy that is incompatible with a normal daily life.

Cost was not taken into account when adjuvant trials with IFNs were started in melanoma, in the 1980s. Nowadays, cost is clearly an important argument for decision-makers, since IFNs are expensive and toxicity generates important medical and social expenses. To be acceptable, a costly high-dose IFN regimen must be associated with much better results than low-dose regimens.

APPROACHES EMPLOYED IN CONTROLLED ADJUVANT IFN TRIALS IN MELANOMA

Most controlled adjuvant IFN trials[1–3,8–12,16–18] were designed in the period 1983–1992, at which time it was very difficult to answer the questions posed above, or to formulate hypotheses about the ideal target group and the optimal regimen.

High-risk populations

Basically, three high-risk melanoma populations were studied.

1. *Patients with clinically detectable node metastases.* These were studied in the WHO 16 trial[9,10] and the ECOG 1684 trial,[2] which can be grouped together, since only a minority without clinically detectable nodes (33%) were included.
2. *Patients without clinically detectable nodes.* These were studied in the French Cooperative Group trial,[3] the Austrian Cooperative Group trial[8] and the Scottish trial.
3. *Both clinically node-positive and primary node-negative melanoma patients.* These were studied in the SWOG trial[16] and the NCCTG trial.[11]

Principles of treatment

Four basic principles of adjuvant treatment were assessed in controlled adjuvant trials.

1. High-dose 'chemotherapy-like' principle
This is based on the assumption that a cytotoxic effect is more likely to be observed with maximally tolerable doses. However, such doses can be proposed only for a short period (3 months) or a limited longer period (12 months) in patients with a major risk – mainly stage III AJCC patients.

- ECOG 1684:[2] IFNα-2b, 20 MU/m^2 i.v. days 1–5 × 4 weeks, followed by 10 MU/m^2 three times a week (TIW) × 11 months, versus control.
- ECOG 1690: IFN-α2b, high dose as above, versus a low dose of 3 MU TIW, versus control.
- NCCTG:[11] IFNα-2a, 20 MU/m^2 TIW × 3 months, versus control.
- EORTC 18952: IFNα-2b, 10 MU s.c. days 1–5 × 4 weeks, followed by either 10 MU s.c. TIW × 11 months or 5 MU s.c. TIW × 23 months, versus control.
- ECOG 1697: IFN-α2b, 20 MU/m^2 5 days a week × 4 weeks, versus control.

2. 'Early-phase treatment' principle
This is based on the assumption that the immunomodulatory effects of IFNs are more likely to be useful at an early stage of melanoma, before true nodal tumours develop. Low doses of IFN were thus proposed for primary melanoma without clinically detectable nodes.

- French Cooperative Group trial:[3] 3 MU TIW × 1.5 years, versus control.
- Austrian Cooperative Group trial:[8] 3 MU TIW × 1.5 years, versus control.
- Scottish trial: 3 MU TIW × 2 years, versus control.
- EORTC 18871: IFNα-2b, 1 MU every 2 days × 1 year, versus IFN-γ, versus control.

3. 'Longest possible treatment' principle

This is based on the assumption that the immunomodulatory effects of low doses of IFN can be efficient even at a late stage of the disease when patients have developed nodal tumours, provided that the treatment is prolonged for years.

- WHO 16:[9,10] IFNα-2a, 3 MU s.c. TIW × 3 years, versus control.
- ECOG 1690: IFNα-2b, 3 MU s.c. TIW × 2 years, versus high doses (cf above), versus control.

A combination of principles 1 and 3 has also been evaluated: high doses of IFN during a short time, followed by a long treatment with low-dose IFN in patients in AJCC stage III.

- EORTC 18952: IFNα-2b, 10 MU s.c. days 1–5 × 4 weeks, followed by either 5 MU s.c. TIW × 23 months or 10 MU s.c. TIW × 11 months, versus controls, versus high doses (cf above).

INTERPRETATION OF RESULTS OF ADJUVANT IFN TRIALS IN MELANOMA

Analysis of results and comparisons between trials are difficult for several reasons.

1. Only a few trials have provided final results.[2,3,8,11,13]
2. The nodal status of patients is ambiguously defined. It was clearly defined by clinical examination in European trials: palpable nodes versus no palpable nodes. It was defined by elective node dissection in past ECOG trials (E1684) and variously by clinical or surgical staging in NCCTG trials. Sentinel node dissection is presently increasingly utilized in American trials. The same patient can be considered as node-negative in one trial and as node-positive in another.
3. The staging system is confusing, since AJCC stage III and WHO stage II describe the same group of patients. Furthermore, none of these staging systems clearly state whether the involvement of the nodes has to be established on clinical data or surgical

pathology evaluation, where studies potentially utilizing histological data, immunophenotypic data or molecular data must be considered.
4. Patients with primary tumours with a Breslow thickness over 4 mm were included in two different categories of trials. These patients were enrolled in trials addressing melanoma over 1.5 mm without clinically detectable nodes. They were also enrolled in trials addressing node-positive patients – first because primary melanomas over 4 mm are known to be often associated with histologically positive nodes, and second because the risk of recurrence is close to that of node-positive patients.

DEFINITION OF A LOW-DOSE REGIMEN

The question of what is a low dose or a high dose of IFN is very subjective. Depending on whether it is determined by the dose itself, the toxicity, the difficulty in the management of patients, the impact on patients' quality of life, or the cost, the definition of low and high doses can be very different. In adjuvant trials, 1 MU IFN-α is usually considered as a 'very low' dose, 3 MU as a 'low dose', 5 MU as a 'low intermediate' dose and 10 MU or more as a 'high' dose. For IFN-γ, a dose of 0.2 mg/day is usually considered as 'low'. From a practical point of view, we consider that this classification can be simplified.

Low-dose regimens are those that are well tolerated and can easily be prolonged over a very long period (more than a year). All regimens using less than 6 MU IFN-α, three times a week can be considered as 'low-dose' regimens. In this regard, a short induction high-dose phase followed by a long low-dose phase is basically a low-dose regimen from a practical and clinical point of view.

High-dose regimens may be limited by toxicity, or require to be closely monitored, and may not be routinely compatible with a normal life if administered for more than a few months. Therefore we consider regimens using 10 MU IFN-α2 or more, administered three times

Table 4.1 Adjuvant therapy of melanoma using IFNs: randomized controlled trials with a low-dose regimen arm

	French group[3]	Austrian group[8]	Scottish group	SWOG 8642[12]	EORTC 18871	WHO 16[9,10]	EORTC 18952	ECOG 1690
Inclusion criteria	Primary CM >1.5 mm without node involvement			Primary CM >1.5 mm and N+	Primary CM >3 mm and N+	Clinically detectable nodes	Primary CM >4 mm and/or N+	
Corresponding AJCC stages	IIA and B	IIA and B		IIA and IIB + III	IIB + III	III	IIB + III	IIB + III
Treatment IFN	IFN-α2a	IFN-α2a		IFN-γ	IFN-α2b versus IFN-γ	IFN-α2a	IFN-α2b	IFN-α2b
Dose	3 MU daily × 3 weeks, then 3 MU TIW	3 MU daily × 3 weeks, then 3 MU TIW			3 MU TIW versus IFN-γ	3 MU TIW	5 MU TIW, after 1 month 10 MU/day	3 MU TIW
Duration (months)	18	12			12	36	24	
Control arm	Observation	Observation			3-arm trial: observation IFN-γ	Observation	3-arm trial: observation higher-dose regimen	3-arm trial: observation high-dose regimen
Number of patients Total	499	311	NP	202	800	474	NP (1000)	642
Treated	253 (244 eligible)	154 (143 eligible)		137 (97 eligible)	NP	238 (218 eligible)	NP	427 (608 eligible)
Main analysis Main endpoint	RFS	RFS						RFS/OS

Table 4.1 continued

	French group[3]	Austrian group[8]	Scottish group	SWOG 8642[12]	EORTC 18871	WHO 16[9,10]	EORTC 18952	ECOG 1690
Results	$p = 0.038$ (sequential analysis)	$p = 0.02$	NP	$p = 0.81$	NP Negative	NP Negative	NP NM	$p = 0.17$[a]
Final analysis Median follow-up	5 years	41 months						52 months
Relapse-free survival	$p = 0.035$ (log-rank) $p = 0.033$ (Cox)	$p = 0.02$		Negative		NP NS[a]		NS for low-dose versus control
Overall survival	$p = 0.59$ (log-rank) $p = 0.046$ (Cox)	NM		Negative		NP NS[a]		Negative
Tolerance	Excellent	Excellent	NP	Excellent	NP	Excellent	NP	NP
Conclusion	Positive	Positive	NP	Negative	NP	Negative	NM	Negative (NS for low-dose versus control)

CM, cutaneous melanoma; N+, node-positive; NM, not mature; NP, not yet published; NS, not significant; OS, overall survival; RFS, relapse-free survival; TIW, three times a week.
[a] Personal communication.

a week for several months, to be high-dose regimens. In this chapter, we shall focus on regimens using less than 6 MU IFN-α, or less than 0.2 mg/day IFN-γ. The development of new methods for delivery of IFN, and the use of drugs that may be able to limit the toxic effects of IFN, might prompt us in the future to reconsider what is a 'low' dose of IFN.

LOW-DOSE IFN IN ADJUVANT TRIALS IN MELANOMA

Different trials using low-dose IFN

Low doses of IFN-α (<6 MU) and IFN-γ have been tested in different groups of melanoma patients. Randomized controlled studies are summarized in Table 4.1. They were based either in the 'Early-phase disease treatment' principle in primary malignant melanoma with a Breslow thickness over 1.5 mm without clinically detectable lymphadenopathy, or on the 'Longest possible treatment' principle in patients with clinically detectable nodes. We shall focus on the first type of trials,[3,8] since the second strategy was shown to be ineffective.[9]

Results of low-dose IFN-α trials in primary melanoma patients without clinically detectable nodes

Low-dose trials
Only two randomized placebo-controlled studies have assessed a low-dose IFN-α regimen in primary melanoma patients: the French Cooperative Group trial[3] and an Austrian Cooperative Group trial.[8] Patients were included on the basis of tumour thickness (>1.5 mm) and absence of clinically detectable lymph node metastases. The proportion of patients with histologically proven lymph node involvement at inclusion was not evaluated, since only patients with clinical evidence of node involvement were biopsied.

After resection of a primary cutaneous melanoma thicker than 1.5 mm, patients without clinically detectable lymph node metastases

were randomly assigned to receive either 3 MU IFN-α2a, three times weekly for 18 months or no treatment. Treatment was started within six weeks[3] or four weeks[8] after primary tumour resection. In the Austrian trial, there was a three-week period of daily injections of 3 MU IFN-α2a. The primary endpoint was the relapse-free interval; overall survival was a secondary endpoint.

French Cooperative Group trial[3]
A statistical sequential procedure was used to adjust the sample size to the minimum required number of patients to show a 15% improvement in relapse-free survival. IFN-α2a demonstrated a significant benefit for relapse-free interval ($p = 0.038$), since a total of 499 patients had been enrolled, 489 of whom were eligible: 245 in the control arm and 244 in the IFN arm. A long-term analysis, after a median follow-up of five years, showed a significant prolongation of relapse-free interval ($p = 0.035$) (Figure 4.1a). After adjustment for the predetermined prognostic factors, the risk of relapse remained significantly lower in the IFNα-2a group ($p = 0.033$), with a hazard ratio of 0.74 (95% confidence interval 0.56–0.98). There was a clear trend toward an increase in overall survival ($p = 0.059$) in IFN-α2a-treated patients compared with the controls (Figure 4.2a). After adjustment for the usually recognized prognostic factors, the risk of death was significantly lower in the IFN-α2a group ($p = 0.046$). There were 100 relapses and 59 deaths among the 244 IFN-α2a-treated patients versus 119 relapses and 76 deaths among the 245 controls. The estimated rates of relapse for years 1, 3 and 5 were 16%, 32% and 43% respectively for the IFN-α2a group, and 20%, 44% and 51% respectively for the control group. The estimated death rates for years 1, 3 and 5 were 2.5%, 15% and 24% respectively for the IFN-α2a group, and 4%, 21% and 32% respectively for the control group (Figure 4.2a). No significant interaction between treatment and sex, age and baseline melanoma characteristics was demonstrated, using a Cox model. In different thickness groups, the same trend in favour of IFN-α2a-treated patients was observed. Only 10%

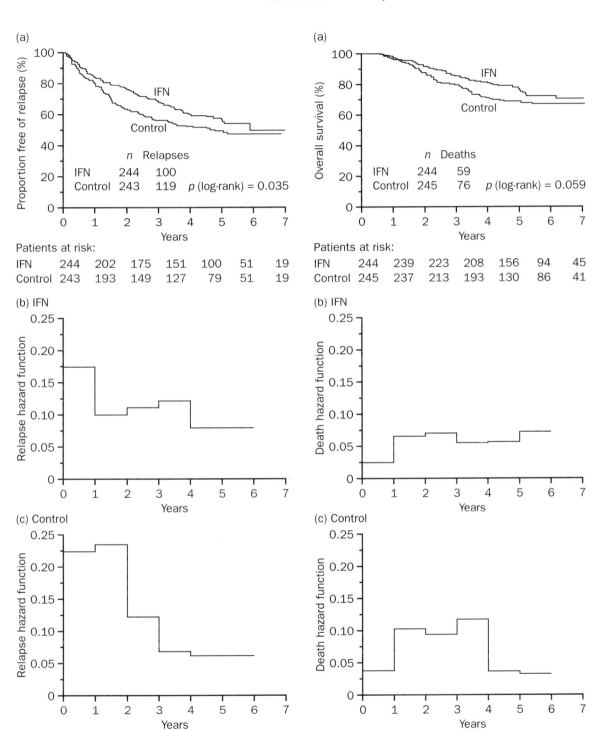

Figure 4.1 Relapse-free survival in French Cooperative Group on Melanoma trial. (a) Kaplan–Meier curves. (b) Hazard ratio of relapse in IFN-treated patients. (c) Hazard ratio of relapse in controls. (From Grob et al.[3])

Figure 4.2 Overall survival in French Cooperative Group on Melanoma trial. (a) Kaplan–Meier curves. (b) Hazard ratio of death in IFN-treated patients. (c) Hazard ratio of death in controls. (From Grob et al.[3])

patients experienced WHO grade 3 or 4 adverse events. There were no drug-related deaths. Treatment was compatible with normal daily life.

Austrian Cooperative Group trial[8]

The Austrian trial enrolled 311 patients: 154 in the IFN-α2a arm and the balance in the observation arm. A significant prolongation of disease-free survival time was observed in treated patients (*p* = 0.02) (Figure 4.3), although no survival data are reported. In a subgroup analysis, the benefit was independent of tumour thickness as calculated by Cox analysis (*p* = 0.001). Death was reported in 17 patients on IFN-α2a and 21 patients on observation, but the median follow-up does not yet permit a meaningful survival analysis. Grade II toxicity requiring dose modification was observed in only 8 patients. Treatment has been discontinued for a median of 11 days for 12 patients and permanently stopped for an additional 5.

LESSONS OF RECENT LOW-DOSE ADJUVANT IFN TRIALS

Clinical impact

- *IFN-α is the first drug to have shown in randomized control studies an adjuvant effect on melanoma: with low doses in an early phase of intermediate-risk disease and high doses in a later high-risk phase.*
- *A low-dose IFN regimen can prolong relapse-free survival in melanoma without clinically detectable nodes.*

Two trials demonstrated a significant benefit in relapse-free survival in stage IIA and IIB melanoma[3,8] treated with 3 MU three times a week during 18 months. The French multicentre trial,[3] which is the only low-dose IFN trial with a median follow-up and a number of events permitting overall survival analysis, also showed a benefit in overall survival after a median follow-up of five years. The effect on survival is borderline-significant using the log-rank test (*p* = 0.059), but significant (*p* = 0.04) when risk factors (age, gender and primary tumour thickness) are taken into account in the Cox model.

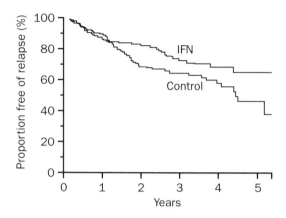

Figure 4.3 Relapse-free survival in the Austrian Melanoma Group trial. (From Pehamberger et al.[8])

- *The tolerance of low-dose IFN-α is excellent and also the quality-of-life assessment is favourable.*

All the adjuvant trials using low-dose IFN-α2a in melanoma,[3,8–10] whatever the disease stage, confirm the excellent tolerance of this regimen. This was expected from reports on 3 MU three times a week in other indications for the agent.[19]

- *The benefit of the low-dose regimen treatment outweighs its toxicity.*

IFN-α2a at the doses used in this regimen was generally well tolerated. Since it was self-administered at home, or with the help of a nurse, treatment was compatible with normal daily life. In the French Cooperative Group trial,[3] the benefit could not be expressed in terms of median survival increase, since the median was not reached. There was a benefit of 9 months in the time to 75% relapse-free survival and of 18 months in the time to 75% overall survival. A Q-TWiST analysis demonstrated a clear benefit for the patient.[13]

Target population

- *Patients with a Breslow thickness over 1.5 mm are suitable targets for adjuvant therapy.*

A nonselected population of melanoma with a Breslow thickness over 1.5 mm is usually not considered as a very high-risk group. In the French trial[3] as well as the Austrian trial,[8] the relapse-free rate at five years in controls was less than 50%. The death rate in controls in the French trial was high, and more than 30% patients were dead at five years. In this regard, patients with melanoma thickness over 1.5 mm are undoubtedly at 'high risk', and thus require adjuvant therapy. Other trials should focus on this group, which combines several advantages for adjuvant therapy: early invasive disease, low tumour load and elevated-risk situation.

- *Adjuvant treatment with low-dose IFN-α is efficient only at an early stage when regional nodes are not yet clinically detectable.*

The two trials[3,8] using 3 MU of IFN-α2a with a favourable impact upon relapse-free survival were performed in patients without clinically detectable nodes. In cases with clinical evidence of lymph node involvement, low-dose[9] IFN-α has had no impact on relapse-free or overall survival, whereas a high-dose schedule, with an i.v. induction phase,[2] has shown improved relapse-free and overall survival. However, it is still difficult to assert that low doses are useless in patients with clinically evident nodal disease. The short high-dose i.v. induction phase might be crucial. Whether or not an induction phase followed by a prolonged 'low-dose' regimen could be effective as well remains an open question. The EORTC 18952 trial (see Table 4.1) may help to answer this question.

- *The clinical status of the regional nodes seems to be a more important determinant of response than the histological status of the nodes.*

In both the French[3] and Austrian[8] low-dose trials, the effect was similar regardless of the tumour thickness, including the thickest melanomas (>4 mm). The sentinel node technique has clearly shown that the probability that tumour cells will be detected in nodes increases with the thickness of the primary tumour.[7] We thus infer that the effect of the low-dose IFN-α2a regimen was similar regardless of the histological status of the nodes. Although low-dose IFN-α2a does not have any impact in patients

with massive nodal disease, as shown by WHO trial No. 16[10] and ECOG 1690,[20] it is probably effective in patients with histologically involved but clinically undetectable nodes. In this regard, it has to be underlined that clinically palpable nodes are true metastatic tumours, able to grow rapidly and to metastasize, whereas little is known about the meaning of the presence of some tumour cells in a node. It is known only that sentinel node positive patients relapse more frequently and more rapidly than do sentinel node negative patients. The low-dose IFN-α2a regimen provides us with a new argument that the presence of some tumour cells in the nodes is a completely different situation from clinically detectable nodes. Indeed, low-dose IFN-α2a seems to be effective in the presence of tumour cells in the nodes, but not when a true tumour has developed.

- *In primary melanoma with a Breslow thickness over 4 mm, low doses seem to provide a better risk–benefit ratio than high doses.*

In the French[3] and Austrian multicentre[8] trials, low doses of IFN-α were also apparently advantageous in tumours with Breslow thickness over 4 mm, although the analysis in this subgroup was not significant, because of the low number of cases. Conversely, in the ECOG 1684 trial,[2] high doses of IFN-α did not give any benefit in a subgroup of primary melanoma patients with thickness over 4 mm without node involvement, although the number of patients in this group was too limited to allow any definitive conclusion to be drawn. Similarly, in the NCCTG trial,[11] no benefit was obtained with high-dose IFN-α in primary melanoma thicker than 1.7 mm without nodes, whereas a favourable trend was found in patients with positive nodes. Taking all these data into account, there is no reason to use a toxic high-dose IFN-α regimen in stage IIB primary melanoma, and a well-tolerated low-dose regimen is at least relatively nontoxic.

IFN regimen

- *Efficacy seems to require a minimal dose, even at an early stage.*

Very low doses (<3 MU) are probably not effective as adjuvant therapy of intermediate- to high-risk melanoma. In the EORTC trial 18871, very low doses of IFN-α2b every two days were compared with observation and with IFN-γ every two days. The interim results do not seem to show any advantage for very low doses of IFN-α.

- *A short induction high-dose phase is apparently not necessary in the early phase of primary melanoma.*

There was no *high-dose* induction phase in the IFN trials conducted in French and Austrian patients with intermediate-risk melanoma without clinically detectable nodes (as mentioned above, in the Austrian trial, there was a three-week period of daily *low-dose* IFN).

- *The type of IFN-α (IFN-α2a or IFN-α2b) may not be crucial.*

Successful reduction of relapse rates has been obtained with IFN-α2a in early primary melanoma[3,8] and with IFN-α2b in patients with more advanced disease,[2] although this has not been confirmed in a second trial.[20] This could be interpreted as being due to a 'stage specificity' of the two types of IFN-α. This apparent 'stage specificity' of the two types of IFN-α is more likely to result from differences in dose (low versus high) and regimen (induction phase versus no induction phase) than from the subtle chemical differences between the two molecules.

- *The impact of low doses of IFN-α in an adjuvant setting might be related to the duration of the treatment.*

It is important to determine the kinetics of the IFN effect upon the hazard ratio for relapse or death during low-dose[3] and high-dose[2] regimens. These hazard ratios give information about the time course of the IFN-α effect: the time of maximum activity and the duration of the treatment effect. With the high-dose IFN-α schedule in patients with node metastases, these hazard ratio curves suggest that all the effect was obtained during the first months.[2]

Conversely, with the low-dose regimen in patients with early invasive melanoma, the kinetics of activity is apparently quite different. In the multicentre French trial,[3] hazard ratio curves suggested that IFN-α reduced relapse risk during the first two and three years, with maximum effect close to treatment discontinuation (Figures 4.1b, c). After this period, the risk apparently returned to that of the no-treatment group. The hazard of death was decreased in IFN-treated patients from the second to the fourth year[3] (Figures 4.2b, c). This is reasonable, since death is expected to occur often one or two years after relapse. In other words, an 18-month treatment with low doses of IFN seems to delay the natural history of the disease. Curiously enough, although the hazard ratios were not published in the Austrian trial,[8] the relapse-free survival curves in IFN-treated patients and in controls diverge approximately 15 months after randomization when IFN-α has been discontinued. This would suggest different kinetics of IFN activity, although both the French cooperative and Austrian cooperative trials have used the same low-dose IFN-α regimen in similar patients. These speculations have yet to be confirmed, but it is possible that a longer treatment with low-dose IFN would prolong the impact on survival in melanoma patients without lymph node metastases. This well-tolerated low-dose regimen prolonged over 18 months would probably be acceptable for patients, as has been shown in the three-year schedule of the WHO trial 16.[9,10]

Cost-effectiveness

The cost-effectiveness ratio of adjuvant therapy with low-dose IFN-α2a in stage IIA and B melanoma is within the lower range for widely accepted therapies. A cost-effectiveness analysis of the results of the French trial evaluated the 10-year cost per year gain to be around US$7000 and the lifetime cost per year gain around US$2000.[13] This is one-seventh of the same evaluation for a high-dose regimen in node-positive patients.[14] For comparison, it is one-tenth to one-fifth of the cost of systematic mammography for women aged over 50 or the cost of renal dialysis at home, one-twentieth to one-tenth of the cost of captopril for moderate hypertension, and one-hundredth of the cost of liver transplantation or systematic mammography for women aged below 50.

STATE OF THE ART

- *3 MU IFN-α2a during 18 months is a well-tolerated cost-effective adjuvant treatment for primary melanoma thicker than 1.5 mm without clinically detectable nodes.*

This includes patients with AJCC stage IIA or IIB or WHO stage I melanoma thicker than 1.5 mm. It potentially also includes AJCC stage III melanoma, where stage III means clinically undetectable but histologically positive nodes as assessed by elective or sentinel node dissection. Indeed, inclusion in the French[3] and Austrian[8] low-dose trials was based on clinical assessment of nodes. Recently, elective node dissection has been validated as a prognostic marker, and sentinel node evaluation has been proven to have increased prognostic precision. There is no reason why the results of low-dose trials should be different, whatever the results of sentinel node dissection (see above). A patient with a tumour thicker than 1.5 mm and a positive sentinel node dissection contrasting with a normal clinical examination remains a good candidate for a low-dose regimen.

- *In patients with clinically detectable nodes, low doses are not effective, and a high-dose IFN-α2b regimen can be proposed (see Chapter 5).*

This includes patients with AJCC stage III melanoma when staging is based on clinical evaluation of nodes.

FUTURE PROSPECTS

The results of the low-dose IFN-α adjuvant trials in early and intermediate-risk melanoma must be confirmed. The impact on overall survival has to be confirmed by a longer follow-up of the Austrian study. The exact duration of the adjuvant effect has to be defined in more mature data, following 10-year follow-up.

The major questions: ideal dose and duration of treatment

- Would the addition of a short high-dose i.v. IFN-α induction phase be useful in early melanoma? An ECOG trial is currently starting to investigate a one-month high-dose i.v. regimen alone versus controls, and may provide information on this question.
- Would a low but higher dose of IFN-α (so-called 'intermediate dose', i.e. 5–6 MU) be more effective and more cost-efficient in early melanoma? The three-arm EORTC 1895 trial compares observation versus an induction phase plus IFN-α2b, 5 MU three times a week for two years or 10 MU s.c. three times a week for one year in stage IIB and III patients. A separate analysis in the subgroup of IIB patients (T4N0M0) may provide further information about the effect of intermediate doses in patients without clinically detectable nodes.
- Would a longer treatment be more effective and cost-efficient? The hazard ratio curves in the French trial[3] suggest that a longer treatment would provide a more sustained benefit. This has yet to be demonstrated in a randomized trial.
- Would a long-acting form of IFN be as efficient as a three times weekly regimen? New sustained-release forms (PEG-IFNs) are being developed and are available for clinical evaluation.

Recognition of responders to IFN-α before start of treatment

Is there any marker? For the moment, no tumour or immunological marker has emerged. Our results (to be published) suggest that a simple haematological profile may provide useful information to help in selecting responders.

Selection of an adjuvant regimen on the basis of sentinel node dissection

Will sentinel node dissection give more information than simple palpation in selecting patients who will respond? In this regard, the results of the French[3] and Austrian[8] trials do not suggest that patients with histological involvement of the nodes should react differently from node-negative patients. In terms of IFN regimen choice, sentinel node-positive patients cannot be immediately assimilated with clinically node-positive patients. If a low dose is efficient in sentinel node-positive patients, the risk/benefit ratio is likely to be better than that with a high dose regimen. At least, this must be evaluated in a comparable study in sentinel node-positive patients.

Combination of adjuvant treatment

Bearing in mind that no chemotherapy has ever shown an effect, the question here is whether a combination of IFNs with vaccines would be more efficient. Some trials have explored this hypothesis, in the ECOG and US Intergroup with GM2 vaccination.

Sequence of successive treatments

Once it has been demonstrated that low doses of IFN are effective in primary tumours, and high doses are efficient in patients with clinically detectable nodal metastases, two new questions are posed.

- Following early adjuvant treatment with low-dose IFN-α when apparently free of nodal metastases, should a patient be given high-dose IFN-α adjuvant therapy when nodal metastases develop? For chemotherapy, the answer would be negative. However, the clinical development of nodal metastases does not mean that low-dose IFN-α therapy was not effective. It could be that low-dose IFN has delayed the recurrence, and that high-dose IFN-α therapy may provide an additional benefit.
- If the two regimens cannot be administered with cumulative benefit in the same patient, the major question is whether patients are better treated early with low-doses IFN-α, or late with a high-dose regimen when they develop clinically evident nodal metastases. Which strategy would be the best: a well-tolerated regimen in a large number of individuals (after removal of a melanoma greater than 1.5 mm in thickness) or a less easily tolerated regimen in a smaller number (who develop clinically evident nodes)?

CONCLUSIONS

From a clinical point of view, IFN at a dose of 3 MU three times a week is the first well-tolerated regimen to demonstrate an adjuvant effect in melanoma patients, but it appears that it has to be started early before nodal metastases become clinically detectable.

From a conceptual point of view, several principles have been widely accepted in the last few decades:

1. A drug had to be effective in the treatment of metastases for it to be reasonable to test it in an adjuvant setting.
2. The use of the highest tolerable doses is the best schedule in the therapy of cancer.
3. Adjuvant therapy must be tested first in very high-risk patients, i.e. patients who have been treated for a significant tumour load.

Although many questions are still unanswered, the efficacy of a low-dose IFN-α regimen in an adjuvant setting in early melanoma demonstrates the following:

- A drug proven to be poorly efficient in a metastatic setting can be efficacious in an adjuvant setting.
- Small doses of an immunomodulatory drug can achieve important clinical effects.
- An adjuvant therapy can show major benefit in early invasive tumours, but may fail when started at a more advanced stage.

REFERENCES

1. Nathan E, Mastrangelo MJ, Adjuvant therapy for cutaneous melanoma. *Semin Oncol* 1995; **22:** 647–61.
2. Kirkwood J, Strawdermann MH, Ernstoff MS et al, Interferon alfa-2b adjuvant therapy of high risk resected cutaneous melanoma: the Eastern Cooperative Oncology Group Trial EST 1684. *J Clin Oncol* 1996; **14:** 7–17.
3. Grob JJ, Dreno B, De La Salmoniere P et al, Randomised trial of interferon alpha-2A as adjuvant therapy in resected primary melanoma thicker than 1.5 mm without clinically detectable node metastases. *Lancet* 1998; **351:** 1905–10.
4. Taylor JL, Grossberg E, The effects of interferon-α on the production and action of other cytokines. *Semin Oncol* 1998; **1:** 23–9.
5. Dianzani F, Antonelli G, Mechanisms of action of the interferons: biological basis. In: *Clinical Applications of the Interferons* (Stuart-Harris R, Penny R, eds). Chapman and Hall: London, 1997: 19–31.
6. Kirkwood J, Studies of interferons in the therapy of melanoma. *Semin Oncol* 1991; **18**(Suppl 7): 83–90.
7. Morton D, Wen DR, Wong JH et al, Technical details of intraoperative lymphatic mapping for early melanoma. *Arch Surg* 1992; **127:** 392–9.
8. Pehamberger H, Soyer HP, Steiner A et al, Adjuvant interferon alfa-2a treatment in resected primary stage III cutaneous melanoma. *J Clin Oncol* 1998; **16:** 1425–9.
9. Cascinelli N, Evaluation of efficacy of adjuvant therapy with IFN-alpha 2a in melanoma patients with regional node metastases. *Proc Am Soc Clin Oncol* 1995; **14:** 410 (abst).
10. Cascinelli N, Bufalino R, Morabito A, Results of adjuvant interferon study in WHO melanoma programme. *Lancet* 1994; **343:** 913–14.
11. Creagan ET, Dalton RJ, Ahmann DL et al, Randomized, surgical adjuvant clinical trial of recombinant interferon alfa 2a in selected patients with malignant melanoma. *J Clin Oncol* 1995; **13:** 2776–83.
12. Bajetta E, Di Leo A, Zampino MG et al, Multicenter randomized trial of decarbazine alone or in combination with two different doses and schedules of interferon alfa-2a in the treatment of advanced melanoma. *J Clin Oncol* 1994; **12:** 806–11.
13. Fagnani F, Lafuma A, Grob JJ et al, Economic analysis of adjuvant treatment of melanoma (>1.5 mm, no lymph node metastases) with IFN alpha 2A. *Proc Am Soc Clin Oncol* 1998; **17:** 1622 (abst).
14. Hillner BM, Kirkwood JM, Atkins MB et al, Economic analyses of IFN alpha 2b in high risk melanoma based on projection from ECOG 1684. *J Clin Oncol* 1997; **15:** 2351–8.
15. Cole BF, Gelber RD, Kirkwood JM et al, Quality-of-life-adjusted survival analysis of interferon alfa-2b adjuvant treatment of high-risk resected cutaneous melanoma: an Eastern Cooperative Oncology Group Study. *J Clin Oncol* 1996; **14:** 2666–73.
16. Meyskens FL, Kenneth J, Kopecky J et al, Randomized trial of adjuvant human interferon gamma versus observation in high-risk cutaneous melanoma: a Southwest Oncology Group study. *J Natl Cancer Inst* 1995; **87:** 1710–13.
17. Nathanson L, Interferon adjuvant therapy of melanoma. *Cancer* 1996; **78:** 944–7.
18. Demierre MF, Koh K, Adjuvant therapy for cutaneous malignant melanoma. *J Am Acad Dermatol* 1997; **36:** 747–64.
19. Hagenbeek A, Carde P, Meerwaldt JH et al, Maintenance of remission with human recombinant interferon alfa-2a in patients with stages III and IV low-grade malignant non-Hodgkin's lymphoma. *J Clin Oncol* 1998; **16:** 41–7.
20. Kirkwood JM, Ibrahim J, Sondak V et al, Preliminary analysis of the E1690/S9111/C9190 Intergroup postoperative adjuvant trial of high- and low-dose IFNα2b (HDI and LDI) in high-risk primary or lymph node metastatic melanoma. *Proc Am Soc Clin Oncol* 1999; **18:** 537A (Abst 2072).

5

Adjuvant therapy of melanoma

Sanjiv S Agarawala, John M Kirkwood

INTRODUCTION

With the twentieth century drawing to a close, metastatic melanoma (American Joint Committee Classification, AJCC, stage IV) is still incurable in most cases. The rapid rise in the incidence of cutaneous melanoma in the USA and other countries makes it imperative to devise strategies that will improve diagnosis, refine prognostic markers, and, most importantly, eradicate micrometastatic disease in those patients who are deemed potentially surgically curable. The latter has been the basis for an ongoing search for an effective adjuvant therapy that will improve the relapse-free and overall survival of patients with clinically localized melanoma.

The prognosis of primary cutaneous melanoma is determined at the primary site by the depth of the lesion measured in millimeters using an ocular micrometer, and regionally by the presence of lymph node involvement, determined either by clinical findings or histopathologic microscopic examination. This is reflected in the AJCC and the TNM system, where localized melanomas are divided into stages IA (<0.76 mm, T1), IB (0.76–1.5 mm, T2), IIA

(1.51–4 mm, T3), and stage IIB (>4 mm, T4). Regional lymph node involvement is classified as stage III (N1). Among localized cutaneous melanomas, the highest risk for systemic relapse exists for patients with stage IIB disease (five-year survival 57%; ten-year survival 44%).[1] The outlook for patients with stage III disease is even worse, with five-year survivals of 10–46%, depending upon the number of nodes involved.

It is the latter two groups of patients that have been the major focus of clinical trials conducted by the major cooperative groups in the USA and Europe in the quest for an immunologic therapy that will improve survival. This chapter summarizes recent and ongoing postsurgical adjuvant efforts in this area using interferons and vaccines.

THE INTERFERONS

Isaacs and Lindeman[2] first described the interferons (IFNs) in 1957. Originally named for their inhibitory properties in terms of viral replication, they are now known to be complex polypeptides that demonstrate a vast array of biologic properties, including the modulation of cellular proliferation, immune modulation and antiangiogenesis, in vitro and in vivo.

Two major types of IFN exist: type I and type II. Type I IFNs include IFN-α, IFN-β, IFN-τ and IFN-ω. They are closely related, share a common receptor and are encoded by genes on chromosome 9. Type II IFN is IFN-γ, which interacts with a distinct receptor and is encoded by genes on chromosome 12. The type I IFNs have well-defined effects upon the phenotype and function of T cells, natural killer (NK) cells and monocytes, and thereby modulate the immune system. Although the immunomodulatory properties of type II IFN exceed those of type I IFNs in vitro and in experimental animal models, the former has yet to demonstrate the benefits reported with the type I IFNs in clinical trials against human cancer, including melanoma.

Of the six IFNs currently marketed in the USA, two subspecies of IFN-α, IFN-α2a (Roferon-A, Roche Laboratories, Nutley, NJ) and IFN-α2b (Intron A, Schering Plough Corporation, Kenilworth, NJ) have been most extensively investigated in the therapy of melanoma. IFN-α2b (Intron A) has recently received FDA approval for the adjuvant therapy of high-risk melanoma in a schedule developed by the Eastern Cooperative Oncology Group (ECOG trial E1684). The use of maximally tolerated doses of IFN-α has been advocated to provide maximal immunologic and cytostatic effects, as well as to minimize the impact of anti-IFN antibodies. To test this hypothesis, trials using high doses of IFN-α with or without an induction intravenous phase, have been conducted by the ECOG and other cooperative groups.

Tables 5.1 and 5.2 summarize the details of trials of adjuvant therapy of melanoma using IFNs.

Table 5.1 Summary of interferon trials for adjuvant therapy of melanoma

High-dose trials
- High-risk melanoma:
  With induction phase:
    E1684
    E1690

  Without induction phase:
    NCCTG trial

- Intermediate-risk melanoma:
    E1697

Low-dose trials
- High-risk melanoma:
    WHO 16

- Intermediate-risk melanoma:
    French
    Austrian

Intermediate-dose trials
- High-risk melanoma:
    EORTC
    Scandinavian Melanoma Group

HIGH-DOSE IFN-α TRIALS

High-dose IFN-α for one year with an intravenous induction phase

ECOG trial E1684

On the basis of a phase I–II trial of intravenously (i.v.), intramuscularly (i.m.) and subcutaneously (s.c.) administered IFN-α2b conducted by our group,[3] the ECOG trial E1684 was designed to test the hypothesis that maximally tolerated doses of IFN-α2b administered for one year would be effective in prolonging relapse-free and overall survival in patients with surgically resected, high-risk melanoma. This trial randomized, to treatment or observation,

Table 5.2 Adjuvant IFN-α and IFN-γ trials in high-risk melanoma

Trial	Years	Accrual	Agent	Dose schedule	Treatment duration	Outcome analysis[a]
ECOG E1684[4]	1984–1989	287	IFN-α2b	20 MU/m^2 i.v. daily, 5 days a week 10 MU/m^2 s.c., 3 times a week	4 weeks 48 weeks	OS, $p = 0.047$ RFS, $p = 0.004$
NCCTG 83–7052[10]	1984–1989	262	IFN-α2a	20 MU/m^2 i.m., 3 times a week	12 weeks	OS, RFS $p = $ NS
WHO 16[21]	1990–1993	944	IFN-α2a	3 MU s.c. daily, 3 times a week	36 months	OS, RFS $p = $ NS
SWOG 8942[11]	1988–1989	134	IFN-γ	0.1 mg s.c., 3 times a week	12 months	OS, RFS $p = $ NS
ECOG E1690[9]	1990–1995	642	IFN-α2b	(A) 20 MU/m^2 i.v. daily, 5 days a week 10 MU/m^2 s.c., 3 times a week or (B) 3 MU s.c. daily, 3 times a week	4 weeks 48 weeks 24 months	RFS, $p = 0.03^b$ OS, $p = $ NS OS, RFS $p = $ NS
ECOG E1694	1995–1998	851	IFN-α2b vs GMK vaccine	(A) 20 MU/m^2 i.v. daily, 5 days a week 10 MU/m^2 s.c., 3 times a week or (B) GMK s.c. weekly × 4, then every 3 months	12 months 96 weeks	Concluded 14 October 1999
EORTC 18–871	1	800	IFN-α2b	(A) 1 MU 3 times a week (B) 0.2 mg s.c. 3 times a week (C) Observation	1 year 1 year	Pending
ECOG E1697	1998	1444	IFN-α2b	20 MU/m^2 daily, 5 days a week	4 weeks	Active

[a] OS, overall survival; RFS, relapse-free survival; $p = $ NS, not statistically significant.
[b] Preliminary analysis at 52 months, Cox.[9]

287 patients with either deep primary (T4, AJCC stage IIB) melanomas or primary melanoma of any thickness with either concurrent or subsequent metastases to regional lymph nodes (TxN1, AJCC stage III), between 1984 and 1990. All patients entering this study had received primary wide excision, and regional lymphadenectomy. Patients were designated 'high-risk' by virtue of the presence of pathologically proven regional lymph node metastases (89%) or deep primary lesions in the absence of regional lymph node involvement (11%).

At seven years of follow-up, there was a statistically significant prolongation of median survival from 2.8 to 3.8 years, and of relapse-free interval from 1.0 to 1.7 years (p_1 = 0.02 and 0.002 respectively).[4] This benefit was most pronounced among the 249 stage III subjects, who comprised 89% of the population entering this study (p = 0.006 and 0.0006 for median survival and relapse-free survival respectively).[5] The small subset of patients with stage IIB (node-negative) disease failed to show benefit, but a treatment interaction was identified in this group, with an imbalance in the distribution of cases with primary ulceration. This finding, coupled with the small numbers in this subset, precludes any firm conclusions from E1684 in regard to this group of patients. This landmark trial was the basis for FDA Oncologic Drug Advisory Committee recommendation of a licensure for IFN-α2b (Intron A) as the first adjuvant therapy of melanoma following surgical resection in patients with stage IIB or stage III melanoma.

An intriguing observation drawn from analysis of the hazard function curves for relapse in the treated and observed groups is the dramatic separation, occurring early in the first month of therapy. This has led to speculation that the i.v. induction phase is of critical importance to this regimen, and has spurred efforts to test this induction regimen alone in patients with lower-risk (stage IIA) disease (see below).

Not surprisingly, substantial toxicity was noted with this full-year regimen employing maximal tolerable dosages. Grade 3 or 4 (ECOG toxicity scale) events requiring dose modification and/or delays were required at least once in 50% of patients during the i.v. induction phase and in 48% of patients during the s.c. maintenance phase. Notably, most treatment delays occurred in the first four months of the regimen, after which toxicity-related treatment modifications were unusual. Constitutional and neurologic toxicities were subjectively most troublesome to patients. Leukopenia (25%) and biochemical abnormalities of liver function (15%) were most frequently the basis of dose modification, but tended to be transient and reversible. Fatal hepatotoxicity and liver failure occurred in two patients early in the trial. While both patients had evidence of antecedent liver disease, the importance of appropriate monitoring of liver function tests (weekly during induction and monthly for three months, then quarterly during maintenance) cannot be overemphasized.

The modest relapse-free and overall survival benefit seen in this trial make patient quality of life an important consideration. The impact of this therapy upon quality of life was evaluated in a retrospective quality-adjusted analysis of time spent without symptoms or toxicity (Q-TWiST) study.[6] The concept of Q-TWiST was developed by Goldhirsch et al[7] in 1989 to assess the 'trade-off' between side-effects and benefits of therapy. The time spent for patients during and after treatment, with treatment-related toxicity, relapse and TWiST were analyzed with weighting of the time spent in each of the intervals according to accepted indices. After 84 months of follow-up, the group of patients receiving IFN-α2b gained a mean of 8.9 months without relapse (p = 0.03) and 7 months of overall survival time (p = 0.02) compared with the observation group. The treated group experienced at least one episode of severe treatment-related toxicity over a period of time that averaged less than 5.8 months. The net result was that the IFN-α2b-treated group had more quality-of-life adjusted survival time than the observation group, and this was the outcome of analyses regardless of the relative valuations placed on time with toxicity and time with relapse.

The high-doses of IFN-α2b administered in this trial make patient and/or insurer costs a major concern. An economic analysis of the E1684 regimen was recently published by Hillner et al.[8] The projected incremental cost in 1996 US dollars per life-year gained in the IFN cohort of patients ranged from $13 700 after 35 years to $32 600 at seven years (the median follow-up of E1684). The benefits of IFN projected over a lifetime yield incremental costs per life-year or quality-adjusted life-year that are both less than $16 000. This figure is less than the rigorous Canadian benchmark of $20 000 per quality-of-life-year gained, and is comparable to other accepted adjuvant therapies of breast and colorectal cancer. Given the significant and durable benefit of this therapy, with 37% of treated patients continuously disease-free at five years as opposed to 26% in the observation group, this therapy has been rapidly adopted as the standard therapy for resected high-risk melanomas in the USA and several other countries.

Intergroup trial ECOG 1690

To confirm and extend the preliminary results of the E1684 trial, the E1690 intergroup trial was initiated in 1990. This randomized three-arm study compared the same high-dose regimen of IFN-α2b, described above, or a low-dose regimen of IFN-α2b, 3 MU s.c. three times a week as pursued by the WHO in Europe, versus observation. As this trial was initiated prior to the maturity of E1684, the control arm remained observation. Targeted accrual of 642 patients was completed in June 1995. Entry criteria for this study were the same as for E1684, except for the elimination of the requirement for elective lymphadenectomy for patients with clinically node-negative disease (pT4cN0). Primary end-points were relapse-free survival (RFS) and overall survival (OS), utilizing the log-rank statistic comparing the high-dose and low-dose arms versus observation.

Between 1990 and 1995, 642 patients entered the study, with 608 evaluable patients at 52 months median follow-up, as this was unblinded in 1998. The study population categorized by stage of disease comprised 162 T4cN0, 68 T1–4pN1cN0, 83 T1–4cN1 and 326 recurrent N+. At an interim analysis conducted in October 1998, more than 90% of the events specified in

the protocol had occurred. An improvement in RFS for the high-dose arm over observation (hazard ratio 1.28; $p = 0.05$) was noted, with a consistent benefit in the node-negative and node-positive patients with two to three and four or more positive nodes. Improvement in RFS was not significant for the low-dose arm. Neither the high-dose arm nor the low-dose arm was associated with an improvement in OS as compared with observation.

The outcomes for the observation groups of E1684 and E1690 are substantially different, with the latter trial significantly improved ($p = 0.001$). This may be related to the larger pT4cN0 group (25% versus 11%), or to the smaller recurrent (51% versus 66%) and cN+ groups in E1690. Asymmetrical crossover usage of IFN-α2b in patients relapsing from the observation arm has been shown, and an analysis of the 'salvage' treatment has demonstrated that recipients of IFN-α2b benefitted to a significant degree – often having had regional nodal relapse that when resected was identical to the setting for which the original trial was aimed.

A further analysis of the outcome for patients who experienced locoregional as opposed to distant and visceral relapses has indicated that the greatest benefit of IFN-α2b occurred among those patients with locoregional (surgically potentially curable) disease.[9]

High-dose intramuscular IFN-α2a without an induction phase: NCCTG 83–7052

The NCCTG study 83–7052 was designed to test the role of high-dose IFN-α administered for a three-month period in patients with stage II and III melanoma. Eligibility for this trial was similar to that for the E1684 and 1690 trials discussed above, except that some patients with AJCC stage IIA disease were also allowed to be entered. Two hundred and sixty-two patients with resected stage IIA/B melanoma greater than 1.69 mm depth or stage III disease were randomized to treatment or observation. Elective lymphadenectomy was not a requirement for study entry, and about 50% of patients had clinically node-negative (stage II) disease.

Important differences between this and the E1684 treatment regimen were the schedule and route of administration. IFN-α2a (Roferon) was administered at a dose of 20 MU/m²/day i.m. three times a week for 12 weeks. Analysis at maturity in 1995 revealed no significant impact upon survival or relapse-free interval overall. However, a trend to benefit was noted among the patients with clinical stage III (node-positive) disease who received IFN-α2a.[10] The total prescribed dose of IFN in this trial was 720 MU/m², compared with 1840 MU/m² in the ECOG E1684 trial, and the actual fraction of planned dosage administered in this trial was less than that administered in the E1684 trial. It is tempting to consider that the higher early and/or more prolonged dose administered in E1684 may partly explain the difference in outcomes of these two high-dose trials, although this is speculation at present.

HYBRID INTERMEDIATE-DOSE REGIMENS OF IFN-α

Interest in testing the role of a more intense induction therapy followed by the maintenance treatment regimen that proved successful in the ECOG E1684 trial, coupled with efforts to reduce toxicity, have led the European Organization for Research and Treatment of Cancer (EORTC) to devise hybrid regimens of subcutaneously administered therapy.

The EORTC have recently commenced a study (18-952) testing the impact of intermediate doses of IFN-α2b administered over one or two years, as compared with observation, upon relapse-free interval and survival of high-risk melanoma. The induction phase of this regimen is 10 MU (flat dose) given s.c. five days per week for four weeks followed by a maintenance phase of either 10 MU s.c. three times a week for 12 months or 5 MU s.c. three times a week for 24 months. This three-arm study has been planned to accrue 1000 patients with high-risk resected melanoma, including patients with nodal disease with or without extracapsular extension. The goal is to evaluate the impact of two lower-dosage, less toxic regimens that do not include the i.v. component of E1684. Since the study lacks a high-dose arm that would replicate the E1684 trial, it will be difficult to interpret the results if they are negative.

The Scandinavian Melanoma Cooperative Group is conducting a similar three-arm study in high-risk melanoma, with the difference that the maintenance treatment dose is 10 MU s.c. three times a week for both treatment arms – one given for 12 months and the other for 24 months (arms B and C respectively). The total dosage of IFN-α2b to be delivered in arm B of this trial is 50% of that in the E1684 trial, and that in arm C is 95% of that administered in the E1684 trial. Both the EORTC study and the Scandinavian study include a quality-of-life assessment.

HIGH-DOSE BRIEF-COURSE INTRAVENOUS IFN FOR 'INTERMEDIATE RISK' MELANOMA

The group of patients with T3cN0 (Breslow depth 1.5–4 mm, AJCC stage IIA) melanoma is several-fold larger than the 'high-risk' stage III population considered eligible for E1684 and E1690. Because of their somewhat better prognosis, they have often been overlooked in adjuvant therapy trials. Data from the University of Alabama and the Sydney Melanoma Unit indicate five- and ten-year survivals of 72.5% and 62% for this group as a whole. Of patients with the new diagnosis of melanoma, 31% fall into this category. In terms of the recent (1998 US) melanoma incidence of 40 300 cases, approximately 12 400 new cases fall into stage IIA, and of these at least 3400 will die of their disease. It is evident that an effective adjuvant therapy for this group of patients would be of major importance.

High-dose IFN-α has not yet been investigated for this subset of patients – partly because of reluctance to expose patients with a relatively more favourable prognosis to the toxicity and expense of 12 months' treatment. The NCCTG trial (83-7052) discussed above included patients with this category of disease, but lacked sufficient power to draw any meaningful conclusions for this subset. Low-dose IFN-α has been applied for this group of patients in European trials that are discussed in Chapter 4.

The early and marked separation of the relapse-free survival curves and hazard plots for treatment versus observation noted in the E1684 trial has led us and others to hypothesize that the peak serum levels of the induction regimen may have been of paramount importance in obtaining benefit. Also, a short induction regimen alone is attractive and feasible in this group of patients with intermediate prognosis for relapse-free and overall survival at five to ten years. With this in mind, the ECOG has initiated a trial designed to test the role of high-dose IFN-α in patients with stage IIA disease (E1697). Based upon data from E1684 discussed above, patients will be assigned to receive either the induction phase of E1684 (20 MU/m^2, Monday through Friday for four weeks) or observation. Accrual began in early 1999, with a total of 1444 patients anticipated from the USA (ECOG) and Canada (NCI Canada) over a two- to three-year period. This trial has been designed with a power to detect a 7% increase in cure fraction and/or survival, and is stratified for use of current prognostic assessment utilizing sentinel node mapping and selective nodal biopsy to define disease stage.

In summary, the adjuvant therapy of patients with melanoma has recently shown significant survival and relapse-free interval impact for the intravenous and subcutaneous administration of maximally tolerable dosages of recombinant IFN-α2b in a trial of the ECOG. While this represents a toxic therapy, corollary analyses of its impact upon quality of life using Q-TWiST methods and cost–efficacy analyses all argue for the benefit and utility of this intervention, especially for node-positive patients at highest risk of relapse with resectable melanoma. A corroborative trial has been completed, and data from the preliminary analysis of data from the E1690 Intergroup trial corroborate the benefit of the E1684 regimen in relation to continuous relapse-free survival. More recent trials applying lower doses of IFN-α2b, and IFN-α2a for longer periods of time, have not yet reached the maturity (median follow-up of seven years) that was present for E1684 at its first publication, but these suggest a measurable impact upon disease relapse for lower-risk groups of node-negative patients with intermediate depths of tumor invasion (see Chapter 4). The lower risk and longer time-course of stage II melanoma make it necessary to await more mature data to draw final conclusions from these trials. The transience of benefits with lower-dose regimens suggests that the next step in trial development along this line will be to pursue longer (potentially indefinite) therapy.

With the advent of depot forms of interferon (IFN-α2a and IFN-α2b), it is to be anticipated that trials designed to deliver cumulative (concentration × times) doses that may exceed those reached in prior trials, with lower toxicity and perhaps greater efficacy, lie in the future.

The analysis of known immunologic and antiproliferative as well as anti-angiogenic mechanisms of IFN-α2 is now important in relation to the recent (E1690) and current (E1694) Intergroup trials. It is anticipated that as the mechanism of therapeutic benefit and surrogates for response to IFN are identified, candidate patients who will have improved likelihood of response may be chosen without the liability of toxicity among those who are unable to benefit from therapy. In addition, the advent of molecular markers of disease (see Chapter 1) will define more appropriate target populations.

CURRENT AND FUTURE DIRECTIONS

Analysis of mechanism of action of IFN-α, alone and in combination

The antitumor mechanism of type I IFNs has been suggested to be direct and antiproliferative, immunomodulatory and antivascular. These putative mechanisms have each been supported by preclinical laboratory in vitro analyses, although there exist little data drawn from careful analysis of clinical trials in the human cancer to support any conclusion at the present time.

Antiproliferative evaluation of the IFNs against human tumour cells in vitro have generally failed to correlate with clinical response, except perhaps in selected hematologic neoplasms such as hairy cell leukemia. Melanoma has been well documented to be deficient in the expression of MHC class I antigens known to be important for T-cell recognition and effector response. Our analyses have demonstrated the upregulation of MHC class I antigens[11] in tumor samples obtained from patients with stage III melanoma. Furthermore, significant shifts in the distribution of T-cell subsets in the blood have been documented among recipients of IFN-α, as well as IFN-α and IFN-γ.[12] These observations support the hypothesis that the impact of IFN therapy occurs upon the host effector system, although this has not previously been possible to dissect at the level of T-cell responses to MHC class I restricted epitopes that have been defined over the past few years.

IFN in relation to T-cell-defined vaccines for melanoma

The analysis of T-cell responses to melanoma has defined a series of peptide antigens that fall into well-defined categories:

- differentiation antigens (i.e. these associated with organelles of melanization);[13]
- more highly cancer-restricted antigens (cancer–testis antigens as defined by Old);[14]
- antigens that result as a consequence of mutation of normal cellular genes such as CDK4.[15,16]

The precision of modern T-cell immunology permits us to anticipate an analysis of the mechanism of IFN action in terms of host immune response to these peptide antigens, where it is conceivable that the host response to antigens of melanoma may be augmented either through the upregulation of MHC class I antigens (HLA-ABC), or costimulatory molecules, or through the function of IFN-α, as a dendritic cell potentiating cytokine (dendrokine).

The pursuit of IFN as a potentiator of T-cell response to defined antigens in human cancer is in its infancy, and while preclinical rationale for this approach is strong, there are no current clinical data to allow a synthesis or conclusions in regard to the potential benefit of such an approach, nor in regard to the timing, dosage and schedule optimization.

IFN in relation to B-cell (antibody-inducing) approaches to adjuvant therapy for melanoma

Among the vaccines that have been evaluated for adjuvant therapy of high-risk resected melanoma in randomized controlled trials to date, none has yet shown benefit that approaches that observed with IFN-α. However, serological study of patients with melanoma has shown increased frequency of antibody response to the GM2 molecule, a glycolipid expressed on most melanoma cells. This is the most immunogenic among the gangliosides of melanoma in careful studies by Livingston and Old over the past 20 years at Memorial Hospital.[17] After careful development of a vaccine comprising purified GM2 and BCG, given in conjunction with immunomodulatory doses of cyclophosphamide, Livingston conducted a small phase III trial of GM2–BCG/cyclophosphamide versus BCG/cyclophosphamide, which revealed a trend toward improved relapse-free but not overall survival.[18] This study showed that among patients who developed anti-GM2 IgM antibody responses (nearly all responses to this vaccine were IgM), relapse-free survival was significantly prolonged. The GM2 vaccine was thereafter scaled up commercially (GMK, Progenics, Inc.) modified by conjugation to a carrier (KLH) to increase its immunogenicity, along with the use of a newer saponin adjuvant (QS21 (Aquila Pharmaceuticals) to induce IgG as well as IgM in an increased fraction of immunized subjects. The phase III trial data regarding GM2 was the best-developed for a defined vaccine antigen of melanoma, and was selected by the Melanoma Committee of the ECOG as the next phase III trial option, in comparison with IFN-α, in 1994. Trial E1694 tests 96 weeks of vaccination against GMK in comparison with 52 weeks of high-dose IFN-α2b exactly as administered in E1684 and E1690. The trial commenced in 1996, and projects accrual of 851 patients with stage IIB/III melanoma by mid-1999 to detect a potential 10% improvement of RFS over IFN.

Combinations of IFN-α and GM2 vaccination

The synthesis of any GM2 vaccine-associated benefit and the benefit of IFN-α observed in E1684 and E1690 is an obvious goal. This provided the basis for design of a phase II trial of GMK vaccination in combination with IFN-α at high dose. This trial, launched in selected sites of the ECOG and at Memorial Sloan-Kettering in 1997, accrued 106 patients to three arms testing GMK alone, versus GMK given concurrently with IFN-α at high dose (as the most facile bimodality combination), versus GMK followed after one month of vaccination with IFN-α at high dose (in order to allow immunization to commence prior to any lymphopenic response that might inhibit or abrogate the GM2 immunization). The preliminary results of this trial[9,19] reveal that no significant inhibitory interaction exists when measured in terms of anti-GM2 IgM/IgG. These results pave the way to consideration of combinations of GMK and IFN-α as disease outcome data become available from the GMK phase III trial E1694.

Combinations of IFN-α2b and radiotherapy

Regional failure of melanoma has been recognized as a major problem for patients with locally advanced disease, especially at the regional nodal basin. Extracapsular extension has been problematic in patients with head and neck melanoma. Patients have therefore been treated with hypofractionated radiotherapy in a non-randomized historically referenced trial at the MD Anderson Cancer Center.[20] The ECOG has recently initiated a trial comparing IFN-α2b at high dosage (as in E1684) versus IFN-α2b plus hypofractionated radiotherapy, as suggested from the experience at MD Anderson. This study targets 150 patients (75 per treatment arm) with extracapsular extension of melanoma, and will provide answers to the question regarding the role of radiotherapy in regionally advanced melanoma, as well as the effects of the combination of IFN-α and radiotherapy for patients who have both high regional failure rates and high distant relapse risk.

CONCLUSIONS

The era of empirical development of chemotherapy, biologic therapy and combined-modality approaches to melanoma and other diseases is now emerging into an era in which the therapeutic application of molecular mediators such as the cytokines (including IFN-α) may be understood in terms of their mechanisms. With the availability of ganglioside vaccines capable of stimulating antibody responses to potentially relevant melanoma antigens and peptide vaccines selected and optimized in terms of T-cell responses, the opportunity to intervene specifically to induce an improved host immune response against melanoma is at hand. The strategies of molecular therapy under evaluation now will demand rigorous laboratory as well as clinical trial designs to be developed, and will optimally build upon the data that have already been acquired in relation to the IFNs, as the cornerstone of adjuvant trial development in this field. As laboratory surrogates for the detection of the disease are understood (molecular detection using RT-PCR as reviewed in Chapter 1), and immunologic methods of reliable precise measurement of host response (e.g. ELISPOT and tetramer flow cytometry assays for antigen-specific T cells at a population level), laboratory progress in adjuvant therapy of melanoma will accelerate progress in the clinic.

The systematic development of trials of IFN-α from phase I–II to III, and its application, first of all in measurable metastatic disease in resectable and then in high-risk and intermediate-risk adjuvant settings, provide a paradigm for the evaluation of new biologic agents, particularly for vaccines. As we have moved from a focus upon survival prolongation to the evaluation of relapse-interval prolongation as clinical endpoints for trials, intermediate endpoints of increasing interest and potential relevance, including the modulation of MHC and tumor antigens as well as host immune responses, may become the most appropriate correlates of disease outcome in our current trials. The adoption of more precise laboratory end-points may allow the application of newer biologic agents to expose only the beneficiaries of these therapies to treatment. Laboratory analyses will permit us to more rapidly combine the available agents at our disposal, in a rational and constructive manner to improve the results of therapy.

REFERENCES

1. Buzaid AC, Ross MI, Balch CM et al, Critical analysis of the current American Joint Committee on Cancer Staging System for Cutaneous Melanoma and proposal of a new staging system. *J Clin Oncol* 1997; **15**: 1039–51.
2. Isaacs A, Lindemann JJ, Virus interference: the interferon. *Proc R Soc Lond* 1957; **147**: 258–67.
3. Kirkwood JM, Ernstoff MS, Davis CA et al, Comparison of intramuscular and intravenous recombinant alpha-2 interferon in melanoma and other cancers. *Ann Intern Med* 1985; **103**: 32–6.
4. Kirkwood JM, Strawderman MH, Ernstoff MS et al, Interferon alfa-2b adjuvant therapy of high-risk resected cutaneous melanoma: the Eastern Cooperative Oncology Group trial EST 1684. *J Clin Oncol* 1996; **14**: 7–17.
5. Kirkwood JM, Strawderman MH, Ernstoff MS et al, Adjuvant therapy of high-risk melanoma: the role of high-dose interferon α-2b. In: *Adjuvant Therapy of Cancer VIII* (Salmon SE, ed). Lippincott-Raven: Philadelphia, 1997: 251–7.
6. Cole BF, Gelber RD, Kirkwood JM et al, A quality-of-life-adjusted survival analysis of interferon alfa-2b adjuvant treatment for high-risk resected cutaneous melanoma: an Eastern Cooperative Oncology Group study (E1684). *J Clin Oncol* 1996; **14**: 2666–73.
7. Goldhirsch A, Gelber RD, Simes RJ et al, Costs and benefits of adjuvant therapy in breast cancer: a quality-adjusted survival analysis. *J Clin Oncol* 1989; **7**: 36–44.
8. Hillner BE, Kirkwood JM, Atkins MB et al, Economic analysis of adjuvant interferon alfa-2b in high-risk melanoma based on projections from ECOG 1684. *J Clin Oncol* 1997; **15**: 2351–8.
9. Kirkwood JM, Ibrahim J, Sondak V et al, Preliminary analysis of the E1690/S9111/C9190 Intergroup postoperative adjuvant trial of high- and low-dose IFNα2b (HDI and LDI) in high-risk primary or lymph node metastatic melanoma. *Proc Am Soc Clin Oncol* 1999; **18**: 537A (Abst 2072).
10. Creagan ET, Dalton RJ, Ahmann DL et al, Randomized, surgical adjuvant clinical trial of recombinant interferon alfa-2a in selected patients with malignant melanoma. *J Clin Oncol* 1995; **13**: 2776–83.
11. Kirkwood JM, Sosman J, Ernstoff M et al, E2690: a study of the mechanism of IFN alfa-2b in high risk melanoma in the ECOG/Intergroup trial E1690. *Proc Am Assoc Cancer Res* **1995; 36**: 641.
12. Ernstoff MS, Gooding W, Nair S et al, Immunological effects of treatment with sequential administration of recombinant interferon gamma and alpha in patients with matastatic renal cell carcinoma during a phase I trial. *Cancer Res* 1992; **52**: 851–6.
13. Maeurer MJ, Storkus WJ, Kirkwood JM, Lotze MT, New treatment option for patients with melanoma: review of melanoma-derived T-cell epitope-based peptide vaccines. *Melanoma Res* 1996; **6**: 11–24.
14. Old LJ, Cancer immunology: the search for specificity. *Cancer Res* 1981; **41**: 361–75.
15. Wolfel T, Hauer M, Schneider J et al, A p161NK4a-insensitive CDK4 mutant targeted by cytolytic T lymphocytes in a human melanoma. *Science* 1995; **269**: 1281–4.
16. Storkus WJ, Kirkwood JM, Tuting T, Vaccine trials in high-risk melanoma: induction of effector T-cell responses to melanoma. In: *Molecular Diagnosis and Treatment of Melanoma* (Kirkwood JM, ed). Marcel Dekker: New York, 1998.
17. Livingston PO, The case for melanoma vaccines that induce antibodies. In: *Molecular Diagnosis and Treatment of Melanoma* (Kirkwood JM, ed). Marcel Dekker: New York, 1997.
18. Livingston PO, Wong GYC, Adluri S et al, Improved survival in stage III melanoma patients with GM2 antibodies: a randomized trial of adjuvant vaccination with GM2 ganglioside. *J Clin Oncol* 1994; **12**: 1036–44.
19. Chapman PB, Morrissey D, Ibrahim J et al, Eastern Cooperative Oncology Group phase II randomized adjuvant trial of GM2-KLH + QS21 (GMK) vaccine ± high dose interferon-α2b (HD IFN) in melanoma (MEL). *Proc Am Soc Clin Oncol* 1999; **18**: 538A (Abst 2078).
20. Ang KK, Byers RM, Peters LJ et al, Regional

radiotherapy as adjuvant treatment for head and neck malignant melanoma. *Arch Otolaryngol Head Neck Surg* 1990; **116:** 169–72.

21. Cascinelli N, Bufalino R, Morabito A, MacKie R, Results of adjuvant interferon study in WHO melanoma programme. *Lancet* 1994; **343** 913–14.

6

Prostatic carcinoma

Michael R Curtis, John A Heaney, Robert J Amdur, Alan R Schned, Robert Harris, Marc S Ernstoff

INTRODUCTION

Despite serious questions about the value of screening for prostate cancer,[1,2] the disease is still the most common cancer in men, with an estimated 184 500 new cases of prostate cancer in the USA in 1999, and about 39 200 prostate cancer-related deaths.[3] Advocates of 'watchful waiting', treating patients only with non-curative intent, suggest that 5- and 10-year disease-specific survival rates are similar in men treated expectantly to those treated with curative therapy.[4–6] Others will point to prostate cancer cause-specific mortality rates at 10 years of up to 51–63% with conservative therapy,[7,8] compared with rates of 6–15% with radical prostatectomy and radical radiotherapy.[9,10] A definitive, randomized, controlled study comparing 'watchful waiting' with curative therapy has not been carried out, so physicians and patients are left to sort through the conflicting literature to determine the best plan of treatment for the individual patient with prostate cancer. Data from a recently initiated national study of radical prostatectomy versus observation trial (PIVOT) for early-stage prostate cancer (confined to the gland) will not be available for some time to come.

The key to understanding why there is no therapeutic strategy uniformly accepted for prostate cancer begins with an appreciation that there is enormous heterogeneity of prostate tumor tissue. In reviewing the slides of a radical prostatectomy specimen, one frequently will see multiple Gleason grade patterns in the same specimen adjacent to, or intermingled with, benign glands. Animal models and tissue culture studies confirm that disparate populations of tumor cells exist in an individual tumor.[11,12] Other differences identified within an individual deposit of tumor are seen at ultrastructural and molecular levels, and include variable expression of hormone receptors, growth factor receptors, oncogenes and tumor suppressor genes.[13–15] Some tumors will exhibit neuroendocrine differentiation,[16] while others will show features similar to transitional cell carcinoma.[17] In this context, early-stage prostate cancer can be thought of in three categories:

- indolent disease that will never metastasize and does not need treatment;
- aggressive disease that has already metastasized microscopically and will not be cured by definitive local treatment;

- cancers that have the potential to metasta-size but have not at the time of diagnosis, and can be cured with local therapy.

Thus it is not surprising that for certain patients non-curative management will be the most beneficial therapy, while other patients will be best served by an aggressive, multimodality approach.

Amid this confusion remains the concept that prostate cancer, like other malignancies, has a natural progression over time from curable local disease to metastatic life-threatening cancer.[18] This perspective, combined with a dramatic increase in the number of new cases diagnosed annually, has led to a concomitant increase in the number of radical prostatectomies performed. Lu-Yao et al[19] reported that 5.75 times the number of radical prostatectomies were performed in the USA in 1990 as compared with 1984. Medicare data indicate that this number has risen 2.5 times from 1990 to 1994.[20] Accompanying this rise in treatment by radical prostatectomy is an increase in radiation therapy for stages A–C prostate cancer.[10,21]

Radical surgery will lead to five-year disease-free survival rates, as defined by undetectable levels of prostate-specific antigen (PSA), of up to 91% when the disease is pathologically organ-confined.[22] Despite the hope that earlier diagnosis of prostate cancer would lead to a higher rate of curative surgery, there has been a persistently high incidence of non-organ-confined disease with radical prostatectomy. Up to one-half of prostatectomy specimens from patients with cancer confined to the gland by clinical staging criteria will have extracapsular disease.[9,23–26] It is well documented that patients with extracapsular or margin-positive disease have higher rates of disease recurrence.[22,27,28]

Traditionally, adjuvant therapy in prostate cancer has consisted of radiation therapy and/or orchiectomy as a supplement to radical prostatectomy when the pathologic examination indicated that prostate cancer was present beyond the margins of surgical resection ('positive margins').[29] The development of reversible medical castration using hormonal therapy, in the face of the disappointingly high rate of extraprostatic involvement, has led to an expanded concept of curative adjuvant therapy.[30–32] While the recent use of preoperative (or preradiotherapy) hormonal therapy, known as *neoadjuvant hormonal therapy* (NHT), began in earnest in the 1980s, it is, in fact, an older therapy rediscovered.[33]

HISTORICAL ASPECTS OF HORMONAL THERAPY OF THE PROSTATE

Hormonal manipulation with the intent to alter the prostate was initiated in 1893 with White[34] performing castration on 111 men with symptoms of outlet obstruction. It is likely that some of their symptoms were secondary to prostate carcinoma and that the relief of obstruction was a result of androgen withdrawal.[35] In the mid 1930s, Gutman et al[36] showed that high levels of acid phosphatase are secreted in prostate cancer, and, in 1941, Huggins and Hodges[37] extended this work to discover that prostate cancer is androgen-dependent. The earliest use of NHT was probably by Vallett,[38] who, in 1944, reported performing orchiectomy followed by radical perineal prostatectomy. Other investigators followed this approach,[39–41] but it fell out of favor by the mid 1950s. Soloway et al[42] suggest that it was abandoned largely because of the morbidity of permanent hormonal therapy without clear evidence that it altered the course of the disease.

In 1969, Scott and Boyd[43] reported a retrospective series of patients with stage C prostate cancer (cancer outside the capsule of the gland but with no distant metastasis) who underwent radical prostatectomy preceded by estrogen therapy, orchiectomy, or both. They noted 5-, 10- and 15-year survivals similar to those in patients with surgically treated stage B1 disease (cancer that is located in one lobe of the gland without extracapsular spread). In the 1970s, estrogen therapy was combined with simultaneous external-beam radiation for the treatment of prostate cancer without apparent benefit.[44–46] In 1984, Green et al[47] reported a higher rate of complete response in a small, non-randomized study, when estrogen therapy was administered for two months prior to, and concurrent with, external-beam radiation. These data, combined with the development of reversible medical castration, led to wider study of NHT in conjunction with radical therapy by the late 1980s.

NEOADJUVANT HORMONAL THERAPY AND RADICAL PROSTATECTOMY

Theoretical rationale for NHT in radical prostatectomy

Like many carcinomas, prostate cancer is a systemic phenomenon. The primary cause of death in prostate cancer is metastatic disease rather than the local lesion.[48] As a general concept, it is appealing to think of the combination of a systemic therapy to treat unrecognized distant micrometastases accompanying a definitive therapy to neutralize the primary tumor. Among the heterogeneous mixture of prostate cancer cells, some cells are 'hormone-sensitive' (androgen-dependent) while others are 'hormone-insensitive' (androgen-independent).[49] One current hypothesis is that the primary tumor, having undergone the most cell divisions, has a higher likelihood of mutations causing androgen independence, while younger, micrometastatic disease is still likely to be androgen-dependent.[48]

The biochemical mechanism of cell death in androgen blockade is a well-described series of events known as programmed cell death or apoptosis.[50] The prostate tumor cells that enter the apoptotic pathway are subject to endonuclease activation and chromatin cleavage. DNA is fragmented within 24 hours by calcium-dependent DNases in an active process requiring ATP. A characteristic ladder of DNA fragments can be seen in agarose gel electrophoresis of genomic DNA.[49] Cell death is not dependent on the stage of the cell cycle,[51] and the reduction in tumor volume in experimental models is from 10–99% of the original tumor burden.[52]

Bruchovsky et al[53] performed pioneering work studying the effects of androgen suppression in the Shionogi mouse mammary tumor model. Twenty days after implantation in nude mice, this androgen-dependent tumor reached an average weight of 6 g. Castration of the animals led to a 90% decrease in tumor weight. Following a short dormant period, the tumor grew to the pre-castration size, despite low levels of androgen receptor and 5-α-reductase, indicating that the tumor grew in an androgen-free state. The investigators observed a marked change in the relative number of androgen-independent cells capable of forming tumor in a limiting-dilution assay used to determine cancer stem cell frequency: there was one stem cell per 4000 cells in the primary tumor compared with one in 200 in the tumor population that recurred. At the point of maximal regression, there was only one stem cell per 70 000 tumor cells. Thus the stem cells, presumably the source of recurrent disease, are relatively depleted at the nadir of tumor size.

These data have important implications for the addition of NHT to the curative therapy of prostate cancer. They suggest that NHT may lead to a regressed tumor with fewer stem cells, but NHT will only be curative if the tumor has not reached an androgen-independent state. Theoretically, the optimal timing of the curative therapy should be at the point of smallest tumor volume, before mutation and clonal selection leads to androgen-independent cells.

The mechanism of the transition from androgen dependence to androgen independence is not yet completely understood. Isaacs and Coffey[52] demonstrated from work in a Dunning rat model that the development of an androgen-independent state appeared to be the result of clonal selection. They showed that both androgen-dependent and androgen-independent cell populations exist initially, but that, following androgen withdrawal, the androgen-independent cell population grows selectively. Other investigators have proposed that autocrine secretion of growth factors by the tumor cells promotes this transition,[54] or that it may come about following a somatic point mutation of the androgen receptor.[55] More recently, Landstrom et al[56] suggested that the underlying cause of androgen-independent tumor growth might be a reduction of the number of tumor cells being depleted by apoptosis, rather than an increase of cell proliferation rate.

While the majority of metastatic androgen-independent prostate cancers express androgen receptor, mutations in the receptor can be identified in at least half of the patients.[57] If suppression of apoptosis proves to be the critical factor in the development of androgen independence, it is likely to be related to expression of the proto-oncogene *bcl-2* and its inhibitor *bax*. *bcl-2* is a proto-oncogene that encodes for a protein, Bcl-2, that inhibits apoptosis,[58–60] while *bax* encodes for a protein, Bax, that accelerates rates of cell death.[61] Multiple studies in late stage prostate cancer show *bcl-2* overexpression in androgen-independent tissue.[62,63] In vitro and in vivo studies have shown that overexpression of the Bcl-2 oncoprotein protects prostate cancer cells from apoptotic stimuli and correlates with tumor transition to androgen independence.[64] The mechanism of cell death suppression by Bcl-2 protein may be through the prevention of sustained increase in cytoplasmic and nuclear calcium. Recent clinical studies from radical prostatectomy specimens have shown that overexpression of Bcl-2 protein is an independent predictor of biochemical relapse.[65]

The presence of wild-type *p53*, a tumor suppressor gene, is also required for cell cycle regulation and apoptosis.[66,67] There is a functional interaction between *p53* and *bcl-2* that indicates that *p53* will downregulate *bcl-2*.[67–69] Immunohistochemical staining for Bcl-2 and p53 protein expression in radical prostatectomy specimens has shown that the combination of mutant *p53* and overexpression of *bcl-2* is associated with a threefold increase in the risk of biochemical relapse compared with patients who are negative for these markers.[65] More work needs to be done in this area to understand the relationships between hormonal manipulation and prostate cancer cell death.

CHOICES OF HORMONAL THERAPY USED IN NHT TRIALS

Diethylstilbestrol (DES)

The traditional form of 'medical castration' has been carried out with the use of the estrogen, diethylstilbestrol (DES), which inhibits release of luteinizing hormone (LH) from the anterior pituitary. Following the administration of DES, the Leydig cells of the testes lose their stimulus to produce testosterone, and castrate levels of testosterone are reached in one or two weeks. In vitro studies suggest that DES also has direct cytotoxic effects and promotes apoptosis.[70] In a randomized Veterans Administration study of placebo, orchiectomy and DES for clinical stage C or D prostate cancer reported in 1967, the DES group had significantly higher cardiovascular morbidity and mortality.[35,71] DES has the advantage of being an oral agent, and it is extremely inexpensive. With the advent of the luteinizing hormone-releasing hormone (LHRH) agonists, DES has fallen out of favor largely because of these significant cardiovascular side-effects. However, at a Veterans Administration hospital recently, it has been substituted for LHRH agonists owing to financial constraints,[72] and low doses have been used in some NHT trials.[73] Low-dose coumadin may prevent the hypercoagulable complications associated with DES use.[74]

Luteinizing hormone-releasing hormone (LHRH) agonists

Based on the pioneering work by Schally et al,[75] the identification of the decapeptide synthetic analogs of LHRH has led to a new class of hormonal therapy. These analogs, which are 100 times more powerful than the naturally occurring form, cause an initial surge of LH and follicle-stimulating hormone (FSH) release and an increase in serum testosterone. However, with chronic administration, there is uncoupling of gonadatrophin-releasing hormone receptors from their effectors, intracellular sequestration of the receptors, and depletion of the stores of gonadotrophins.[76,77] The resulting fall in LH and FSH leads to castrate levels of testosterone. Because of the transient increase in testosterone, or 'flare', LHRH agonists are usually given with an antiandrogen in the setting of metastatic disease. Presently in the USA, LHRH agonists come as one-, three- or four-month subcutaneous depot injections of leuprolide (Lupron) or goserelin acetate (Zoladex). Both buserelin (Suprefact) and triptorelin (Decapeptyl) are widely used in Europe, but an application for approval by the US Food and Drug Administration (FDA) has not been submitted. One other LHRH analog, naferelin acetate (Synarel), is available in the USA, and is administered twice daily by nasal inhalation. However, it has been approved by the FDA only for use in patients with endometriosis.

Antiandrogens

In patients with previously untreated metastatic prostate cancer, a large, randomized, prospective intergroup study showed an advantage in both time to progression and overall survival when the nonsteroidal antiandrogen flutamide was used with leuprolide, as compared with the administration of leuprolide alone.[32] Since this study was reported in 1989, in virtually all trials of NHT, antiandrogens are administered along with LHRH agonists to block the weakly androgenic steroid production of the adrenal cortex (dehydroepiandrosterone and androstenedione). This combined androgen blockade (CAB) is also referred to as maximal androgen deprivation (MAD) or maximal androgen blockade (MAB). One meta-analysis, combining 22 randomized trials, failed to show a survival benefit of CAB over conventional castration (medical or surgical) in patients with advanced disease.[78] However, this analysis has been subject to criticisms, and a subsequent meta-analysis does show a significant survival advantage.[79] This controversy continues, with the recent publication of a study comparing orchiectomy with and without flutamide showing no advantage to CAB, and a subsequent meta-analysis, including this study, demon-

strating small but significant advantage to CAB.[80,81]

'Antiandrogens' refers to a group of androgen-receptor blockers, and the exogenous synthetic forms are divided into steroidal and nonsteroidal antiandrogens. The steroidal antiandrogen cyproteranone acetate (Androcur) is a hydroxyprogesterone derivative that both binds the androgen receptors and has progestational activity.[82] Cyproteranone has been used widely in Europe for advanced prostate cancer as well as in a recent prospective NHT trial in Canada.[83]

Three nonsteroidal antiandrogens are available in the USA: flutamide (Eulixen), bicalutamide (Casodex) and Nilutamide (Nilandron). Flutamide was the first commercially available nonsteroidal antiandrogen, and it acts as a competitive inhibitor for dehydrotestosterone and testosterone T-receptor protein binding. Because of the relative affinities of dehydrotestosterone, testosterone and flutamide, high concentrations of flutamide are required to block androgens from the androgen receptor. To maintain high levels of the oral agent, dosing of flutamide is three times daily. Gastrointestinal distress, primarily diarrhea, can occur in up to 15% of patients, and, in some cases, may lead to withdrawal of therapy.[35] Bicalutamide is a five- to tenfold more potent antiandrogen than flutamide, with probably equal efficacy and a lower side-effect profile.[84,85] It has the additional advantage of once-daily dosing. However, data concerning the use of bicalutamide in NHT are limited. Nilutamide is chemically similar to flutamide and is widely used in Europe, but its use poses the risk of night blindness and interstitial pneumonitis in some patients.[35] Nilutamide is also once-daily dosing, and is the least expensive of the antiandrogens. There are insufficient data to state definitively that any one of the antiandrogens is superior to another.

Other agents

Estramustine phosphate (Emcyt) has both estrogenic and cytotoxic properties.[35] It has been shown experimentally to exhibit antimicrotubule properties, and it is cytotoxic in cells that are capable of dividing.[86] Estramustine is used extensively in Europe for the treatment of advanced disease, but it produced disappointing results in a National Prostatic Cancer Project trial.[87] Estramustine has been used recently along with acetylsalicylic acid in a prospective randomized trial of NHT in Europe.[88] Encouraging results have been seen in the treatment of metastatic prostate cancer using the combination of estramustine with vinblastine, etoposide or paclitaxel.[89]

CLINICAL OBJECTIVES OF NHT

The primary clinical objectives of NHT are to treat both local and systemic occult disease by eliminating androgen-sensitive micrometastatic disease with hormonal manipulation, followed by surgical removal of the primary tumor with its residual hormonally unresponsive cells.[90] The ultimate goal of NHT is to improve disease-free and overall cancer-specific survival. There are multiple prospective, randomized clinical trials currently underway in pursuit of this goal. The more immediate, 'surrogate' goal of NHT, for which there are now data, is to determine whether NHT will 'downstage' tumors at surgical resection and decrease the rates of capsular penetration and of positive margins.

Data on NHT in clinical stage B prostate cancer

Does NHT decrease the likelihood of extra-organ disease and does it decrease the rate of positive margins? Combining five non-randomized trials of NHT in clinical stage B prostate cancer where the final pathologic data are known, 164 of 205 patients (80%) remained stage B at final pathology.[91–95] These results compared favorably with contemporary radical prostatectomy series, which show that up to half of clinical stage B patients are found to

have pathologic stage C disease at radical prostatectomy.[9,23–26] The rate of positive surgical margins likewise was decreased in these NHT studies, with, for example, Solomon et al[92] reporting 13.2% positive margins in contrast to non-randomized controls of 46.7%. Despite these encouraging results, all authors called for prospective randomized, controlled studies, which are now underway and producing preliminary results.

Table 6.1 shows published data from three prospective, randomized, controlled trials of NHT prior to radical prostatectomy. Two large studies, reported by Soloway et al[95] and Labrie et al[83] randomized a total of 416 patients either to three months of leuprolide and flutamide followed by radical prostatectomy or to immediate radical prostatectomy. Labrie et al[83] found 77% organ-confined disease in the NHT group, in contrast to 51% in the control group, while Soloway et al[95] saw the organ-confined rate increase from 22% in the controls to 53% in the NHT group. The rate of positive surgical margins also improved, with Labrie et al[83] showing a decrease from 34% to 8%, and Soloway et al[95] a decrease from 48% to 18%. Van Poppel et al[88] used estramustine for six weeks preoperatively, and found 82.3% organ-confined disease in the intervention group and 67.6% in those going directly to surgery. The European Study Group on Neoadjuvant Treatment randomized 159 patients in a similar format to three months of goserelin and flutamide or immediate radical prostatectomy. The positive margin rate of 13% in the NHT arm compared favorably with a rate of 36% in the control arm.[96] Van Poppel et al,[88] Fair et al,[90] Klotz et al[97] and Pederson et al[98] all reported decreases approaching 50% in the rate of positive margins in the NHT group compared with controls.

Will this decreased rate of positive margins influence cause-specific survival? Despite initial enthusiasm for this approach, the answer will not be known until long-term, follow-up studies are available. However, interim data from one non-randomized and two randomized trials reporting no improvement in rate of PSA relapses at 12–26 months have dampened early enthusiasm.[73,99,100]

Table 6.1 Prospective randomized trials of NHT in clinical stage B carcinoma						
Authors and year		Number of patients	Treatment	Duration	Pathologic stage B (%)	Margin-positive (%)
Van Poppel et al[88] (1995)	Cases	36	Estramustine and aspirin	6 weeks	82.3	19.4
	Controls	37	Control	6 weeks	67.6	45.9
Soloway et al (1995)	Cases	138	Luprolide and flutamide	3 months	53	18
	Controls	144	Control	3 months	22	48
Labrie et al[83] (1994)	Cases	75	Luprolide and flutamide	3 months	77	8
	Controls	59	Control	3 months	51	35

Trials of NHT in clinical stage C prostate cancer

The results of trials with the goal of 'downstaging' clinical stage C tumors to pathologic stage B are controversial. Non-randomized trials are particularly flawed by the inaccuracies of clinical staging. Morgan and Myers[101] reviewed 232 cases of clinical stage C prostate cancer at the Mayo Clinic, and found that, *without* NHT, 51 patients (22%) had organ-confined disease. While experience with endorectal-coil MRI is improving the accuracy of clinical staging, it is still an imprecise diagnosis.[102] Moul[33] recently reviewed 303 patients from the literature who were treated with NHT for clinical stage C disease, and found that 30% had pathologic stage B disease. This number clearly is not very favorable when viewed in the light of the data of Morgan and Myers,[101] and the real issue of clinical overstaging remains problematic.

The randomized, controlled studies of Labrie et al[83] and Van Poppel et al[88] have included small numbers of clinical stage C patients, with conflicting results. In 27 patients, Labrie et al[83] found 41.6% pathologic stage B disease in the untreated group and 73.3% in the NHT group. Van Poppel et al[88] studied 54 patients, and found equivalent numbers with pathologic stage B disease, but there was a higher rate of margin positivity in the NHT patients. It is likely that only large randomized trials, perhaps including the use of endorectal-coil MRI, will determine if NHT will play a role in clinical stage C prostate cancer.

Other effects of NHT

NHT decreased the volume of the prostate by 30–50% in all studies.[33] Initial reports also indicated that it facilitated the surgical procedure both subjectively and with reduced blood loss.[103] In contrast, in the randomized trials of

Soloway et al[99] and Van Poppel et al,[88] no significant decrease in blood loss or operative times between the NHT and control arms was reported. When asked to rate the technical difficulty of the prostatectomy, surgeons in the Soloway et al[99] study found the NHT group to have a higher percentage of more difficult dissections. However, there was no increase in complications in the NHT group.

Additionally, NHT will bring about a sharp drop in prostate-specific antigen (PSA) levels. Oesterling et al[104] reported a 98.5% decrease in the PSA of 21 patients whose average androgen deprivation therapy was two months. Schulman and Sassine[91] suggested that the degree of PSA drop may select patients with organ-confined disease who would benefit most from radical prostatectomy. However, Soloway et al[99] and McLeod et al[105] have not demonstrated a correlation between positive margins and nadir PSA level. There are insufficient data to draw firm conclusions at this time.

How long should the NHT be given? Most North American trials use three months of maximal androgen deprivation, while Van Poppel et al[88] used six weeks. In a prospective, nonrandomized trial, Gleave et al[73] used an ultrasensitive assay to measure PSA. They evaluated 50 patients with clinically localized prostate cancer who underwent eight months of NHT with either cytoproteranone acetate and low-dose DES, or an LHRH agonist and flutamide. They found that 22% of the cases reached an undetectable PSA after three months, 42% after five months, and 84% after eight months. Only 4% of the patients had positive surgical margins. While the true significance of this finding is not yet known, it suggests that extended NHT may lead to an optimal decrease in tumor volume. Further study of this approach is certainly warranted.

NHT and pathology

As indicated by the discrepant results of the controlled trials, not only is clinical staging subject to inaccuracies, but pathologic staging is dependent on the presence or absence of capsu-lar invasion, which itself can be a subjective determination. It is not known if the true determination of the extent of the disease is made more difficult by NHT, nor is it clear if variations in tissue processing between NHT studies make comparison of results unreliable.[33] Using cytokeratin immunohistochemistry, Zheng et al[106] found a significant number of cases in which extra-organ and margin involvement was detected. This was overlooked on conventional hematoxylin- and eosin-stained sections in patients who received NHT. It is well established that NHT causes dramatic changes in the histopathologic appearance of both benign and malignant tissues, including glandular atrophy, nuclear pyknosis, cytoplasmic vacuolation, squamous metaplasia, and a relative increase in the stroma.[107–112] Because of these changes, many pathologists will not assign a grade to prostate cancer in a patient who received NHT.[113] Only long-term follow-up data will clarify these questions.

Conclusions about NHT and radical prostatectomy

1. NHT will decrease prostate volume 30–50% and decrease PSA to potentially undetectable levels.
2. Clinical stage B tumors appear to have consistently lower rates of extra-organ disease and positive surgical margins in seven prospective, randomized trials. The optimal length of preoperative NHT treatment has not been determined.
3. Not enough information is available on the effect of NHT in clinical stage C tumors.
4. NHT is still under investigation, and long-term benefit of disease-free survival and disease-specific survival is not yet known.

NHT AND DEFINITIVE RADIOTHERAPY FOR PROSTATE CANCER

Radiation therapy is broadly accepted as a modality in the curative management of the patient with localized prostate cancer. Multiple series of patients receiving external-beam irradiation with intent to cure have suggested long-term control and survival rates similar to series of radical prostatectomy.[114–117] In the era of PSA testing, two recent studies suggest that, with definitive radiotherapy, the freedom from biochemical failure can range from 50% to 70% at five to six years following treatment.[116,117] Critics point to a series from Stanford that reported that 80% of consecutively treated patients given external-beam irradiation have rising PSA levels at five-year follow-up.[118] With all of these studies, legitimate questions can be raised about selection bias, clinical staging inaccuracies, and both the definition and significance of a rising PSA level. Looking for ways to improve cure rates, there is now great interest in the potential benefits of NHT associated with definitive radiation therapy.

Theoretical rationale for NHT in radiation therapy

Tumor size at the time of radiation therapy has been shown to correlate with the success or failure of radiation treatment,[119,120] and androgen deprivation is well known to reduce tumor volume in most patients.[33] These findings gave rise to the hypothesis that androgen deprivation preceding, and during, radiation therapy leads to improved control of the primary tumor.[121] Further support for this hypothesis comes from the understanding that androgen deprivation leads to apoptosis of the tumor, which might enhance cell killing by radiation therapy.[122,123] Zeitman et al[124] have shown that castration in animal models prior to radiation substantially increases tumor sensitivity to radiation without a comparable increase in normal sensitivity.

Clinical trials of NHT with radiation therapy

In the early 1980s, the Radiation Therapy Oncology Group (RTOG) began phase I and II trials of NHT with definitive radiation therapy. These initial studies, which focused on the possibility of post-irradiation potency and the tolerance of short-term hormonal alterations with respect to acute reactions to pelvic irradiation, established the toxicity of megestrol, DES, and goserelin acetate with flutamide.[119–121] A phase III randomized cooperative trial, coordinated by the RTOG, compared NHT and radiation with radiation therapy alone. This study, which accrued 471 patients with locally advanced prostate cancer from 1987 to 1991, was designed before PSA testing was widely available; PSA testing was added later to the follow-up. Patients with clinically defined stage B–D tumors of at least 25 cm³, and including regional lymph node involvement below the common iliac chain determined by computed tomography (CT), were assigned either to receive two months of goserelin acetate and flutamide prior to and during radiation, or to go directly to radiation. Interim results, published in 1995 at a median follow-up of 4.5 years, showed a significant improvement in the local progression rates (46% versus 71%) in the group that received NHT. Likewise, progression-free survival, defined as a PSA of 4.0 or less, was greater in the NHT group (36%) than in the control arm (15%).[122] Gomez et al[125] have also shown a significant improvement in biopsy-negative disease at 24-month follow-up, with NHT continuing for 6 months after curative radiation therapy. Long-term survival data are not yet available, nor is it clear what the significance is of a post-irradiation PSA level between 0 and 4.0.[126] Nonetheless, these surrogate markers indicate that NHT treatment for the patient who chooses radiation therapy with curative intent may be of considerable benefit.

Use of NHT preceding three-dimensional (3D) conformal radiotherapy for localized carcinoma of the prostate may improve the therapeutic ratio and thus lead to a reduction in the morbidity of treatment. Forman et al[127] prospectively evaluated twenty patients with CT scans before and after three months of leuprolide therapy. Both pre- and post-hormone CT scans were entered into a standardized 3D treatment planning system. An overall 37% reduction in prostate size translated directly into field size measurement reductions: the volumes of the bladder and rectum receiving maximal radiation were reduced by 21% and 23% respectively.[127] Theoretically, this potential reduction in toxicity of treatment also could allow for an escalation of the radiation dose without increased morbidity. Yang et al[128] reported similar reductions in prostate size, but cautioned that the reduction in rectum and bladder subject to treatment is not related linearly to the reduction in prostate size. The variable size of the rectum and bladder were found to be important factors in normal tissue radiation exposure, as well as sagging of the bladder following NHT.

Which patients will do well with curative radiation therapy? Without NHT, a preoperative PSA level less than 15 ng/ml is the most important predictor of biochemical freedom from relapse at three-year follow-up.[129] From the treatment arm of the RTOG cooperative trial, 57 patients had immunohistochemical staining for p53 protein performed on their biopsy specimens, and abnormal p53 protein expression was correlated strongly with treatment failure, independently of tumor grade and clinical stage.[130]

Conclusions about NHT and curative radiation therapy

1. Use of NHT preceding, and concurrent with, definitive radiation therapy is well tolerated and has in vitro and in vivo experimental support.
2. NHT appears to increase the therapeutic ratio of radiation therapy, and potentially can decrease morbidity.
3. Preliminary data suggest that progression-free survival is greater in patients receiving NHT, but the long-term effect on disease-specific survival is unknown.

RADIATION AS ADJUVANT THERAPY FOR RADICAL PROSTATECTOMY

Like most of the issues in prostate cancer therapy, the use of radiation therapy as an adjuvant treatment in patients with pathologically documented extra-organ disease at radical resection is controversial. The introduction of serum PSA levels as a mechanism to follow the clinical course of patients receiving radical treatment has exposed the fact that studies reporting low rates of clinical failure (5–15%) following radical prostatectomy may, in fact, have substantially higher rates of biochemical failure (31–35%).[9,131,132] While the significance of asymptomatic biochemical failure is not yet clear, there are convincing data that patients with lymph node involvement, positive margins or seminal vesicle involvement will have higher rates of clinically significant disease recurrence.[22,28,133] Does this group of patients benefit from adjuvant radiation therapy?

The argument for adjuvant radiation therapy in patients with unfavorable pathology begins with the observation that the recurrence of local disease traditionally has been a harbinger of the development of distant metastasis. If improvement in local control is demonstrated with adjuvant radiation therapy then perhaps the local disease will be less likely to be a source of distant metastasis, and will lead to an improvement in morbidity and mortality.[26] Those arguing against adjuvant radiation for margin-positive disease point out that a positive pathologic margin does not necessarily mean there is residual tumor in the pelvis. They note that only 10–20% of patients with margin-positive disease will have an elevated PSA level in the immediate postoperative period.[133–135] Furthermore, an elevated postoperative PSA may be the result of distant metastasis rather than locally persistent disease.

Clinical studies of local control before the PSA era

To address the issue of potential benefit from adjuvant radiation therapy, the first important question is whether it improves local control. Unfortunately, there is a paucity of controlled studies that address this question. In the pre-PSA era, studies depended on the detection of local recurrence or distant metastasis as evidence of treatment failure. Lightner et al[136] have shown that even experienced personnel will not be able to distinguish consistently with digital rectal exam between those patients with biopsy-proven recurrent local disease and those with undetectable postoperative PSA levels. Furthermore, these early studies include different surgical and radiotherapy techniques, incomplete information on nodal status, and non-controlled study populations. Of 12 non-randomized, comparative studies,[137–148] all suggested that local control was improved with adjuvant radiation. Six of these larger, comparative studies reported that local disease failure decreased from 17–30% without radiation to 0–6% with radiation. One of these studies[144] suggested a survival advantage to adjuvant radiation, but reexamination of this study has raised questions about that conclusion.[145]

Studies in the PSA era

There are three studies that did not have PSA data prior to initiating adjuvant radiation therapy but that reported on it in follow-up.[26,29,149] Zeitman et al[26] treated 68 patients with negative lymph nodes, but positive margins or extracapsular disease, and reported a four-year 77% freedom from biochemical relapse. They defined failure as a detectable PSA in a patient in whom it had been either undetectable or unknown, or any rise in PSA in a patient who had detectable postoperative levels. When they compared these results to series at other institutions that reported results with radical prostatectomy alone,[131,132] they found that patients who received adjuvant therapy for positive margins had a 64% freedom from biochemical relapse at four years, in contrast to a 34% freedom from biochemical relapse rate in the prostatectomy-alone series. Patients with seminal vesicle involvement also appeared to benefit, with an improvement to 43% freedom from biochemical relapse in contrast to 24–36% in the prostatectomy-alone groups.[26] Petrovich et al[149] and Freeman et al[29] reported similar results. The major criticism of these studies is that, without the pre-radiotherapy PSA levels, some of the patients may not have had residual dis-

ease following the surgery, and thus did not need additional therapy.

In a study in which pre-radiotherapy PSA levels were known, Morgan and Myers[101] compared 17 pathologic stage C patients who received adjuvant radiation with 33 patients who did not receive this treatment. At a minimum 12 month follow-up, 94% of the adjuvant group had an undetectable PSA, compared with 64% of those without adjuvant treatment. Lange et al[146] treated 29 patients with radiation therapy for rising PSA levels from 9 to 95 months after radical prostatectomy. Of this group, 43% saw a decrease in PSA to undetectable levels, including 31% of patients with D1 disease and 100% of those with positive surgical margins.

The largest study in the PSA era that evaluated adjuvant radiation therapy was reported by McCarthy et al.[147] In this study, 95 patients treated with adjuvant radiation for stage C disease had (i) an undetectable PSA (32 patients), (ii) a persistently elevated PSA (20 patients), or (iii) an initially undetectable PSA that later increased (43 patients). At an average 52-month follow-up, 79% of patients in group A were without evidence of biochemical failure, while group C had a 63% rate of freedom from biochemical relapse at 72-month follow-up. The patients with a persistently elevated PSA did not respond so well: only 40% were without biochemical evidence of relapse at 52 months. Although the follow-up was not identical and the study was not randomized, one possible implication of this study is that an inferior PSA response is seen in margin-positive patients when adjuvant radiation therapy is delayed until the PSA begins to rise. However, this difference may not be real, since it may represent overtreatment of some patients never destined to develop a rising PSA. The other suggestion is that patients in whom the PSA does not reach an undetectable level may not benefit significantly from adjuvant radiotherapy.

In an effort to identify those patients most likely to benefit from adjuvant radiation therapy, Wu et al[150] reported on a series of 53 patients who were referred for adjuvant radiotherapy following radical prostatectomy due to a detectable PSA. They used multivariate analysis to attempt to identify factors that predict a likelihood of significant benefit from adjuvant radiotherapy. In their analysis, they considered the last PSA level before radiotherapy (pre-RT PSA) and whether the PSA became undetectable after radical prostatectomy. They also looked at PSA doubling time following radical prostatectomy, radiotherapy dose, Gleason score, capsular penetration, surgical margin status and seminal vesicle involvement. In univariate analysis, both the presence of an undetectable PSA after radical prostatectomy and the pre-RT PSA were significant predictors of response to adjuvant radiotherapy, with a decrease of the PSA to undetectable levels. However, in multivariate analysis, only pre-RT PSA predicted who would become biochemically disease-free. Wu et al[150] concluded that 'postprostatectomy radiotherapy is unlikely to be curative when administered to patients whose PSA level is persistently elevated after radical prostatectomy, or those with PSA levels greater than 2.5 ng/ml at the time of radiotherapy'.

A stepwise multivariate logistic analysis has been performed by Forman et al,[151] who generated a model in which adjuvant radiotherapy treatment outcome can be predicted. From a review of 50 patients receiving postoperative radiotherapy for an elevated PSA, the model is driven by clinical stage, pre-RT PSA, Gleason score and initial response to treatment. The model correctly classified 80% of patients and, with 92% specificity, identified the patients who would fail and potentially require alternative therapies.

Two important issues remain unresolved: (i) how is biochemical relapse defined, and (ii) what is the significance of a rising PSA in the patient who has received radiotherapy? Haab et al[152] used an ultrasensitive PSA assay to study prospectively a mixed group of 17 patients who received adjuvant radiotherapy for rising PSA levels. While 6 of 17 patients responded with an undetectable PSA level, all patients in the group experienced a subsequent rise in PSA at a mean of 10.6 months.

Conclusions about radiation as an adjuvant for radical prostatectomy

1. In patients with persistent pelvic disease following radical prostatectomy, local control appears to be improved by adjuvant radiation therapy.
2. No survival benefit has yet been shown with adjuvant radiation therapy.
3. Preliminary data suggest that a low or undetectable pre-RT PSA may identify the patients most likely to benefit from adjuvant radiation therapy.

ADJUVANT HORMONAL THERAPY

By the mid to late 1990s, hormonal manipulation in the adjuvant setting was theoretically appealing, but, like many prostate cancer therapeutic strategies, it has not proved of benefit to survival. Like NHT, the objective of adjuvant hormonal therapy is to use systemic treatment to delay both tumor recurrence rates and disease-specific mortality rates. The breast cancer model provides the theoretical rationale and template for adjuvant hormonal treatment of prostate cancer. It has been well demonstrated in the Early Breast Cancer Trialists' Collaborative Group[153] that short-term adjuvant hormonal blockade with tamoxifen will reduce the annual recurrence rates by up to 26% and mortality rates by up to 25%. A significant reduction in the odds ratio was seen for both node-positive and node-negative patients. Because most prostate cancer is also hormonally sensitive, extrapolating the breast cancer experience suggests possible benefit of hormonal blockade in the patient with early prostate cancer.[154]

In 1986, Zincke et al[155] proposed that adjuvant hormonal therapy might delay disease progression in patients treated by radical prostatectomy. Retrospective data in a non-randomized study suggested that patients with stage C disease after radical prostatectomy who underwent immediate surgical castration have decreased local and systemic progression but no improvement in survival.[156] In patients with stage D1 disease, Zincke et al[157] reported an improvement in overall survival in patients who are treated with radical prostatectomy and immediate orchiectomy compared with patients treated by radical prostatectomy alone. Pilepich et al[158] reported that administration of an LHRH agonist following definitive radiation therapy delayed both time to PSA relapse and time to progression. Owing to the morbidity of medical and surgical castration, and a lack of well-established benefit, immediate hormonal therapy in the strictly adjuvant setting is not widely practiced.

Antiandrogens are ideal theoretical candidates as adjuvant therapy because they are generally well tolerated, and side-effects, particularly involving libido and sexual function, are minimal in most patients. However, one of the many unanswered concerns is whether early treatment with androgen blockers will bring on the hormone-refractory state earlier in the course of disease than in the untreated patient. Another major question surrounds patient selection for hormonal adjuvant therapy: While the patient with micrometastatic disease might benefit from early hormonal treatment, how can this patient be selected from the patient with minimal local disease who could potentially be better treated by pelvic radiation?[113]

There are few mature data to answer these questions. In 1995, Andriole et al[159] reported preliminary results of a randomized controlled trial of the 5α-reductase inhibitor finasteride (Proscar) in 120 men with rising PSA levels following radical prostatectomy. Finasteride is best known for its use in benign prostatic hyperplasia (BPH), and is not strictly an 'antiandrogen'. It acts by inhibiting the conversion of testosterone to the more active form, dihydrotestosterone (DHT), by the type 2 isoenzyme of 5α-reductase. By lowering DHT, finasteride has been shown to inhibit the growth of the prostate in BPH. Because it does not significantly lower testosterone levels, side-effects involving libido and sexual function are minimal.[160,161] It has also been shown to inhibit growth in PC3 and DU145 human prostate cancer cell lines.[162]

The men enrolled in the study by Andriole et al[159] had heterogeneous clinical situations, but all had undergone radical prostatectomy, had no evidence of local recurrence, had negative bone scans, and had PSA levels between 0.6 and 10.0 ng/ml. They received either 10 mg finasteride for 12 months or placebo, followed by 12 months in which all received finasteride 10 mg. The results of patient PSA levels after 12 months of placebo versus finasteride are shown in Figure 6.1. There was a 7-month delay in the rise in PSA levels among the treated group, and this lag behind the rise in the control group persisted through the 24 months of the study. Survival data are not yet available, but it is important to note that, of 13 patients treated with medical or surgical castration following a median length of 13 months of finasteride, 12 still appeared to be hormonally responsive as manifested by drops in PSA levels. The one patient who did not respond had already developed overt metastatic disease prior to castration.

In 1995, men undergoing radical prostatectomy with curative intent began enrolling in a prospective, randomized, controlled trial of monotherapy with the antiandrogen bicalutamide versus placebo. Clinical progression and disease-specific survival will ultimately be addressed by this study, and, before these data mature, time to PSA failure will be evaluated as well. However, as of the late 1990s, adjuvant hormonal therapy must be regarded as experimental and of unproved benefit.

COMBINATION ADJUVANT RADIOTHERAPY WITH ADJUVANT HORMONAL THERAPY

There has been little study of adjuvant radiotherapy combined with adjuvant hormonal therapy. Wiegel et al[163] compared 56 advanced stage patients treated with adjuvant radiotherapy. Of this group, 27 were treated with immediate orchiectomy in addition to the radiotherapy. The 10-year overall survival rate was 63% in the radiotherapy-alone group, and 92% in the radiotherapy-plus-orchiectomy group. The authors hypothesize that the radiotherapy

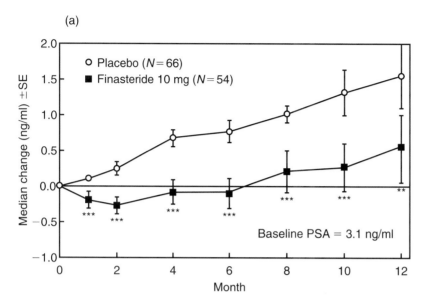

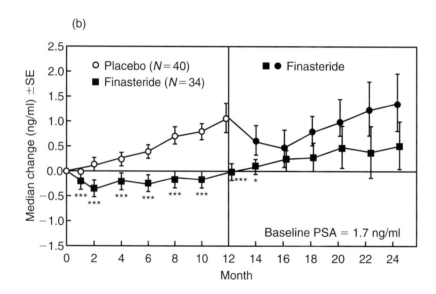

Figure 6.1 Serum PSA (median change from baseline) in patients treated with 10 mg finasteride or placebo for (a) 12 months (** $p \leqslant 0.01$, *** $p \leqslant 0.001$, versus placebo) and (b) 24 months (* $p < 0.05$, ** $p < 0.01$, *** $p < 0.001$, versus placebo). SE, standard error.

may have treated local disease while the adjuvant hormonal therapy eliminated the micrometastatic distant metastasis. Most of the patients in this study were treated in the pre-PSA era, and the sample size was small, non-randomized and retrospective, but the data are encouraging. Gong et al[164] have used combined androgen blockade for six months postoperatively, combined with radiation therapy midway through this period. They suggest that the combined approach leads to a significant improvement in disease-free survival when compared with radiation therapy alone.

IDENTIFYING THE NEED FOR ADJUVANT THERAPY

With no adjuvant therapy proven to increase disease-specific survival, are there ways to identify patients at higher risk for treatment failure and thus candidates for experimental adjuvant therapies? Partin et al[165] created a multifactor model for identifying men who are at high risk of recurrence, based on PSA, radical prostatectomy Gleason score and pathologic stage. Bauer et al[15] suggested that p53 and Bcl-2 protein expression predict for higher risk of recurrence after radical prostatectomy, independently of Gleason score and stage, while Moul et al[166] showed that cathepsin and epidermal growth factor receptor immunoreactivity do not predict for higher risk of recurrence. p53 protein immunoreactivity has also been shown to be associated with a higher incidence of locally persistent disease following definitive radiotherapy.[167] DNA ploidy has been proposed to be a significant predictor for clinical progression-free survival.[168] It is hoped that these potential markers, as well as the cell adhesion molecule E-cadherin,[169] matrix metalloproteinases,[170] urokinase,[171,172] angiogenesis factors,[173] and many others currently under study, will soon be able to identify with a high degree of certainty the individual patient at higher risk of recurrence, and therefore the one who will benefit from adjuvant therapy.

FUTURE DIRECTIONS

It is likely that the coming decade will see an explosive increase in adjuvant therapies for prostate cancer. Rapid advances in molecular biology and translational clinical research will be augmented by increased public interest in prostate cancer, with an aging population in the industrialized world. Not only has the advent of PSA testing led to an increase in prostate cancer diagnoses, but it serves as a surrogate biomarker to evaluate the effectiveness of new therapies before long-term survival data are available.

Chemopreventive agents as adjuvant therapy

One area of rapid development in prostate cancer research with potential applications as an adjuvant therapy is chemoprevention. Prostate cancer is an excellent theoretical candidate for chemoprevention because of the long latency between initiation and clinically significant disease. Likewise, there is frequently a long latency period between biochemical failure and clinical recurrence following definitive therapy. Perhaps patients at high risk of recurrence will one day be placed on adjuvant chemopreventive therapy.

Two prime candidates for chemopreventive adjuvant therapy of prostate cancer are analogs of vitamin A (retinoids) and analogs of vitamin D (deltanoids). Since the discovery of the steroid receptor superfamily, there has been a rapid advance in the attempt to develop new agents for the chemoprevention of cancer.[174,175] The intracellular receptors for the retinoids and deltanoids, as well as classic steroids, all belong to a superfamily involved in the selective regulation of transcription of specific genes that control cell differentiation and proliferation. Retinoids have the ability to exert a hormone-like control of normal cellular differentiation and proliferation in essentially all epithelia that are target sites for the development of invasive carcinoma. Furthermore, retinoids can restore normal cellular differentiation to dysplastic epithelium.[176,177] Deltanoids induce differentiation of both murine and human leukemia cells, and are potent regulators of gene expression.[178,179] Since the process of carcinogenesis is characterized fundamentally by a loss or arrest of cellular differentiation, Sporn and Roberts[176] have suggested that the retinoids could be used as physiologic, rather than cytotoxic, agents to arrest or reverse the process of carcinogenesis. This approach has been validated in many studies in experimental animals,[180] and there are now significant clinical data to indicate that it is also applicable to humans.[181] Animal studies with deltanoids have shown similar results.[182]

Retinoids and deltanoids in prostate cancer

Recent data suggest a significant role for retinoids and deltanoids in the chemoprevention of prostate cancer. A prospective epidemiological study indicates that, in humans, a low level of vitamin A is associated with a higher risk of developing prostate cancer,[183] but studies correlating vitamin A consumption and prostate cancer risk are conflicting.[184] In vitro studies of all-*trans*-retinoic acid (ATRA) and 13-*cis*-retinoic acid (isotretinoin) have shown inhibition of PSA secretion and expression at mRNA and protein levels, increased differentiation, and decreased tumorigenic potential in human prostate cell lines.[185–187] Three studies have demonstrated that dietary fenretinide, a synthetic retinoid, significantly decreases the development of prostate cancer in rat and mouse carcinogenesis models.[188–190]

Vitamin D deficiency has been hypothesized to be a risk factor for prostate cancer.[191] This has been supported by findings that mortality rates from prostate cancer are correlated inversely with the availability of ultraviolet light,[192] and that mean serum 1,25-dihydroxyvitamin D_3 (1,25-$(OH)_2D_3$) levels were lower in patients subsequently developing prostate cancer.[193] In vitro studies with 1,25-$(OH)_2D_3$ have demonstrated the presence of vitamin D receptor in human prostate tissues and cell lines, and suggested an antiproliferative and a differentiating action.[193] Deltanoids have been shown to inhibit proliferation of human breast cancer cell lines,[194] but they have not been studied thoroughly for their potential usefulness in suppressing prostate carcinogenesis.

Antiangiogenic agents

Angiogenesis is well recognized as an important component of tumor growth and metastasis. Inhibition of tumor-induced angiogenesis was proposed by Folkman in 1971.[195] Angiogenesis has been associated with prostate cancer,[196] and is perhaps modulated by urokinase-type plasminogen activator.[197] A detailed review of therapeutic strategies to inhibit angiogenesis can be found elsewhere,[198] but particular mention of suramin is appropriate because it has undergone clinical trials in advanced prostate cancer and potentially could have applications to adjuvant therapy.

Suramin is a polysulfonated naphthylurea initially developed as an agent against African trypanosomiasis. While it has multiple mechanisms of action, it is primarily a growth factor antagonist and inhibitor of enzymes involved in the catabolism of glycans.[199,200] In treating prostate cancer, it has led to a 75% decrease in PSA levels among patients with advanced hormone refractory disease[200–202] and is currently under study in prospective randomized trials. Its use is limited by significant side-effects, including direct toxic effects on the adrenal gland and thrombocytopenia. Suramin has not been recommended for approval by the US FDA, and data from randomized studies are being reassessed. Because of its potentially high therapeutic index and the theoretical lower rate of drug resistance, suramin, or another antiangiogenic agent with an improved side-effect profile, is an attractive candidate for adjuvant therapy of prostate cancer.

Other future adjuvant therapies

Understanding the biology of prostate cancer may lead to better strategies for adjuvant therapy. There has been a growing list of autocrine and paracrine growth pathways identified in prostate cancer cells, including interleukin-6 (IL-6), epidermal growth factor (EGF)-like substances, and transforming growth factor β (TGF-β).[203–205] IL-6 receptors and secreted endogenous IL-6 have been identified in prostate cancer cells, and may function as an autocrine growth factor.[206] TGF-β may have both stimulatory and inhibitory effect on cell growth.[206] In the Dunning rat prostate cancer model, TGF-β is able to inhibit EGF-dependent growth.[205] AT-3 cells, a cell line established from the Dunning rat prostate cancer, can be caused to attach or detach from six-well plates when exposed to different media conditions and different concentrations of TGF-β.

Furthermore, AT-3 cells are able to produce TGF-β in a latent form, suggesting that this cytokine may also function as an autocrine or paracrine growth factor. The use of agents or antibodies that block alternative growth factor autocrine/paracrine pathways may be a useful therapeutic strategy.

A number of molecular and cellular markers for the biological behavior of prostate cancer have been identified. Of these, the expression of HER2/Neu protein is of particular interest. The *HER2/neu* proto-oncogene (also known as c-*erbB-2*) encodes for a 185–190 kDa protein (HER2/Neu, or c-ErbB-2) with tyrosine kinase activity.[207] While *HER2/neu* cell transformation in the rat is through a point mutation, the transforming activity of *HER2/neu* in humans is thought to be related to the overexpression of HER2/Neu protein.[208] Gene amplification and protein overexpression have been demonstrated in a variety of human adenocarcinomas, including approximately 30% of breast and ovarian carcinomas, and they correlate with metastasis and poor prognosis.[209,210] While HER2/Neu protein expression is well documented in ovarian and breast carcinoma, its expression and role in prostate cancer has not been well documented until recently.[211,212] Kuhn et al[211] found that 34% of 53 primary prostate cancers and 0 of 9 benign prostatic hypertrophy samples expressed HER2/Neu protein. Sadasivan et al[212] found that none of 15 samples of benign prostatic tissues expressed HER2/Neu protein, but 9/25 prostate cancers were positive. Overexpression of HER2/Neu protein seemed to correlate with poor prognostic factors, such as high grade, late stage, increased ploidy and high percentage of cells in S phase. Although it is too soon to say whether HER2/Neu protein will have significant prognostic implications, it may be useful as a target for antibody therapy.

Immune responses have been identified to mutated oncogene products,[213] and autologous antibody and T-cell immunity have been identified in patients with breast and ovarian cancers expressing HER2/Neu protein.[214,215] Antibody and T-cell responses were noted to both the intracellular and extracellular domain peptides of HER2/Neu protein. These data suggest that autoimmunity to HER2/Neu protein is present and might possibly be exploited for therapeutic benefit.

A humanized bispecific antibody (MDXH210) to HER2/Neu protein and the high-affinity IgG receptor (FcγR1a) on monocytes, macrophages, dendritic cells and activated granulocytes has been shown to be safe in prostate cancer patients, and is currently under evaluation in hormone-refractory metastatic disease. A humanized monoclonal antibody to HER2/Neu protein (Herceptin) has been found to have activity in breast cancer, and is now under evaluation in prostate cancer.

Preliminary evidence suggests that a host response to prostate cancer exists in men. In four primary prostate cancers, 7–19% of the tumor cell suspensions comprised tumor-infiltrating lymphocytes (TILs).[216] TIL were expanded from 1.8×10^3 to 6.9×10^4, depending on the conditions used. Although the phenotypic analysis showed a majority of CD3+ cells, natural killer (NK) activity and low level of lymphokine-activated killer (LAK) activity were demonstrated in all four prostate samples. In one case, TILs demonstrated killing against autologous tumor. Additional evidence for the role of immune therapy comes from the observation that LAK cells generated from rats bearing the Dunning prostate tumor R-3227 AT-3 can reduce the number of lung metastases as well as causing regression of established metastases.[217] In addition, a number of reports suggest that NK activity correlates with stage of prostate cancer in men and with the success of treatment.[218]

Finally, T-cell mediated immunity has been demonstrated in the Dunning rat model. Moody and Isaacs[219] transfected the MAT LyLu subline of the Dunning rat prostate cancer with the gene for IL-2, and found that animals rejected tumor cell inoculums containing both wild-type and transfected cells. These animals also were able to reject a subsequent challenge of wild-type prostate cancer cells two weeks later.

Prostate-specific antigen (PSA), a kallikrein-like serine protease produced by epithelial cells of prostatic tissue, catalyzes the liquefaction of seminal coagulum.[220,221] PSA is highly specific for prostate cancer cells, which makes it an attractive protein target for immune recognition. Furthermore, it is now known that intracellular proteins undergo immunologic processing by the cell, and subsequently can be recognized by immune effector cells.

Patients with advanced prostate cancer are likely to produce anti-PSA IgG antibody.[222] We have confirmed this finding in three patients with elevated serum PSA and known metastatic prostate cancer. An endogenous IgG antibody response to PSA supports the role of T-cell-mediated immune responses to prostate cancer. Additional support for this concept comes from the observation that PSA may function as a T-cell mitogen. We tested peripheral blood mononuclear cells from three men with metastatic prostate cancer, and found that two of them had significant mitogenic responses to PSA following eight days of stimulation. The mitogenic capabilities of PSA and its ability to elicit an endogenous IgG antibody response provide a rationale for exploring PSA-derived immunodominant peptides as agents for active specific immunity.

Recently, we and others have identified PSA-derived immunodominant peptides that can bind to HLA-A2.[223,224] With the advent of prostate-specific vaccines, it is exciting to postulate that the force of the immune system can be brought to bear on the prevention and treatment of prostate cancer.[225]

Subsequent to our report, two studies have suggested that prostate cancer vaccines can cause clinical responses and that T-cell-mediated therapies to prostate cancer may have significant utility. Murphy et al[226] conducted a trial of intravenous dendritic cell vaccine in prostate cancer patients. They reported that 7/10 patients responded to DCs pulsed with the prostate-specific membrane antigen-derived peptide PSM-P2. Valone et al[227] have reported strong T-cell proliferative and weak antibody responses to prostate tissue-specific antigen when this antigen was loaded to DCs in vitro and given intravenously to prostate cancer patients.

SUMMARY

Adjuvant therapy for prostate cancer presently consists primarily of hormonal manipulation surrounding surgical and radiation therapies with curative intent. With rapid advances in the understanding of prostate tumor biology, strategies of adjuvant therapy for prostate cancer are entering the molecular age. Clinical applications of molecular therapies to prostate cancer are still early in their development, but a real potential exists that there will soon be therapies with proven benefit for the individual patient with prostate cancer. Finally, we may be able to answer Willet Whitmore's famous query, 'When treatment is possible, is it necessary, and when it is necessary, is it possible?'[228]

REFERENCES

1. Chodak GW, Questioning the value of screening for prostate cancer in asymptomatic men. *Urology* 1993; **42:** 116–18.
2. United States Preventative Task Force, *Guide to Clinical Preventive Services*, 2nd edn. Williams and Wilkins: Baltimore, 1995: 119–34.
3. American Cancer Society Web Page, Cancer Facts and Figures, 1999.
4. Cespedes RD and Thompson Jr IM, Screening for prostate cancer. In: *Prostate Cancer* (Ernstoff MS, Heaney JA, Peschel RE, eds). Blackwell: Melden, MA, 1998: 76–90.
5. Fleming C, Wasson JH, Albertsen PC et al, A decision analysis of alternative treatment strategies for clinically localized prostate cancer. Prostate Patient Outcomes Research Team. *J Am Med Assoc* 1993; **269:** 2650–8.
6. Johansson JE, Adami HO, Andersson SO et al, High 10-year survival rate in patients with early, untreated prostatic cancer. *J Am Med Assoc* 1992; **267:** 2191–6.
7. Aus G, Hugosson J, Norlén L, Long-term sur-

vival and mortality in prostate cancer treated with noncurative intent. *J Urol* 1995; **154**: 460–5.

8. Albertsen PC, Fryback DG, Storer BE et al, Long-term survival among men with conservatively treated localized prostate cancer. *J Am Med Assoc* 1995; **274**: 626–31.

9. Zincke H, Bergstralh EJ, Blute ML et al, Radical prostatectomy for clinically localized prostate cancer: long-term results of 1,143 patients from a single institution. *J Clin Oncol* 1994; **12**: 2254–63.

10. Dearnaley DP, Radiotherapy of prostate cancer: established results and new developments. *Semin Surg Oncol* 1995; **11**: 50–9.

11. Noble RL, Development of androgen-stimulated transplants of Nb rat carcinoma of the dorsal prostate and their response to sex hormones and tamoxifen. *Cancer Res* 1980; **40**: 3551–4.

12. Horoszewicz JS, Leong SS, Kawinski E et al, LNCaP model of human prostatic carcinoma. *Cancer Res* 1997; **43**: 4049–58.

13. Raghavan D, Adjuvant systemic therapy of prostate cancer. *Semin Oncol* 1995; **22**: 633–40.

14. Harper ME, Goddard L, Glynne-Jones E et al, An immunocytochemical analysis of TGF-α expression in benign and malignant prostatic tumors. *Prostate* 1993; **23**: 9–23.

15. Bauer JJ, Sesterhenn IA, Mostofi FK et al, Elevated levels of apoptosis regulator proteins p53 and bcl-2 are independent prognostic biomarkers in surgically treated clinically localized prostate cancer patients. *J Urol* 1996; **156**: 1511–16.

16. Davis NS, diSant'Agnese PA, Ewing JF et al, The neuroendocrine prostate: characterization and quantitation of calcitonin in the human prostate gland. *J Urol* 1989; **142**: 884–8.

17. Montie JE, Wood DP Jr, Venderburg S et al, The significance and management of transitional cell carcinoma of the prostate. *Semin Urol* 1990; **7**: 262–8.

18. Walsh PC, Prostate cancer kills: strategy to reduce deaths. *Urology* 1994; **44**: 463–6.

19. Lu-Yao GL, McLerran D, Wasson J et al, An assessment of radical prostatectomy: time trends, geographic variation, and outcomes. *J Am Med Assoc* 1993; **269**: 2633–6.

20. *SEER Cancer Statistics Review 1973–1993*. National Cancer Institute: Bethesda, MD, 1996.

21. Meetlin C, Jones GW, Murphy GP, Trends in prostate cancer care in the United States, 1974–1990: observations from the patient care evaluation studies of the American College of Surgeons Commission on Cancer. *Cancer* 1993; **43**: 83–92.

22. Catalona WJ, Smith DS, 5-year tumor recurrence rates after anatomical radical retropubic prostatectomy for prostate cancer. *J Urol* 1994; **152**: 1837–42.

23. Lerner SE, Seay TM, Blute ML et al, Prostate specific antigen detected prostate cancer (clinical stage T1C): an interim analysis. *J Urol* 1996; **155**: 821–6.

24. Noldus J, Stamey TA, Histological characteristics of radical prostatectomy specimens in men with a serum prostate specific antigen of 4 ng/ml or less. *J Urol* 1996; **155**: 441–3.

25. Wasson JH, Cushman CC, Bruskewitz RC et al, A structured literature review of treatment for localized prostate cancer. *Arch Fam Med* 1993; **2**: 487–93.

26. Zeitman AL, Coen JJ, Shipley WU et al, Adjuvant irradiation after radical prostatectomy for adenocarcinoma of prostate: analysis of freedom from PSA failure. *Urology* 1993; **42**: 292–9.

27. Epstein JI, Carmichael MJ, Pizov G et al, Influence of capsular penetration on progression following radical prostatectomy: a study of 196 cases with long-term followup. *J Urol* 1993; **150**: 135–41.

28. Mukamel E, deKernion JB, Dorey F et al, Significance of histological prognostic indicators in patients with carcinoma of the prostate. *Br J Urol* 1990; **65**: 46–50.

29. Freeman JA, Lieskovsky G, Cook DW et al, Radical retropubic prostatectomy and postoperative adjuvant radiation for pathological stage C (PCN0) prostate cancer from 1976 to 1989: intermediate findings. *J Urol* 1993; **149**: 1029–34.

30. Labrie F, Dupont A, Cusan L et al, Downstaging of localized prostate cancer by neoadjuvant therapy with flutamide and lupron: the first controlled and randomized trial. *Clin Invest Med* 1993; **16**: 499–509.

31. The Leuprolite Study Group. Leuprolite vs stilbestrol for metastatic prostate. *N Engl J Med* 1984; **311**: 1281.

32. Crawford DA, Eisenberger MA, McLeod DG et al, A controlled trial of leuprolide with and without flutamide in prostatic cancer. *N Engl J Med* 1989; **321**: 419–24.

33. Moul JW, Neoadjuvant hormonal therapy for clinically localized prostate cancer. In: *Urology Annual 1996* (Rous SN, ed). Blackwell Science:

Boston, 1996: 47–56.

34. White JW, The present position of the surgery of the hypertrophied prostate. *Ann Surg* 1893; **18:** 152.

35. McLeod DG, Prostate cancer: past, present, and future. In: *Prostate Cancer* (Dawson NA, Vogelzang NJ, eds). Wiley-Liss: New York, 1994: 1–18.

36. Gutman EB, Sproul EE, Gutman AB, Significance of increased phosphatase activity of bone at the site of osteoblastic metastases secondary to carcinoma of the prostate gland. *Am J Cancer* 1936; **28:** 485–95.

37. Huggins C, Hodges CV, Studies of prostatic cancer: 1. Effect of castration, estrogen, and androgen injections on serum phosphatases in metastatic carcinoma of the prostate. *Cancer Res* 1941; **1:** 293–7.

38. Vallett BS, Radical perineal prostatectomy subsequent to bilateral orchiectomy. *Delaware St Med J* 1944; **16:** 1–9.

39. Colston AC, Brendler H, Endocrine therapy in carcinoma of the prostate; preparation of patients for radical perineal prostatectomy. *J Am Med Assoc* 1947; **134:** 848–53.

40. Parlow AL, Scott WW, Hormone control therapy as a preparation for radical perineal prostatectomy in advanced carcinoma of the prostate. *NY J Med* 1947; **49:** 629–34.

41. Sullivan JJ, Hartwig CH, The use of estrogen therapy preliminary to radical perineal prostatoseminal vesiculectomy in carcinoma of the prostate. *J Urol* 1953; **70:** 499–502.

42. Soloway MS, Hachiya T, Civantos F et al, Androgen deprivation prior to radical prostatectomy for T2b and T3 prostate cancer. *Urol Suppl* 1994; **43:** 52–6.

43. Scott WW, Boyd HL, Combined hormonal control therapy in radical prostatectomy in the treatment of selected cases of advanced carcinoma of the prostate: a retrospective study based upon 25 years of experience. *J Urol* 1969; **101:** 86.

44. Bagshaw MA, External radiation therapy for carcinoma of the prostate. *Cancer* 1980; **45:** 1912–21.

45. Narayan P, Lange PH, Current controversies in the management of carcinoma of the prostate. *Semin Oncol* 1980; **7:** 460–7.

46. Schroeder FH, Belt EL, Carcinoma of the prostate: a study of 213 patients with stage C tumors treated by total perineal prostatectomy. *J Urol* 1975; **114:** 257–60.

47. Green N, Bodner H, Broth E et al, Improved control of bulky prostate carcinoma with sequential estrogen and radiation therapy. *Int J Radiat Oncol Biol Phys* 1984; **10:** 971–6.

48. Fair WR, Aprikian A, Sogani P et al, The role of neoadjuvant hormonal manipulation in localized prostatic cancer. *Cancer Suppl* 1993; **71:** 1031–8.

49. Cher ML, Carroll PR, Small EJ, Shinohara K, Neoadjuvant androgen deprivation before radical prostatectomy: current status and trial design. In: *Prostate Cancer* (Dawson NA, Vogelzang NJ, eds). Wiley-Liss: New York, 1994: 175–83.

50. Hsieh W-S, Simons JW, Systemic therapy of prostate cancer. New concepts from prostate cancer tumor biology. *Cancer Treat Rev* 1993; **19:** 229–60.

51. Kyprianou N, English HF, Isaacs JT, Programmed cell death during regression of PC-82 human prostate cancer following androgen ablation. *Cancer Res* 1990; **50:** 3748–53.

52. Isaacs JT, Coffey DS, Adaptation vs. selection as the mechanism responsible for the relapse of prostatic cancer to androgen ablation therapy as studied in the Dunning R-3327-H adenocarcinoma. *Cancer Res* 1981; **41:** 5070–5.

53. Bruchovsky N, Rennie PS, Coldman AJ et al, Effects of androgen withdrawal on the stem cell composition of the Shionogi carcinoma. *Cancer Res* 1990; **50:** 2275–82.

54. Kim JH, Sherwood ER, Sutkowski DM et al, Inhibition of prostatic tumor cell proliferation by suramin: alterations in TGF alpha-mediated autocrine growth regulation and cell cycle distribution. *J Urol* 1991; **146:** 171–6.

55. Newmark JR, Hardy DO, Tonb D et al, Androgen receptor gene mutations in human prostate cancer. *Proc Natl Acad Sci USA* 1992; **89:** 6319–23.

56. Landstrom M, Damber JE, Bergh A, Prostatic tumor regrowth after initially successful castration therapy may be related to a decreased apoptotic cell death rate. *Cancer Res* 1994; **54:** 4281–4.

57. Taplin ME, Bubley GJ, Shuster TD et al, Mutation of the androgen-receptor gene in metastatic androgen-independent prostate cancer. *N Engl J Med* 1995; **332:** 1393–8.

58. Hockenbury D, Nunez G, Milliman C et al, Bcl-2 is an inner mitochondrial membrane protein that blocks programmed cell death. *Nature* 1990; **348:** 334.

59. Bissonnette RP, Echeverri F, Mahboubi A, Green DR, Apoptotic cell death induced by c-myc is inhibited by bcl-2. *Nature* 1992; **359:** 552.

60. Korsmeyer SJ, Bcl-2 initiates a new category of oncogenes: regulators of cell death. *Blood* 1992; **80:** 879.

61. Krajewski S, Krajewska M, Shabaik A et al, Immunohistochemical determination of in vivo distribution of Bax, a dominant inhibitor of Bcl-2. *Am J Pathol* 1994; **145:** 1323–6.

62. McDonnell TJ, Troncoso P, Brisbay SM et al, Expression of the protooncogene bcl-2 in the prostate and its association with emergence of androgen-independent prostate cancer. *Cancer Res* 1992; **52:** 6940–4.

63. Colombel M, Symmans F, Gil S et al, Detection of the apoptosis-suppressing oncoprotein bcl-2 in hormone-refractory human prostate cancer. *Am J Pathol* 1993; **143:** 390–400.

64. Raffo AJ, Perlman H, Chen M-W et al, Overexpression of bcl-2 protects prostate cancer cells from apoptosis in vitro and confers resistance to androgen depletion in vivo. *Cancer Res* 1995; **55:** 4438–45.

65. Bauer JJ, Sesterhenn IA, Mostafi KF et al, p53 nuclear protein expression is an independent prognostic marker in clinically localized prostate cancer patients undergoing radical prostatectomy. *Clin Cancer Res* 1995; **1:** 1295–300.

66. Lane DP, p53, guardian of the genome. *Nature* 1992; **358:** 15.

67. Oren M, The involvement of oncogenes and tumor suppressor genes in the control of apoptosis. *Cancer Metastasis Rev* 1992; **11:** 141–8.

68. Chiou S, Rao L, White E, bcl-2 blocks p53-dependent apoptosis. *Mol Cell Biol* 1994; **14:** 2556–63.

69. Miyashita T, Harigai M, Hanada M, Reed JC, Identification of a p53-dependent negative response element in the bcl-2 gene. *Cancer Res* 1994; **54:** 3131–5.

70. Roberson CN, Roberson KM, Padilla G et al, Diethylstilbestrol induces apoptosis in human androgen-insensitive prostatic cancer cells in vitro. *Proc Am Urol Assoc Suppl* 1996; **155:** 343 (abst).

71. Veterans Administration Cooperative Urological Research Group (VACURG): Treatment and survival of patients with cancer in the prostate. *Surg Gynecol Obstet* 1967; **124:** 1401.

72. Martoccia D, Mastandrea F, Lockhart J, Persky L, Estrogen substitution for (LHRH) agonists: immediate effect on PSA. *Proc Am Urol Assoc Suppl* 1996; **155:** 578 (abst).

73. Gleave ME, Goldenberg SL, Jones EC et al, Biochemical and pathological effects of 8 months of neoadjuvant androgen withdrawal therapy before radical prostatectomy in patients with clinically confined prostate cancer. *J Urol* 1996; **155:** 213–19.

74. Fleshner N, Klotz L, A phase 1–2 trial of DES plus low dose coumadin in advanced prostate cancer. *Proc Am Urol Assoc Suppl* 1996; **155:** 610 (abst).

75. Schally AV, Kastin AJ, Coy DH, LH-releasing hormone and its analogues: recent basic and clinical investigation. *Int J Fertil* 1976; **1:** 1–12.

76. Hazum E, Conn PM, Molecular mechanism of gonadotropin releasing hormone (GnRH) action. I. The GnRH receptor. *Endocr Rev* 1988; **9:** 379–86.

77. Huckle WR, Conn PM, Molecular mechanism of gonadotropin releasing hormone action. II. The effector system. *Endocr Rev* 1988; **9:** 387–6.

78. Prostate Cancer Trialists' Collaborative Group. Maximum androgen blockade in advanced prostate cancer: an overview of 22 randomized trials with 3283 deaths in 5710 patients. *Lancet* 1995; **346:** 265–9.

79. Caubet J-F, Tosteson TD, Dong EW et al, Meta-analysis of published randomized clinical trials for MAB in prostate cancer. *Proc Am Soc Clin Oncol* 1996; **15:** 254 (abst).

80. Eisenberger MA, Blumenstein BA, Crawford ED et al, Bilateral orchiectomy with or without flutamide for metastatic prostate cancer. *N Engl J Med* 1998; **339:** 1036–42.

81. Bennett CL, Tosteson TD, Schmitt B et al, Maximum androgen-blockade with medical or surgical castration in advanced prostate cancer: a meta-analysis of nine published randomized controlled trials and 4128 patients using flutamide. *Prostate Cancer Prostatic Dis* 1998; **5:** 1–5.

82. Goldenberg SL, Bruchovsky N, Use of cyproterone acetate in prostate cancer. *Urol Clin North Am* 1991; **18:** 111.

83. Labrie F, Cusan L, Gomez J-L et al, Down-staging of early stage prostate cancer before radical prostatectomy: the first randomized trial of neoadjuvant combination therapy with flutamide and a luteinizing hormone-releasing hormone agonist. *Urol Symp* 1994; **44:** 29–37.

84. Schellhammer P, Sharifi R, Block N et al, Maximal androgen blockade for patients with metastatic prostate cancer: outcome of a con-

trolled trial of bicalutamide versus flutamide, each in combination with luteinizing hormone-releasing hormone analogue therapy. Casodex Combination Study Group. *Urology* 1996; **47:** 54–60.

85. Vogelzang NJ, Kennealey GT, Recent developments in endocrine treatment of prostate cancer. *Cancer* 1992; **70:** 966–76.

86. Sterns ME, Tew KD, Antimicrotubule effects of estramustine, an antiprostatic tumor drug. *Cancer Res* 1985; **45:** 3891–4.

87. Schmidt JD, Scott WW, Gibbons R et al, Chemotherapy programs of the National Prostatic Cancer Project (NPCP). *Cancer* 1980; **45:** 1937–46.

88. Van Poppel H, De Ridder D, Elgamal AA et al, Neoadjuvant hormonal therapy before radical prostatectomy decreases the number of positive surgical margins in stage T2 prostate cancer: interim results of a prospective randomized trial. *J Urol* 1995; **154:** 429–34.

89. Hudes GR, Nathan FE, Khater C et al, Paclitaxel plus estramustine in metastatic hormone-refractory prostate cancer. *Semin Oncol* 1995; **22:** 41–5.

90. Fair WR, Aprikian AG, Cohen D et al, Use of neoadjuvant androgen deprivation therapy in clinically localized prostate cancer. *Clin Invest Med* 1993; **16:** 516–22.

91. Schulman C, Sassine AM, Neoadjuvant hormonal deprivation before radical prostatectomy. *Clin Invest Med* 1993; **16:** 523–31.

92. Solomon MH, McHugh TA, Dorr RP et al, Hormone ablation therapy as neoadjuvant treatment to radical prostatectomy. *Clin Invest Med* 1993; **16:** 532–8.

93. MacFarlane MT, Abi-Aad A, Stein A et al, Neoadjuvant hormonal deprivation in patients with locally advanced prostate cancer. *J Urol* 1993; **150:** 132–4.

94. Aprikian AG, Fair WR, Reuter VE et al, Experience with neoadjuvant diethylstilboestrol and radical prostatectomy in patients with locally advanced prostate cancer. *Br J Urol* 1994; **74:** 630–6.

95. Soloway MS, Sharifi R, Wajsman Z et al, Randomized prospective study comparing radical prostatectomy alone versus radical prostatectomy preceded by androgen blockade in clinical stage B2 (T2bNxM0) prostate cancer. *J Urol* 1995; **154:** 424–8.

96. Debruyne FMJ, Forster G, Schulman CC et al, European study of neoadjuvant combined androgen deprivation therapy in T2–3, N0, M0 prostatic carcinoma. *Proc Am Urol Assoc Suppl* 1996; **155:** 645 (abst).

97. Klotz LH, Goldenberg LS, Bullock MJ et al, Neoadjuvant cyproterone acetate (CPA) therapy prior to radical prostatectomy reduces tumour burden and margin positivity without altering 6 and 12 month post-treatment PSA: results of a randomized trial. *Proc Am Urol Assoc Suppl* 1996; **155:** 399 (abst).

98. Pedersen KV, Lundberg S, Jugosson J et al, Neoadjuvant hormonal treatment with triptorelin versus no treatment prior to radical prostatectomy: a prospective randomized multicenter study. *Proc Am Urol Assoc Suppl* 1995; **153:** 391 (abst).

99. Soloway MS, Sharifi R, Wajsman Z et al, Randomized prospective study – radical prostatectomy alone vs radical prostatectomy preceded by androgen blockade in cT2b prostate cancer – initial results. *Proc Am Urol Assoc Suppl* 1996; **155:** 555 (abst).

100. Fair WR, Cookson MS, Stroumbakis N et al, Update on neoadjuvant androgen deprivation therapy (ADT) and radical prostatectomy in localized prostate cancer. *Proc Am Urol Assoc Suppl* 1996; **155:** 667 (abst).

101. Morgan WR, Myers RP, Endocrine therapy prior to radical retropubic prostatectomy for clinical stage C prostate cancer. Pathologic and biochemical response. *J Urol* 1991; **145:** 316 (abst).

102. Harris RD, Schned AR, Heaney JA, Staging of prostate cancer with endorectal MR imaging: lessons from a learning curve. *Radiographics* 1995; **15:** 813–29.

103. Sassine AM, Schulman CC, Neoadjuvant hormonal deprivation before radical prostatectomy. *Eur Urol* 1993; **24**(2): 46.

104. Oesterling J, Andrews PE, Suman VJ et al, Preoperative androgen deprivation therapy: artificial lowering of serum prostate specific antigen without downstaging the tumor. *J Urol* 1993; **149:** 779–82.

105. McLeod DG, Coffield S, Johnson CF et al, Serum PSA levels and the rate of positive surgical margins in radical prostatectomy specimens preceded by androgen blockade in clinical B2 ($T_2bN_xM_0$) prostate cancer. *Proc Am Urol Assoc Suppl* 1996; **155:** 650 (abst).

106. Zheng W, Bazinet M, Begin LR et al, Histological changes induced by neo-adjuvant androgen ablation may result in the underde-

tection of positive surgical margins and capsular involvement by prostate cancer. *Proc Am Urol Assoc Suppl* 1996; **155:** 554 (abst).

107. Schned AR, Gormley EA, Florid xanthomatous pelvic lymph node reaction to metastatic prostatic adenocarcinoma. *Arch Pathol Lab Med* 1996; **120:** 96–100.

108. Armas OA, Aprikian AG, Melamed J et al, Clinical and pathobiological effects of neoadjuvant total androgen ablation therapy on clinically localized prostatic adenocarcinoma. *Am J Surg Pathol* 1994; **18:** 979–91.

109. Murphy WM, Soloway MS, Barrows GH, Pathologic changes associated with androgen deprivation therapy for prostate cancer. *Cancer* 1991; **68:** 821–8.

110. Têtu B, Srigley JR, Boivin J-C et al, Effect of combination endocrine therapy (LHRH agonist and flutamide) on normal prostate and prostatic adenocarcinoma: a histopathologic and immunohistochemical study. *Am J Surg Pathol* 1991; **15:** 111–20.

111. Van de Voorde WM, Elgamal AA, Van Poppel HP et al, Morphologic and immunohistochemical changes in prostate cancer after preoperative hormonal therapy: a comparative study of radical prostatectomies. *Cancer* 1994; **74:** 3164–75.

112. Hellstrom M, Haggman M, Nordin B et al, Neoadjuvant GnRH-therapy and radical prostatectomy: effects on tumour volume and density. *Proc Am Urol Assoc Suppl* 1996; **155:** 667 (abst).

113. Klein EA, Hormone therapy for prostate cancer: a topical perspective. *Urology* 1996; **47:** 3–12.

114. Kupelian P, Levin H, Zippe C, Klein E, A contemporary series of external beam radiotherapy versus radical prostatectomy for localized prostate cancer: a single institution experience. *Proc Am Urol Assoc Suppl* 1996; **155:** 556 (abst).

115. Coleman CN, Beard CJ, Kantoff PW et al, Rate of relapse following treatment for localized prostate cancer: a critical analysis of retrospective reports. *Int J Radiat Oncol Biol Phys* 1993; **28:** 303–13.

116. Zagars GK, Pollack A, Radiation therapy for T1 and T2 prostate cancer: prostate-specific antigen and disease outcome. *Urology* 1995; **45:** 476–82.

117. Hanks GE, Lee WR, Schultheiss TE, Clinical and biochemical evidence of control of prostate cancer at 5 years after external beam radiation. *J Urol* 1995; **154:** 456–9.

118. Stamey TA, Ferrari MK, Schmid H-P, The value of serial prostate specific antigen determinations 5 years after radiotherapy: steeply increasing values characterize 80% of patients. *J Urol* 1993; **150:** 1856–9.

119. Pilepich MV, Krall JM, Sause WT et al, Prognostic factors in carcinoma of the prostate – analysis of RTOG study 75–06. *Int J Radiat Oncol Biol Phys* 1987; **13:** 339–49.

120. Pilepich MV, Buzydlowski JW, John MJ et al, Phase II trial of hormonal cytoreduction with megestrol and diethylstilbestrol in conjunction with radiotherapy for carcinoma of the prostate: outcome results of RTOG 83-07. *Int J Radiat Oncol Biol Phys* 1995; **32:** 175–80.

121. Pilepich MV, John MJ, Krall JM et al, Phase II Radiation Therapy Oncology Group study of hormonal cytoreduction with flutamide and Zoladex in locally advanced carcinoma of the prostate treated with definitive radiotherapy. *Am J Clin Oncol* 1990; **13:** 461.

122. Pilepich MV, Krall JM, Al-Sarraf M et al, Androgen deprivation with radiation therapy compared with radiation therapy alone for locally advanced prostatic carcinoma: a randomized comparative trial of the Radiation Therapy Oncology Group. *Urology* 1995; **45:** 616–23.

123. Akakura K, Bruchovsky N, Goldenberg SL et al, Effects of intermittent androgen suppression on androgen-dependent tumors. Apoptosis and serum prostate-specific antigen. *Cancer* 1993; **71:** 2782–90.

124. Zeitman AL, Prince EA, Nakfoor BM et al, Permanent tumor eradication by radiation is enhanced by prior androgen withdrawal in two experimental models. *Proc Am Urol Assoc Suppl* 1996; **155:** 509 (abst).

125. Gomez J-L, Laverdiere J, Cusan L et al, Impact of neoadjuvant and adjuvant antiandrogen therapy associated with curative radiation therapy in early stage prostate cancer: preliminary report of a randomized study. *Proc Am Urol Assoc Suppl* 1996; **155:** 400 (abst).

126. Critz FA, Levinson AK, Williams WH et al, Is an undetectable nadir PSA a reasonable goal following irradiation for prostate cancer? *Proc Am Urol Assoc Suppl* 1996; **155:** 557 (abst).

127. Forman JD, Kumar R, Haas G et al, Neoadjuvant hormonal downsizing of localized carcinoma of the prostate: effects on the volume of normal tissue irradiation. *Cancer Invest* 1995; **13:** 8–15.

128. Yang FE, Chen GT, Ray P et al, The potential for

normal tissue dose reduction with neoadjuvant hormonal therapy in conformal treatment planning for stage C prostate cancer. *Int J Radiat Oncol Biol Phys* 1995; **33**: 1009–17.

129. Lee WR, Hanks GE, Schultheiss TE et al, Localized prostate cancer treated by external-beam radiotherapy alone: serum prostate-specific antigen-driven outcome analysis. *J Clin Oncol* 1995; **13**: 464–9.

130. Grignon D, Caplan R, Sarkar F et al, P53 suppressor gene mutations predict for failure following combined neoadjuvant total androgen ablation and external beam radiation therapy for locally advanced prostate cancer: a study based on RTOG protocol 8610. *Proc Am Urol Assoc Suppl* 1995; **153**: 293 (abst).

131. Frazier HA, Robertson JE, Humphrey PA, Pulson DF, Is prostate-specific antigen of clinical importance in evaluating outcome after radical prostatectomy. *J Urol* 1993; **149**: 516–18.

132. Stein A, deKernion JB, Smith RB et al, Prostate specific antigen levels after radical prostatectomy in patients with organ confined and locally extensive prostate cancer. *J Urol* 1992; **147**: 942–6.

133. Epstein J, Carmichael N, Walsh PC, Adenocarcinoma of the prostate invading the seminal vesicles: definition and relation of tumor volume, grade and margin of resection to prognosis. *J Urol* 1993; **149**: 1040–5.

134. Morgan WR, Zincke H, Rainwater LM et al, Prostate specific antigen values after radical retropubic prostatectomy for adenocarcinoma of the prostate: impact of adjuvant treatment (hormonal and radiation). *J Urol* 1991; **145**: 319–23.

135. Hudson MA, Catalona WJ, Effect of adjuvant radiation therapy on prostate specific antigen following radical prostatectomy. *J Urol* 1990; **143**: 1174–7.

136. Lightner DJ, Lange PH, Reddy PK, Moore L, Prostate-specific antigen and local recurrence after radical prostatectomy. *J Urol* 1990; **144**: 921–6.

137. Hanks GE, Dawson AK, The role of external beam radiation therapy after prostatectomy for prostate cancer. *Cancer* 1986; **58**: 2406–10.

138. Lange PH, Moon TD, Narayan P et al, Radiation therapy as adjuvant treatment after radical prostatectomy: patient tolerance and preliminary results. *J Urol* 1986; **136**: 45–9.

139. Jacobson GM, Smith JA Jr, Stewart JR, Postoperative irradiation for pathologic stage C prostate cancer. *Int J Radiat Oncol Biol Phys* 1987; **13**: 1021–4.

140. Gibbons RP, Cole BS, Richardson RG et al, Adjuvant radiotherapy following radical prostatectomy: results and complications. *J Urol* 1986; **135**: 65–8.

141. Meier R, Mark R, Royal LS et al, Postoperative radiation therapy after radical prostatectomy for prostate carcinoma. *Cancer* 1992; **70**: 1960–6.

142. Walsh P, Adjuvant radiotherapy after radical prostatectomy: Is it indicated? *J Urol* 1987; **138**: 1427–8.

143. Ray GR, Bagshaw MA, Freiha F, External beam radiation salvage for residual or recurrent local tumor following radical prostatectomy. *J Urol* 1984; **132**: 926–9.

144. Anscher MS, Prosnitz LR, Postoperative radiotherapy for patients with carcinoma of the prostate undergoing radical prostatectomy with positive surgical margins, seminal vesicle involvement and/or penetration through the capsule. *J Urol* 1987; **138**: 1407–12.

145. Paulson DF, Moul JW, Robertson JE et al, Postoperative radiotherapy of the prostate for patients undergoing radical prostatectomy with positive margins, seminal vesicle involvement and/or penetration through the capsule. *J Urol* 1990; **143**: 1178–82.

146. Lange PH, Lightner DJ, Medini E et al, The effect of radiation therapy after radical prostatectomy in patients with elevated prostate specific antigen levels. *J Urol* 1990; **144**: 927.

147. McCarthy JF, Catalona WJ, Hudson MA, Effect of radiation therapy on detectable serum prostate specific antigen levels following radical prostatectomy: early versus delayed treatment. *J Urol* 1994; **151**: 1575–8.

148. McCarthy JF, Hudson MA, Catalona WJ, Radiation therapy after radical prostatectomy: long-term followup. *Proc Am Urol Assoc Suppl* 1996; **155**: 608 (abst).

149. Petrovich Z, Lieskovsky G, Langholz B et al, Radiotherapy following radical prostatectomy in patients with adenocarcinoma of the prostate. *Int J Radiat Oncol Biol Phys* 1991; **21**: 949–54.

150. Wu JJ, King SC, Montana GS et al, The efficacy of postprostatectomy radiotherapy in patients with an isolated elevation of serum prostate-specific antigen. *Int J Radiat Oncol Biol Phys* 1995; **32**: 317–23.

151. Forman JD, Duclos M, Shamsa F et al, Predicting the need for adjuvant systemic ther-

apy in patients receiving postprostatectomy irradiation. *Urology* 1996; **47:** 382–6.

152. Haab F, Meulemans A, Boccon-Gibo L et al, Effect of radiation therapy after radical prostatectomy on serum prostate-specific antigen measured by an ultrasensitive assay. *Urology* 1995; **45:** 1022–7.

153. Early Breast Cancer Trialists' Collaborative Group, Systemic treatment of early breast cancer by hormonal, cytotoxic, or immune therapy. *Lancet* 1992; **339:** 1–15 and 71–85.

154. McLeod DG, Kolvenbag GJCM, Defining the role of antiandrogens in the treatment of prostate cancer. *Urol Suppl* 1996; **47:** 85–9.

155. Zincke H, Utz DC, Taylor WF, Bilateral pelvic lymphadenectomy and radical prostatectomy for clinical stage C prostate cancer: role of adjuvant treatment for residual cancer and in disease progression. *J Urol* 1986; **135:** 1199–205.

156. Cheng WS, Frydenberg M, Berkstralh EJ et al, Radical prostatectomy for pathologic stage C prostate cancer: influence of pathologic variables and adjuvant treatment on disease outcome. *Urology* 1993; **42:** 283–91.

157. Zincke H, Combined surgery and immediate adjuvant hormonal treatment for stage D1 adenocarcinoma of the prostate: Mayo Clinic experience. *Semin Urol* 1990; **8:** 175–83.

158. Pilepich MV, Caplan R, Byhardt RW et al, Phase III trial of androgen suppression using goserelin in unfavorable prognosis of carcinoma of the prostate treated with definitive radiotherapy (report of RTOG Protocol 85-31). *Proc Am Soc Clin Oncol* 1995; **14:** 239 (abst).

159. Andriole G, Lieber M, Smith J et al, Treatment with finasteride following radical prostatectomy for prostate cancer. *Urology* 1995; **45:** 491–7.

160. Gormley GJ, Stoner E, Bruskewitz R et al, The effect of finasteride in men with benign prostatic hyperplasia. *N Engl J Med* 1992; **327:** 1185–91.

161. Stoner E, and Members of the Finasteride Study Group, Three-year safety and efficacy data on the use of finasteride in the treatment of benign prostatic hyperplasia. *Urology* 1994; **43:** 184–94.

162. Bolona M, Muzi P, Biordi L et al, Antiandrogens and 5-alpha-reductase inhibition of the proliferation rate in PC3 and DU145 human prostatic cancer cell lines. *Curr Ther Res* 1992; **51:** 799–813.

163. Wiegel T, Bressel M, Carl UM, Adjuvant radiotherapy following radical prostatectomy – results of 56 patients. *Eur J Cancer* 1995; **31A:** 5–11.

164. Gong M, Ferrari M, Stamey TA, Combined androgen deprivation and radiation therapy for treatment of residual prostate cancer following radical prostatectomy. *Proc Am Urol Assoc Suppl* 1996; **155:** 645 (abst).

165. Partin AW, Yoo J, Carter HB et al, The use of prostate specific antigen, clinical stage and Gleason score to predict pathological stage in men with localized prostate cancer. *J Urol* 1993; **150:** 110–14.

166. Moul JW, Maygarden SJ, Ware JL et al, Cathepsin D and epidermal growth factor receptor immunohistochemistry does not predict recurrence of prostate cancer in patients undergoing radical prostatectomy. *J Urol* 1996; **155:** 982–5.

167. Prendergast NJ, Atkins MR, Schatte EC et al, p53 immunohistochemical and genetic alterations are associated at high incidence with post-irradiated locally persistent prostate carcinoma. *J Urol* 1996; **155:** 1685–92.

168. Hawkins CA, Bergstralh EJ, Lieber MM, Zincke H, Influence of DNA ploidy and adjuvant treatment on progression and survival in patients with pathologic stage T3 (pT3) prostate cancer after radical retropubic prostatectomy. *Urology* 1995; **46:** 356–64.

169. Umbas R, Isaacs WB, Bringuier PP et al, Decreased E-cadherin expression is associated with poor prognosis in patients with prostate cancer. *Cancer Res* 1994; **54:** 3929–33.

170. Pajouh MS, Nagle RB, Breathnach R et al, Expression of metalloproteinase genes in human prostate cancer. *Cancer Res Clin Oncol* 1991; **117:** 145–50.

171. Crowley C, Cohen R, Lucas B et al, Prevention of metastasis by inhibition of the urokinase receptor. *Proc Natl Acad Sci USA* 1993; **90:** 5021–5.

172. Hollas W, Hoosein N, Chung LW et al, Expression of urokinase and its receptor in invasive and non-invasive prostate cancer cell lines. *Thromb Haemost* 1992; **68:** 662–6.

173. Liotta LA, Steeg PS, Stetler-Stevenson WG, Cancer metastasis and angiogenesis: an imbalance of positive and negative regulation. *Cell* 1991; **64:** 327–36.

174. Green S, Chambon P, A superfamily of potentially oncogenic hormone receptors. *Nature* 1986; **324:** 615–17.

175. Evans RM, The steroid and thyroid receptor superfamily. *Science* 1988; **240:** 889–95.

176. Sporn MB, Roberts AB, Role of retinoids in

differentiation and carcinogenesis. *Cancer Res* 1983; **43**: 3034–40.

177. Sporn MB, Carcinogenesis and cancer: different perspectives on the same disease. *Cancer Res* 1991; **51**: 6215–18.

178. Abe E, Miyaura C, Sakagami H et al, Differentiation of mouse myeloid leukemia cells induced by 1-alpha, 25-dihydroxyvitamin D3. *Proc Natl Acad Sci USA* 1981; **78**: 4990–4.

179. Lowe KE, Maiyar AC, Norman AW, Vitamin D mediated gene expression. *Crit Rev Eukaryot Gene Expr* 1992; **2**: 65–109.

180. Moon RC, Mehta RG, Rao KVN, Retinoids and cancer in experimental animals. In: *The Retinoids: Biology, Chemistry, and Medicine*, 2nd edn (Sporn MB, Roberts AB, Goodman DS, eds). New York: Raven Press, 1994: 573–95.

181. Hong WK, Itri LM, Retinoids and human cancer. In: *The Retinoids: Biology, Chemistry, and Medicine*, 2nd edn (Sporn MB, Roberts AB, Goodman DS, eds). New York: Raven Press, 1994: 597–630.

182. Anzano MA, Smith JM, Uskokovic MR et al, 1-alpha, 25-dihydroxy-16-ene-23-yne 26,27-hexafluorocholecalciferol (Ro24-5531), a new deltanoid (vitamin D analogue) for prevention of breast cancer in the rat. *Cancer Res* 1994; **54**: 1653–6.

183. Reichman RE, Hayes RB, Ziegler RG et al, Serum vitamin A and subsequent development of prostate cancer in the first national examination survey epidemiologic follow-up study. *Cancer Res* 1990; **50**: 2311–15.

184. Hsing AW, McLaughlin JK, Schuman LM et al, Diet, tobacco use, and fatal prostate cancer: results from the Lutheran Brotherhood Cohort Study. *Cancer Res* 1990; **50**: 6836–40.

185. Dahiya R, Park, HD, Cusick J et al, Inhibition of tumorigenic potential and prostate-specific antigen expression in LNCAP human prostate cancer cell line by 13-*cis*-retinoic acid. *Int J Cancer* 1994; **59**: 126–32.

186. Dahiya R, Boyle B, Park HD et al, 13-*cis*-retinoic acid-mediated growth inhibition of DU-145 human prostate cancer cells. *Biochem Mol Biol Intl* 1994; **32**: 1–12.

187. Fong C-J, Sutkowski DM, Braun EJ et al, Effect of retinoic acid on the proliferation and secretory activity of androgen-responsive prostatic carcinoma cells. *J Urol* 1993; **149**: 1190–4.

188. Pollard M, Luckert PH, Sporn MB, Prevention of primary prostate cancer in Lobund–Wistar rats by N-(4-hydroxyphenyl)retinamide. *Cancer Res* 1991; **51**: 3610–11.

189. Pienta KJ, Nguyen NM, Lehr JE, Treatment of prostate cancer in the rat with the synthetic retinoid fenretinide. *Cancer Res* 1993; **53**: 224–6.

190. Slawin K, Kadmon D, Park SH et al, Dietary fenretinide, a synthetic retinoid, decreases the tumor incidence and the tumor mass of *ras* + *myc*-induced carcinomas in the mouse prostate reconstitution model system. *Cancer Res* 1993; **53**: 4461–5.

191. Schwartz GG, Hulka BS, Is vitamin D deficiency a risk factor for prostate cancer? (Hypothesis). *Anticancer Res* 1990; **10**: 1307–12.

192. Hanchette CL, Schwartz GC, Geographic patterns of prostate cancer mortality. Evidence for a protective effect of ultraviolet radiation. *Cancer* 1992; **70**: 2861–9.

193. Corder EH, Guess HA, Hulka BS et al, Vitamin D and prostate cancer: a prediagnostic study with stored sera. *Cancer Epidemiol Biomarkers Prev* 1993; **2**: 467–72.

194. Peehl DM, Skowronski RJ, Leung GK et al, Antiproliferative effects of 1,25-dihydroxyvitamin D3 on primary cultures of human prostate cells. *Cancer Res* 1994; **54**: 805–10.

195. Folkman J, Tumor angiogenesis: therapeutic implications. *N Engl J Med* 1971; **285**: 1182–6.

196. Andrawis RI, Nashid NS, Lindquist RR et al, Angiogenesis in prostate cancer and benign prostatic hyperplasia. *Proc Am Urol Assoc Suppl* 1996; **155**: 353 (abst).

197. Evans CP, Elfman F, Parangi S et al, Inhibition of prostate cancer angiogenesis and growth by expression of catalytically inactive urokinase-type plasminogen activator. *Proc Am Urol Assoc Suppl* 1996; **155**: 323 (abst).

198. Hawkins MJ, Clinical trials of antiangiogenic agents. *Curr Opin Oncol* 1995; **7**: 90–3.

199. Stein CA, Suramin: a novel antineoplastic agent with multiple potential mechanisms of action. *Cancer Res* 1993; **53**: 2239–48.

200. Myers C, Cooper M, Stein C et al, Suramin: a novel growth factor antagonist with activity in hormone-refractory metastatic prostate cancer. *J Clin Oncol* 1992; **10**: 881–9.

201. Eisenberg MA, Reyno LM, Jodrell DI et al, Suramin, an active drug for prostate cancer: interim observation in a phase I trial. *J Natl Cancer Inst* 1993; **85**: 611–22.

202. Schurmann MG, Schulze H, Pastor J et al, Relationship of response to suramin treatment and survival in hormonal refractory prostate cancer. *Proc Am Urol Assoc Suppl* 1996; **155**: 611 (abst).

203. Siegall CB, Schwab G, Nordan RP et al, Expression of the interleukin 6 receptor in prostate carcinoma cells. *Cancer Res* 1990; **50:** 7786–8.

204. McKeehan WL, Adams PS, TGF and EGF in vitro. *Cell Devel Biol* 1988; **24:** 243–6.

205. Matuo Y, Nishi N, Takasuka H et al, Production and significance of TGF-beta in AT-3 metastatic cell line established from the Dunning rat prostatic adenocarcinoma. *Biochem Biophys Res Commun* 1990; **166:** 840–7.

206. Sporn MB, Roberts AB, Wakefield LM, Cromrugghe B, TGF. *J Cell Biol* 1987; **105:** 1039–45.

207. Bargmann C, Hung M, Weinberg R, The neu oncogene encodes an epidermal growth factor receptor-related protein. *Nature* 1986; **319:** 226–30.

208. McCann A, Dervan PA, Johnston PA et al, c-erb-2 oncoprotein expression in primary human tumors. *Cancer* 1990; **65:** 88.

209. McKenzie SJ, DeSombre KA, Bast BS et al, Serum levels of HER-2 neu (c-erbB-2) correlate with overexpression of p185neu in human ovarian cancer. *Cancer* 1993; **71:** 3942–6.

210. Valeron PF, Chirino R, Vega V et al, Quantitative analysis of p185(HER-2/neu) protein in breast cancer and its association with other prognostic factors. *Int J Cancer* 1997; **74:** 175–9.

211. Kuhn EJ, Kunot RA, Sesterhenn IA et al, Expression of the c-erb-2 (HER-2/neu) oncoprotein in human prostatic carcinoma. *J Urol* 1993; **150:** 1427–33.

212. Sadasivan R, Morgan R, Jennings S et al, Overexpression of HER-2/neu may be an indicator of poor prognosis in prostate cancer. *J Urol* 1993; **150:** 126–31.

213. Gedde-Dahl T III, Spurkland A, Eriksen JA et al, Memory T cells of a patient with follicular thyroid carcinoma recognize peptides derived from mutated p21 ras (Gln-Leu61). *Int Immunol* 1992; **4:** 1331–7.

214. Disis ML, Calenoff E, McLaughlin G et al, Existing T-cell and antibody immunity to HER-2/neu protein in patients with breast cancer. *Cancer Res* 1994; **54:** 16–20.

215. Ioannides CG, Fisk B, Fan D et al, Cytotoxic T cells isolated from ovarian malignant ascites recognize a peptide derived from the HER-2/neu proto-oncogene. *Cell Immunol Immunother* 1993; **151:** 225–34.

216. Haas GP, Solomon D, Rosenberg SA, Tumor-infiltrating lymphocytes from nonrenal urological malignancies. *Cancer Immunol Immunother* 1990; **30:** 342–50.

217. Tjota A, Shang YQ, Piedmonte MR, Lee CL, Adoptive immunotherapy using lymphokine-activated killer cells and recombinant interleukin-2 in preventing and treating spontaneous pulmonary metastases of syngeneic Dunning rat prostate tumor. *J Urol* 1991; **146:** 177–83.

218. Tarle M, Kovacic K, Kastelan M, Correlation of cell proliferation marker (TPS), natural killer (NK) activity and tumor load serotest (PSA) in untreated and treated prostatic tumors. *Anticancer Res* 1993; **13:** 215–18.

219. Moody DB, Isaacs WB, Interleukin-2 (IL-2) transfected prostate cancer cells generate systemic anti-tumor effect. *Proc Am Assoc Cancer Res* 1991; **32:** 247 (abst).

220. Wang MC, Valenzuela LA, Murphy GP, Chu TM, Purification of a human prostate specific antigen. *Invest Urol* 1979; **17:** 159–63.

221. Lilja H, A kallikrein-like serine protease in prostatic fluid cleaves the predominant seminal vesicle protein. *J Clin Invest* 1985; **76:** 1899–903.

222. Chu TM, Kuriyama M, Johnson E et al, Circulating antibodies to prostate antigen in patients with prostate cancer. *Transplant Proc* 1984; **16:** 481–5.

223. Correale P, Tsang K, Walmsley K et al, Generation of human T-cell lines specific for prostate specific antigen using an oligo-epitope peptide. *Proc Am Assoc Cancer Res* 1996; **37:** 488–9 (abst).

224. Ernstoff MS, Branda M, Cardi G et al, Definition of prostate specific antigen derived peptides that bind HLA-A2 allele. *Proc Am Assoc Cancer Res* 1997; **38:** 399.

225. Gorsch S, Mannheimer E, Phillips D et al, In vivo and in vitro immunologic responses to prostate carcinoma cell lines among prostate cancer patients and healthy controls. *Proc Am Assoc Cancer Res* 1994; **35:** 499.

226. Murphy G, Tjoa B, Ragde H et al, Phase I clinical trial: T-cell therapy for CaP using autologous dendritic cells pulsed with HLA-A0201-specific peptides from prostate-specific membrane antigen. *Prostate* 1996; **29:** 371–80.

227. Valone F, Small E, Peshwa MV et al, Phase I trial of dendritic cell-based immunotherapy with APC8015 for hormone-refractory prostate cancer (HPRC). *Proc Am Assoc Cancer Res* 1998; **39:** 1186a.

228. Whitmore WF Jr, Natural history of low-stage prostatic cancer and the impact of early detection. *Urol Clin North Am* 1990; **17:** 689–97.

7

Renal cell carcinoma

Thomas Schwaab, Jens Atzpodien

INTRODUCTION

Renal cell carcinoma (RCC) was estimated to cause 29 900 new cancer causes and 11 600 cancer deaths in the USA in 1998. It is the seventh leading cause of cancer, and accounts for approximately 3% of all malignancies.[1] After prostate cancer and bladder cancer, it is the third-leading urological malignancy. Its incidence increased significantly by 38% from 1974 to 1990. This is felt to be due – at least in part – to earlier diagnosis with the common use of improved radiological techniques.[2]

CONVENTIONAL TREATMENT STRATEGIES

Although cytotoxic agents are considered to be the chemotherapeutic treatment strategies of choice for solid malignancies, the results to date have been poor in this regard in patients with metastatic RCC. The resistance to these agents has been ascribed to high levels of expression of the multidrug-resistance (*MDR-1*) gene product. This P-glycoprotein – a calcium efflux pump – actively exports cytotoxic drugs out of the tumour cells.[3,4] Inhibitors of P-glycoprotein

do not improve chemotherapeutic effects. A second reason for this chemoresistance may be the low growth fraction and long doubling time of RCC tumour cells.[5]

Only a few chemotherapeutic agents have demonstrated some clinical efficacy; these include vinblastine and fluoropyrimidines, such as 5-fluorouracil (5-FU).[2]

Radiotherapeutic approaches as well as hormonal therapies have not shown significant clinical responses.

IMMUNOTHERAPY

In the 1980s, approximately 60% of patients presenting with metastatic disease died within one year. The five-year survival rate was less than 5%.[6,7] However, advanced RCC, once a disease regarded as incurable, has now become a malignancy that may be associated with cure. Therapy has changed considerably in the last decade, with immunomodulatory strategies evolving as a novel and most promising approach. These changes have brought significant hope to patients suffering from disseminated RCC.

The use of immunoadjuvant therapies to treat cancer dates back to the year 1894, when William Coley[8] discovered that a collection of heat-killed bacteria, known as Coley's toxin, activated the immune system and thus led to tumour regression.

According to the immune surveillance theory of Burnet,[9] the emergence of a malignant tumour results from a failure of the immune system to eliminate newly transformed cells. Everson and Cole[10] were the first to demonstrate that RCC is one of the histological types of tumours most frequently associated with spontaneous regressions. Spontaneous regressions of metastatic disease have been reported in less than 1% of cases, mainly after surgical resection of the primary tumour.[11–14]

Clinical observations show long treatment-free intervals, even in the face of metastatic disease. These clinical features of RCC point to a possible key role of the host immune system in the control of tumour growth and progression.

NEPHRECTOMY AND ADJUVANT IMMUNOTHERAPY

The autologous antitumour immune response mediated by cytotoxic T lymphocytes (CTL) and natural killer (NK) cells is dependent on tumour staging, and is significantly reduced in progressed tumours. This is probably due to the intratumoral production of immunoinhibitory molecules such as transforming growth factor β (TGF-β).

In this context, adjunctive nephrectomy as a debulking strategy might be indicated. This would reduce the amounts of tumour-growth-associated factors, enabling the host to respond to systemic immunotherapy.[2] In fact, patients treated with biologic response modifiers and cytoreductive surgery have shown durable remissions.[15–19]

The majority of immunotherapy protocols are employed as adjuvant therapies after nephrectomy. This is to reduce the tumour burden on the one hand, and to avoid limiting immunotherapy owing to pain, bleeding and infection associated with the primary tumour.

The associated delay in the initiation of immunotherapy in this context may result in clinical deterioration and thus may preclude immunotherapy. A recent pilot study evaluated the use of systemic interleukin-2 (IL-2) therapy with the primary tumour still in place.[16] While no responses were observed in the primary tumours of all 51 patients, 3 patients showed a complete (CR) or partial (PR) response at extrarenal sites. These patients underwent nephrectomy. Two patients had a PR while one patient had an ongoing CR. The authors concluded that systemic therapy with the primary tumour in place may be an alternative treatment for selected patients.

The relative efficacy of initial cytokine treatment followed by nephrectomy versus initial adjuvant nephrectomy followed by cytokines remains unclear.[15] Studies have demonstrated that initial cytokine therapy may improve the prognosis, and does not reduce the chances of response.[17–19]

Since open nephrectomy is associated with a prolonged period of recovery, during which metastatic disease can progress and initiation of immunotherapy is delayed, a recent pilot study investigated the feasibility of laparoscopic cytoreductive surgery in this context. This treatment option was shown to be safe in selected patients. With shorter recovery time, treatment with IL-2 could be initiated significantly earlier than following open nephrectomy.[20]

ADJUVANT CELLULAR THERAPY

The candidates for cellular involvement in antitumour immunity include CTL, macrophages, NK cells and antibody-dependent cell-mediated cytotoxicity (ADCC). Evidence has emerged that in solid tumours, antitumour immune responses are mediated more effectively by T cells than by antibodies.[21] Therefore efforts were made to determine the role of adjuvant cellular therapy as a possible treatment option. Cellular therapy involves the infusion of the patient's own immune effector cells, mainly T lymphocytes, that have been stimulated in vitro with cytokines (e.g. IL-2).

Lymphokine-activated killer cells

In 1980, non-MHC-restricted tumour-cell killing by NK cells was described.[22,23] In vitro cytotoxicity of these NK cells was found to be enhanced by prior stimulation with IL-2, resulting in the generation of lymphokine-activated killer (LAK) cells.[24] These findings resulted in the novel theory of adoptive immunotherapy or LAK-cell therapy. This involves harvesting the patient's peripheral blood lymphocytes by apheresis and incubating them with IL-2 to activate them. The resulting LAK cells are reinfused into the patient combined with high-dose IL-2. Treatment schedules proved to be safe, and only mild toxicities were observed.

An initial randomized trial of IL-2 alone against IL-2 plus LAK cells showed that there were no significant differences in response or survival between the groups.[25] In an additional, randomized, multicentre phase III trial of IL-2 with or without LAK cells, the addition of LAK cells did not improve the response rate above that obtained using IL-2 alone.[26]

A combined assessment of several clinical trials of IL-2 and LAK cells with a total of 461 patients showed an overall response rate of 21%, which was similar to that with IL-2 monotherapy.[27]

In conclusion, the time and effort involved in the preparation of LAK vaccines did not justify their addition to single-agent IL-2 therapy, considering the lack of additional clinical benefits.

Tumour-infiltrating lymphocytes

Tumours are infiltrated by both cytotoxic (CD8[+]) and helper (CD4[+]) T cells. These tumour-infiltrating lymphocytes (TIL) have been shown to have specific antitumour activity, presumably because of their potential for recognizing specific tumour-associated antigens (TAA).[28]

A single-cell suspension of TIL is isolated mechanically and enzymatically from a radical nephrectomy specimen. The cells are expanded in vitro in the presence of IL-2.[29] After two weeks of culture, tumour cells have perished while the TIL continue to proliferate. When there are sufficient numbers of cells, TIL are reinfused into the patient together with IL-2.

Phase I/II trials showed response rates of 13% in 31 patients[30] and 33% in 48 patients,[31] with little toxicity. A combined assessment of 89 patients treated with IL-2/TIL combinations in multiple institutions yielded an overall response rate of 24%.[31]

A recent study in which 55 patients were treated with continuous intravenous infusion of IL-2 plus TIL showed 9.1% CR and 25.5% PR, resulting in an overall response rate of 34.6%. The responses showed a median duration of 14 months. This study concluded that immunotherapy with radical nephrectomy, TIL and IL-2 provides substantial clinical benefit.[32] However, a subsequent multicentre, randomized phase III trial conducted by the same authors demonstrated no improved response rate with a combination therapy of CD8[+] TIL and IL-2 when compared with IL-2 monotherapy.[33]

In conclusion, combined immunotherapy with IL-2 and TIL seems to be a feasible and quite effective approach to the treatment of advanced RCC in selected patients. However, its use is limited because of the necessity to perform a nephrectomy and to isolate sufficient numbers of TIL.

Autolymphocyte therapy

The principle of autolymphocyte therapy (ALT) is to activate autologous, tumour-specific memory T cells. These T lymphocytes, which have previously been exposed to tumour antigens, are selected from peripheral blood leukocytes with anti-CD3 monoclonal antibodies. They are expanded in vitro and stimulated with cytokines to increase their cytolytic activity and multicytokine secretion. To reduce activation of suppressor T cells, the cells are irradiated and then reinfused into the patient.

In 1990, 90 patients were treated on an outpatient basis with only mild toxicity. ALT therapy showed a significant survival advantage when compared with cimetidine therapy alone.[34–37]

Randomized trials comparing ALT therapy with single-agent IL-2 should be indicated, but, to the best of our knowledge, have not been performed.

Priming tumour-specific CTL

Animal models have shown that lymphocytes derived from tumour-draining lymph nodes could be effective against advanced malignancies when activated with *Corynebacterium*.[38]

Similarly, in patients with RCC and melanoma, the first trials used a portion of each patient's tumour mass to prime tumour-specific CTL. Tumour cells were irradiated and mixed with T lymphocytes from draining lymph nodes that had been stimulated in culture with bacillus Calmette–Guérin (BCG). These activated CTL were then reinfused into the patient. They demonstrated autologous antitumour cytolytic activity in vitro, and had high levels of granulocyte–macrophage colony-stimulating factor (GM-CSF) and interferon-γ (IFN-γ) production. In a clinical trial involving 12 patients, 2 CR and 2 PR were observed.[39]

The results for a sufficient number of patients treated in clinical trials have not yet been reported, and specifically randomized trials comparing primed CTL with single-agent IL-2 are still missing. Since this is a very labour-intensive treatment approach, its use will be very limited.

ADJUVANT AUTOLOGOUS TUMOUR VACCINE

The rationale for the use of autologous tumour vaccines (AV) is the attempt to boost the host's immune response specifically against its own tumour. AV can potentially induce a tumour-specific cytolytic T-cell response. For this purpose, tumour cells are harvested from nephrectomy specimens, cultured and reinfused after radiation.

Previous studies with a two-year follow-up time suggested survival benefit for patients treated with AV. No significant side-effects were observed.[40,41] In contrast, five-year follow-up results from a randomized trial comparing AV plus BCG with a control group suggested no survival benefit for this treatment option.[42] Combination of subcutaneous (s.c.) IL-2 with AV did not show any benefit.[43] However, we found an improvement of disease-free survival in a large group of patients (n = 208) treated with Newcastle-virus-modified autologous tumour cells in combination with low-dose IL-2 and IFN-α.[44]

Thus, although quite labour-intensive, the use of AV might be a therapeutic option as a surgical adjuvant treatment alternative.

ADJUVANT BIOLOGIC RESPONSE MODIFIERS

Biological response modifiers are molecules capable of supporting or even initiating an immune response. They represent a broad class of agents that may affect tumour cells or host cells in a variety of ways.

Interferons

The first agent to be used in clinical trials in metastatic RCC was IFN-α.[45] Interferons are a group of naturally occurring proteins with synergistic potent antiproliferative and immuno-modulatory properties. They activate NK cells and macrophages, induce monocyte Fc-receptor expression,[46,47] and influence the numbers of peripheral blood lymphocyte subsets in clinical trials.[48] Additionally, they increase the expression of TAA and enhance the expression of MHC class I and class II antigens on the surface of normal and malignant cells. IFN-α has direct cytotoxic effects on tumour cells.[49,50] IFNs suppress the biosynthesis of interstitial collagenase, an enzyme that is crucial for basement membrane invasion and metastasis by tumour cells.[49] According to antigenic type, the major species are designated IFN-α, -β and -γ.

Interferon-γ

Of all the IFNs, IFN-γ has the strongest in vitro activity against RCC cell lines. However, laboratory activity does not match clinical data. A randomized phase II trial of a low-dose IFN-γ regimen (100 μg/week s.c.) produced an objective response rate of 15%.[51] Another open-label trial investigated the efficacy of 100 μg/m^2/day s.c. in 200 patients, showing an overall response rate of 3%, with excellent dose tolerance.[52] No improved results were produced in clinical trials when compared with IFN-α therapy.[53] Our previous work suggested additional effects by administering IFN-γ sequentially with IFN-α in patients with metastatic RCC.[49,53] Working through different receptors, IFN-α and -γ combined can potentially act synergistically. Studies evaluating this combination will have to be undertaken.

Interferon-α

Since the first clinical trials in 1983 suggesting that IFN-α was effective in metastatic RCC, a large number of studies have been conducted. A combined assessment of 13 clinical trials treating more than 900 patients showed an objective response rate of 18.4%. Response duration ranged from 6 to 10 months.[37,38,54]

Combining data from 29 trials involving over 1000 patients, Wirth et al[55] showed in 1993 an objective response rate of 12%, but the complete remission rate was only 2% and the median response duration of those patients achieving a complete response was only eight months.[55]

Although many trials have been conducted, the optimal dosages and schedules have not yet been determined. This is due to the significant variability in reported response rates with different regimens and patient populations. However, for single-agent IFN-α, the published data suggest that a dose of 10–20 MIU/day produces optimal results.[55]

Certain variables seem to predict the likelihood of response to IFN-α therapy. Asymptomatic patients with a good performance status, prior nephrectomy and non-bulky pulmonary and/or soft tissue metastases have a higher likelihood of response.[37]

Response rates of up to 30% and response durations of over 27 months were reported for a distinct subset of patients who had prior nephrectomy, good performance status and no previous chemo- or radiotherapy.[56,57]

Remarkably, especially patients with pulmonary metastases showed significant responses.

In contrast, patients with unresected RCC, extensive prior treatment and bulky metastases to bone or viscera showed a poor response.[58]

Resistance to IFN therapy may be due in part to the development of neutralizing antibodies.[59]

A recently published trial reported on 335 randomized patients, of whom 167 received IFN-α and 168 received medroxyprogesterone acetate (MPA). For patients treated with IFN-α, the risk of death showed a significant reduction of 28%. The one-year survival rate was improved by 12% and the median survival was improved by 2.5 months. The same study suggested the possibility of patients adapting to IFN treatment, resulting in a decrease of side-effects over time.[60]

A very recent report comparing combination therapy of IFN-α2a and vinblastine with vinblastine alone did not show improved clinical responses for IFN-α-based therapies.[61] However, this trial demonstrated a significant survival benefit for patients treated with IFN-α.

In conclusion, IFN-α has shown some clinical benefits, with remarkably long-lasting responses. It seems to be a promising approach when combined with other treatment options[62,63] (Table 7.1).

Combination of IFN-α and 13-*cis*-retinoic acid

Studies have shown that vitamin A (retinol) and its derivatives can induce differentiation and/or inhibit tumour-cell growth in a variety of preclinical model systems. Antiproliferative effects as well as induction of apoptosis are also attributed to them.[64,65] The manner in which 13-*cis*-retinoic acid (13-CRA) augments the anti-tumour effects of IFN-α is unknown.[66] The combination of IFN-α and 13-CRA demonstrated synergistic antitumour effects in vitro against several RCC cell lines.[67,68]

We have reported previously on the remarkable effects of IFN-α/13-CRA combination therapy in patients failing prior systemic treatment.[69]

In a phase II trial, in which 43 RCC patients

Table 7.1 Clinical results with different interferons in advanced RCC[62]

Interferon	No. of patients	CR[a] No.	CR[a] %	PR[a] No.	PR[a] %	Overall response rate (%)
Leukocyte-IFN (Cantell)	166	9	5	21	13	18
Lymphoblastoid IFN	359	7	2	51	14	16
IFN-α2a	420	6	1	59	14	15
IFN-α2b	239	6	3	33	14	17
IFN-β + IFN-β–serine	95	1	1	6	6	7
IFN-γ	262	4	2	21	8	10

[a]CR, complete response; PR, partial response.

Table 7.2 Chemo/immunotherapy including 13-*cis*-retinoic acid (13-CRA)

Agents used	Ref	No. of patients	CR[a] No.	CR[a] %	PR[a] No.	PR[a] %	Overall response rate (%)
IFN-α + 13-CRA	5	43	3	7	10	23.3	30
IL-2 + IFN-α + 13-CRA	124	47	1	2.1	7	14.9	17
IL-2 + IFN-α + 5-FU + 13-CRA + vinblastine	161	24	4	16.7	6	25	41.6
IL-2 + IFN-α + 5-FU + 13-CRA	162	94	8	8.5	21	22.4	31

[a]CR, complete response; PR, partial response.

were treated in an outpatient setting with 3–9 MIU/day IFN-α2a and 1 mg/kg/day 13-CRA, an objective response rate of 30% was achieved. Three complete and 10 partial responses were observed, with a median response duration of 22 months. Seven of these responding patients were progression-free at >10 to >19 months. Interestingly, major responses were observed in sites generally considered to be resistant to IFN therapy.[5]

In conclusion, the addition of 13-CRA seems to be imperative to increase responses to adjuvant therapies employing IFN-α (Table 7.2).

Interleukin-2

With the cloning of IL-2 and its first use in the clinic, it became clear that immunotherapy was a treatment regimen for patients with metastatic RCC that was capable of producing durable remissions. IL-2 is a cytokine produced by helper T lymphocytes upon antigen or antigen-induced activation of resting T cells. It is a growth and activation factor for both T cells and NK cells.[70] In vivo, IL-2 has been shown to generate LAK cells, enhance NK-cell function, augment alloantigen responsiveness, stimulate growth of T cells with antitumour reactivity, and mediate regression of cancer in experimental animals and selected patients with advanced cancer.[71] It affects tumour growth by activating lymphoid cells in vivo without any effect on tumour promotion or proliferation directly.

Recombinant interleukin-2 (rIL-2) obtained European regulatory approval in 1989 and US Food and Drug Association (FDA) approval in 1992 on the basis of demonstrated safety and efficacy in clinical studies involving 255 RCC patients.[72] IL-2 has a short half-life, and its pharmacokinetics are approximately linear when administered as an intravenous (i.v.) bolus. The resulting serum levels are proportional to the dose level.

High-dose IL-2 regimens administered doses of 600 000 or 720 000 IU/kg by 15-minute infusions every eight hours for as many as 14 consecutive doses during five days, as clinically tolerated, followed by a second identical cycle of treatment scheduled after an approximate 10-day rest, with courses repeated every 6–12 weeks.[2]

The initial cumulative experience with high-dose IL-2 therapy showed a 15% objective response rate. Responding patients usually showed a good performance status. The median duration for all objective responses was 54 months. The median survival for all 255 patients was 16.3 months, with 10–20% alive 5–10 years following treatment.[73,74] These findings confirmed the pivotal role of IL-2 in the treatment of selected patients.

However effective IL-2 is, there are significant side-effects. IL-2 toxicity affects the cardiovascular, renal, hepatic and neurological systems, and its initial use was associated with a mortality rate of 4%.[75] Thus all high-dose IL-2 therapy regimens require inpatient administration and occasionally intensive care unit support. As a result, the cost of therapy can be prohibitive, and many patients are unable to tolerate the therapy because of concomitant medical problems.

In the late 1980s, results proved that the major feature of IL-2 treatment was the durability of complete responses, which was in contrast to any other treatment of RCC.[11] In fact,

high-dose IL-2 provided PRs and CRs remaining progression-free at a median follow-up of five years.[76]

However, the significant toxicity led several investigators to assess the efficacy of IL-2 in lower doses. A randomized phase III trial comparing high- and low-dose IL-2 confirmed that the high-dose regimen was more cardiotoxic and was associated with thrombocytopenia as well as a greater number of infectious episodes. There were no statistically significant differences in the response rates or complete remission rates between those regimens. As a result of these trials, at the Medical School, Hannover, Germany, we among others have transformed treatment with IL-2 to a home therapy setting where it can be given safely without grade III/IV toxicity.[77]

In our institution, we have initiated the administration of 20×10^6 IU/m^2 of rIL-2 in two daily doses. This dosage provided a better bioavailability than single-dose administration.[78] Overall response rates and CR incidence appear similar with bolus, continuous i.v. or s.c. administration.[27]

Patients who had been successfully treated with IL-2 once, but showed recurrence of disease, did not benefit from retreatment with IL-2.[79]

However, IL-2 therapy has proved to be the only treatment option capable of inducing long-lasting remissions in patients with advanced RCC. Thus recombinant IL-2 will most likely continue to be a pillar of any future adjuvant treatment regimen of metastatic RCC (Table 7.3).

Combinations of IL-2 and IFN-β or IFN-γ

IL-2 in combination with other cytokines has been studied in small numbers of patients. Combination of IL-2 and IFN-γ in 33 patients yielded 7 (21%) PRs, which approximates the results of studies using IL-2 monotherapy.[80] Thus the addition of IFN-γ to IL-2 treatment did not prove to be beneficial.

The combination of IL-2 and IFN-β has also been examined. An IL-2 and IFN-β combination

Table 7.3 Summary of clinical results with rIL-2 alone, with rIL-2 plus IFN-α, and with rIL-2 plus lymphokine-activated killer (LAK) cells[27]

	Route of administration[a]	No. of patients	CR[a]		PR[a]		Overall response rate (%)
			No.	%	No.	%	
rIL-2 alone	Total	1712	65	3.8	197	11.5	15.4
	i.v. bolus	733	38	5.2	83	11.3	16.5
	c.i.v.	789	21	2.7	86	10.9	13.5
	s.c.	190	6	3.2	28	14.7	18.6
rIL-2 + IFN-α	Total	1411	62	4.4	229	16.2	20.6
	s.c.	675	34	5.0	109	16.1	21.2
	c.i.v.	556	19	3.4	92	16.6	20.0
	i.v.	180	9	5.0	28	15.6	20.5
rIL-2 + LAK cells	Total	461	29	6.3	68	14.8	21.0
	c.i.v.	245	9	4.0	29	11.8	16.3
	i.v. bolus	216	20	9.3	39	18.1	27.3

[a] i.v., intravenous; c.i.v., continuous i.v. infusion; s.c. subcutaneous.
[b] CR, complete response; PR, partial response.

was administered three times a week as an i.v. bolus injection in 24 patients. Of 22 assessable patients, 6 (27%) exhibited objective responses, including 1 CR and 5 PRs. Therefore moderate-dose intermittent IL-2 plus IFN-β can be administered on an outpatient basis in a safe and tolerable fashion. Antitumour activity is observed with this combination.[81]

Thus the addition of IFN-γ or IFN-β to IL-2 does not represent a significantly beneficial treatment alternative.

Combinations of IL-2 and IFN-α

In murine tumour models, IFN-α and IL-2 demonstrated synergistic effects, establishing a compelling rationale for their combined use in humans.[27,82–85] This synergy probably originates from the combination of IFN-α-induced upregulation of MHC expression and IL-2-induced activation of T lymphocytes and NK cells.

A large number of clinical trials have used a wide range of doses for both agents.[86] The majority of patients treated with an IL-2/IFN-α combination received s.c. IL-2, in contrast with its use as a single agent. When taken collectively, these phase I and II trials yielded response rates of approximately 20% in over 1200 patients with metastatic RCC. Approximately 25% of responding patients experienced complete regressions.[87–119] Treatment schedules, cytokine dosages, patient selection criteria and response criteria differed from study to study. Responses overall have occurred at all disease sites, including bone, primary tumours and visceral metastases.[37]

The comparison of high-dose i.v. IL-2 monotherapy and low-dose s.c. IL-2 in combination with IFN-α did not show any significant differences in overall response rates, time to disease progression or median survival.[88] Side-effects were significantly decreased with the IL-2/IFN-α regimen (Table 7.2).

A recent multicentre randomized trial assessed IL-2 and IFN-α monotherapy as well as IL-2/IFN-α combination therapy. In this trial, 138 patients were treated with continuous i.v. IL-2, 147 received s.c. IFN-α and 140 s.c. received an IL-2/s.c. IFN-α combination. The response rates were 6.5%, 7.5% and 18.6% for the groups receiving IL-2, IFN-α and the IL-2/IFN-α combination respectively. Thus it can be seen that the rates for combination immunotherapy were significantly higher than for either monotherapy. The event-free survival was also significantly improved for patients treated with both agents. However, since there were no significant differences in overall survival among the three groups, this study could not conclude that combined treatment provided a significant advantage.[120]

The same study identified a subgroup of patients who will receive virtually no benefit from this treatment regimen. Patients with more than one metastatic site, liver involvement, and an interval from diagnosis of the primary tumour to the appearance of metastatic disease of less than one year have a greater than 70% probability of rapid progression and poor survival despite therapy.

Selected patients should have Eastern Cooperative Oncology Group status 0 or 1, should have no underlying diseases, and should have good cardiac and pulmonary function.[2]

We identified a pretreatment erythrocyte sedimentation rate of over 70 mm/h and a lactate dehydrogenase (LDH) level of over 280 U/l as independent prognostic factors of major significance. A neutrophil count of over 6000/μl, haemoglobin less than 100 g/l, extrapulmonary metastases and bone lesions were identified as minor prognostic variables.[121] We divided patients according to the identified variables into low-risk, intermediate-risk and high-risk groups. A significant survival advantage for patients receiving s.c. IL-2 in the low- and intermediate-risk groups was observed.

Similar results were reported in a very recent study correlating five risk factors with shorter survival: low Karnofsky performance status (<80%), high serum LDH (>1.5 times the upper limit of normal), low haemoglobin, high serum calcium (>10 mg/dl), and absence of prior nephrectomy were reported in a population of 670 patients.[122]

In patients failing initial treatment with either IL-2 or IFN-α, 'crossover' second-line treatment with the other cytokine did not prove to be beneficial.[123]

IL-2, IFN-α and 13-*cis*-retinoic acid combination therapy

Since combination therapies with IL-2/IFN-α and IFN-α/13-CRA showed promising results, it was indicated to test the feasibility and response rate of a combination of s.c. IL-2, s.c. IFN-α and 13-CRA. Accordingly, a phase II trial assessing this three-drug combination in an outpatient setting reported an overall response rate of 17%. Forty-seven patients were treated without significant toxicities. One CR and seven PRs were observed. Primary tumours were not routinely resected. Interestingly, two patients with an intact primary tumour had complete responses of their metastatic disease followed by nephrectomy, and remained free of disease. A median survival of 17 months and a 42% two-year survival rate were reported[124] (Table 7.2).

Interleukin-12

Preclinical and phase I trials have investigated the biological effects of IL-12 and its antitumour activity in metastatic RCC. IL-12 is thought to induce expression of cytokines and chemokines. Combination of IL-2 and IL-12 has been shown to reduce tumour growth in mice far more effectively than either agent alone.[125] The same study postulated possible antiangiogenic effects for the combination treatment. Phase I trials are currently investigating the safety and efficacy of fixed-dose and dose-escalation s.c. IL-12. Preliminary results did not report tumour regressions, but changes in tumour growth were observed. Induction of IFN-γ

Table 7.4 Chemo/immunotherapy with IL-2, IFN-α and 5-fluorouracil

Ref	No. of patients	CR[a] No.	CR[a] %	PR[a] No.	PR[a] %	Overall response rate (%)
162	24	4	17	6	25	42
121	120	13	10.8	34	28.3	39
155	34	3	9	10	29	38
128	41	7	17.1	9	21.9	39
156	246	26	11	54	22	33
130	54	0		9	16.7	16.7
131	36	0		7	19	19
132	21	1	5	1	5	10
133	19	6	31.6	3	15.8	47.4
157	47	7	14.9	2	4.2	19.1
158	16	0		4	25	25
159	111	0		2	1.8	1.8
160	62	1	1.6	11	17.7	19.3
Total	831	68	8.2	152	(18.5)	26.7

[a]CR, complete response; PR, partial response.

expression was observed, resulting in an enhanced antitumour immune response.[37]

Additional studies evaluating the clinical efficacy of novel cytokine therapies are indicated, and will be of great benefit in the search for more effective treatment options.

COMBINED ADJUVANT CHEMO/IMMUNOTHERAPY

Combined chemo/immunotherapy aims at an additive or synergistic effect by combining two different mechanisms: direct cytotoxic effect of chemotherapeutic agents and the immunostimulatory effects of biologic response modifiers.

An early combination therapy with IFN-α and vinblastine showed an overall response similar to that achieved by IFN-α alone, but demonstrated additional toxicity.[62,126]

IFN-α was also combined with 5-fluorouracil (5-FU), since there is biochemical synergy.[63,127] Response rates of 35% were reported.

Since synergistic effects had been observed for immunotherapy with IL-2/IFN-α and between IFN-α and the fluoropyrimidines (e.g. 5-FU), trials were initiated assessing the efficacy of combination IL-2/IFN-α/5-FU (Table 7.4). We initially treated 35 patients with alternating cycles of combination immunotherapy with IL-2/IFN-α and chemo/immunotherapy with bolus 5-FU/IL-2 in an outpatient setting. The overall response rate was 48%, and the treatment did not show any significant toxicity.[128]

In a prospectively randomized trial comparing chemo/immunotherapy with s.c. IL-2, s.c. IFN-α and i.v. bolus 5-FU with oral monotherapy tamoxifen, we reported an overall response rate of 39% for patients treated with chemo/immunotherapy. We also showed a significantly improved overall survival and disease-free survival for the same patients.[129]

Following these initial studies, we conducted a phase II outpatient trial of s.c. IL-2 and IFN-α with i.v. bolus 5-FU. We observed 13 CRs and 34 PRs in 120 patients, resulting in an overall response rate of 39%. The same study produced an overall response rate of 6% for s.c. IL-2 monotherapy. An overall response rate of 28% was observed for IL-2 and IFN-α combination therapy. Stratification of patients by risk factors disclosed an apparent survival advantage for this combination therapy over that obtained with IL-2 and IFN-α alone or in combination.[121] Notably, this combination protocol yielded 5% long-lasting complete remissions.

A similar study evaluated the same regimen of combined s.c. IL-2/IFN-α/5-FU in patients with poorer performance status. Comparable results regarding risk factors were found. Of the 54 patients treated, 25 had undergone nephrectomy, and these patients showed a response rate of 32%. However, the response rate for all patients was only 16%. Thus the authors concluded that nephrectomy might be an additional favourable variable for successful treatment.[130]

A different study using similar dose schedules reported an overall response rate of 19% in only 36 patients.[131]

Several centres in the USA also investigated this combination of chemo/immunotherapy using various schedules. In a phase I trial with 21 patients, an overall response rate of 10% was reported.[132] A subsequent phase II study with 19 patients observed 3 CRs and 6 PRs, resulting in an overall response rate of 47%.[133] In these studies, the treatment regimen differed considerably from the schedule reported in our initial study. While we used s.c. IL-2, the US centres administered IL-2 intravenously. Additionally, the 5-FU administration schedules were different.

However, in a prospectively randomized trial, we are currently evaluating the effects of additional 13-CRA with IL-2/IFN-α/5-FU chemo/immunotherapy. There seems to be a significant survival benefit for combinations including oral 13-CRA.

In conclusion, the combination of chemotherapeutic agents like 5-FU with the (to date) most effective immunotherapeutic approaches (IL-2 and IFN-α) may very well be the treatment of choice for advanced RCC in the future.

FUTURE PERSPECTIVES

The investigation of new immunotherapeutic strategies to treat metastatic RCC is a rapidly developing field. Approaches are diverse and innovative. Here, we should like to focus on the most promising approaches. However, the reader has to be aware that there is still a bulk of ideas unmentioned.

Cytokine gene therapy

The first studies suggesting a role for gene therapy approaches in cancer treatment were initiated in 1967, and showed enhanced immunogenicity of genetically altered tumours. Lindenmann and Klein[134] reported that vaccination with influenza-virus-infected tumour cell lysates generated enhanced systemic immune responses. As newer techniques of gene transfer have been developed, infection with a virus has been replaced with specific gene transfer in an attempt to more carefully regulate the nature of the genetic alteration in the tumour.

The rationale for genetically altered tumour-vaccine-based immunotherapy of cancer depends on the presence of tumour antigens that can be recognized as foreign by the host immune system. To generate an antitumour immune response, the tumour must present novel antigens not found on normal cells and the immune system has to be appropriately activated to respond to these antigens.

One approach has been to introduce cytokine genes ex vivo into tumour cells via transformation. The rationale of this approach is that cytokines are produced at very high concentrations in the tumour microenvironment. One of the critical features of this therapeutic approach for human cancers is that these lymphokines are produced only at the tumour site, thereby eliciting a strong immune response with no systemic toxicity. A number of trials have been initiated.[135]

A very promising cytokine for this approach is GM-CSF. Small clinical trials showed early infiltration of mononuclear cells at the injection site and increased delayed-type hypersensitivity responses without significant toxicity. One of the four treated patients even showed a PR to the vaccine.[136] These results suggest that adoptive transfer of GM-CSF-secreting tumour cells may stimulate an effective antitumour response.

Another approach is the transfer of IL-2 into tumour cells. In mice injected with IL-2-producing tumour cells, tumour-specific cytolytic activity persisted at high levels.[137] Similar results were observed in in vitro studies for IFN-γ.[138] Unfortunately, this methodology is expensive and labour-intensive, which may limit its clinical application.

Additionally, cytokine genes can be transferred into cultured TIL ex vivo to generate more potent T cells for adoptive transfer. Studies have shown that genetically modified TIL are indeed localized into tumour lesions.[139–141]

Monoclonal and bispecific antibodies)

The role of monoclonal antibodies (mAbs) to RCC is evolving. mAbs that bind to specific tumour antigens can be used for imaging or to deliver cytotoxic agents (e.g. toxins or radioisotopes) to the tumour with greater efficacy than any other anticancer agent.

The G250 antigen has been identified as an RCC-specific antigen. The anti-G250 mAb (mG250) reacts with a majority of RCC tumour cells, but not with normal kidney cells. A phase II study investigating the therapeutic use of ^{131}I-labelled mG250 showed 3 of 15 patients achieving a PR.[142]

Another potential approach employs so-called bispecific antibodies (BsAbs). These comprise two specific parts: one is specific for a distinct tumour antigen while the other is spe-

cific for certain antigens on immune effector cells. Thus effector cells can be targeted to tumour cells in a highly specific manner. These antibodies have been evaluated mainly in patients with metastatic breast and ovarian cancer.[143,144] To the best of our knowledge, no trials of this approach have been initiated in RCC patients.

In the absence of randomized trials enrolling sufficient numbers of patients, it seems too early to assess this approach.

Dendritic cells and specific immunization

Dendritic cells (DC) represent another potential tool for generating tumour-specific CTL. As the most potent antigen-presenting cells, they are currently a major field of investigation in the oncologist's search for potent tumour-specific cancer vaccines.

We have recently reported on the presence of potentially activated DC in RCC tumours and suggested possible interactions between DC and T lymphocytes. We have suggested the possibility of glycolipids as potential immunogenic antigens being presented by DC.[145] This shows that DC may indeed play a role in the antitumour immune response. With recent advances in culture techniques, these major players in immune activation are the subject of extensive clinical research. DC can be pulsed with tumour-specific peptide antigens, whole proteins or RNA encoding peptide antigens.

In vitro studies have shown synergistic effects of DC tumour lysate and IL-2 in stimulating a T-cell-dependent immune response.[37,146,147] Additionally, research in melanoma and prostate carcinoma has demonstrated the potential usefulness of DC cultures for generating an antitumour cellular immune response.[148–150]

A pilot study has demonstrated the efficacy of DC in patients with metastatic RCC. DC were cultured from peripheral blood monocytes and pulsed with autologous tumour antigens derived from cell culture following nephrectomy. They were matured and activated by administering prostaglandin E_2 and tumour necrosis factor α (TNF-α). Subsequently, patients received up to six DC infusions per month.[151-153] This study concluded that DC are capable of stimulating a strong antigen-specific immune response in patients with metastatic RCC, even in the presence of a large tumour burden.

DC represent a very promising way of initiating a highly effective and extremely specific antitumour immune response.

Additionally, genes encoding MHC class I molecules can be transferred into tumour cells by direct injection into an accessible tumour mass. Thus tumour-specific antigens would be presented to T lymphocytes by the tumour cells themselves. Patients with tumours expressing low levels of MHC class I molecules may bene-

fit from this approach. However, most human primary RCC express very high levels of MHC class I. Therefore patients with RCC may not benefit from this strategy, particularly if this approach is used to treat patients with stages I–III (minimal residual) disease.[135]

A phase I trial enrolling 14 patients assessed the injection of the HLA-B7 (MHC class I) gene directly into tumours. Although induction of a cellular immune response was observed, no clinical responses were noted. However, intralesional HLA-B7 gene transfer is feasible and safe.[154]

Future studies will have to evaluate the clinical feasibility and efficacy of these and similar approaches to cancer treatment. However, the first results are promising.

REFERENCES

1. Landis SH, Murray T, Bolden S, and Wingo PA, Cancer statistics, 1998. *CA Cancer J Clin* 1998; **48:** 6.
2. Figlin RA, Renal cell carcinoma: management of advanced disease. *J Urol* 1999; **161:** 381.
3. Warner E, Tobe S, Pei Y, Phase I trial of vinblastine (VBL) with oral cyclosporine-A (CSA) as a multidrug resistance modifier in renal cell carcinoma (RCC). *Proc Am Soc Clin Oncol* 1995; **11:** 204.
4. Lemon S, Meadows B, Fojo A, A phase I study of infusional vinblastine with the P-glycoprotein antagonist PSC 833 in patients with metastatic cancer. *Proc Am Soc Clin Oncol* 1995; **14:** 479.
5. Motzer RJ, Schwartz L, Law TM et al, Interferon alfa-2a and 13-*cis*-retinoic acid in renal cell carcinoma: antitumor activity in a phase II trial and interactions in vitro. *J Clin Oncol* 1995; **13:** 1950.
6. Golimbu M, Joshi P, Sperber A et al, Renal cell carcinoma. Survival and prognostic factors. *Urology* 1986; **27:** 291.
7. Muss HB, Interferon therapy of metastatic renal cell carcinoma. *Semin Surg Oncol* 1988; **4:** 199.
8. Coley WB, Treatment of inoperable malignant tumours with the toxins of erysipelas and the *Bacillus prodigosus*. *Trans Am Surg Assoc* 1894; **12:** 183.
9. Burnet FM, *Immunological Surveillance*. Pergamon Press: Oxford, 1970.
10. Everson TC, Cole WH, *Spontaneous Regression of Cancer*. WB Saunders: Philadelphia, 1966: 11.
11. Bower M, Roylance R, Waxman J, Immunotherapy for renal cell cancer. *Q J Med* 1998; **91:** 597.
12. Freed SZ, Halperin JP, Gordon M, Idiopathic regression of metastases from renal cell carcinoma. *J Urol* 1977; **118:** 538.
13. Snow RM, Schellhammer PF, Spontaneous regression of metastatic renal cell carcinoma. *Urology* 1982; **20:** 177.
14. Vogelzang N, Priest E, Borden L, Spontaneous regression of histologically proved pulmonary metastases from renal cell carcinoma: a case with 5 year follow-up. *J Urol* 1992; **148:** 1247.
15. Rackley R, Novick A, Klein E et al, The impact of adjuvant nephrectomy on multimodality treatment of metastatic RCC. *J Urol* 1994; **152:** 1399.
16. Wagner JR, Walther MW, Linehan WM et al, Interleukin-2 based immunotherapy for metastatic renal cell carcinoma with the kidney in place. *J Urol* 1999; **162:** 43.
17. Yang JC, Biologic therapy with interleukin-2: clinical applications/renal cancer. In: *Biologic Therapy of Cancer*, 2nd edn (DeVita VT, Hellman S, Rosenberg SA, eds). JB Lippincott: Philadelphia, 1995: 262.
18. Kim B, Louie AC, Surgical resection following interleukin-2 therapy for metatstatic renal cell

carcinoma prolongs remission. *Arch Surg* 1992; **127:** 1343.

19. Sella A, Swanson DA, Ro JY et al, Surgery following response to interferon-alpha-based therapy for residual renal cell carcinoma. *J Urol* 1993; **149:** 19.

20. Walther MM, Lyne JC, Libutti SK, Linehan WM, Laparoscopic cytoreductive nephrectomy as preparation for administration of systemic interleukin-2 in the treatment of metastatic renal cell carcinoma: a pilot study. *Urology* 1999; **53:** 496.

21. Greenberg PD, Adoptive T cell therapy of tumours: mechanisms operative in the recognition and elimination of tumor cells. *Adv Immunol* 1991; **49:** 281.

22. Yron I, Wood TA Jr, Spiess PJ, Rosenberg SA, In vitro growth of murine T cells. The isolation and growth of lymphoid cells infiltrating syngeneic solid tumors. *J Immunol* 1980; **125:** 238.

23. Lotze MT Grimm EA, Mazumder A et al, Lysis of fresh and cultured autologous tumor by human lymphocytes cultured in T-cell growth factor. *Cancer Res* 1981; **41:** 4420.

24. Grimm EA, Mazumder A, Zhang HZ, Rosenberg SA, Lymphokine-activated killer cell phenomenon. Lysis of natural killer-resistant fresh solid tumor cells by interleukin 2-activated autologous human peripheral blood lymphocytes. *J Exp Med* 1982; **155:** 1823.

25. Rosenberg SA, Lotze MT, Yang JC et al, Prospective randomized trial of high-dose interleukin-2 alone or in conjunction with lymphokine-activated killer cells for the treatment of patients with advanced cancer. *J Natl Cancer Inst* 1993; **85:** 622 [Erratum: **85:** 1091].

26. Law TM, Motzer RJ, Mazumdar M et al, Phase III randomized trial of interleukin-2 with or without lymphokine-activated killer cells in the treatment of patients with advanced RCC. *Cancer* 1995; **76:** 824.

27. Bukowski RM, Natural history and therapy of metastatic renal cell carcinoma. The role of interleukin-2. *Cancer* 1997; **80:** 1198.

28. Halapi E, Yamamoto Y, Juhlin C et al, Restricted T cell receptor V-beta and J-beta usage in T cells from interleukin-2-cultured lymphocytes of ovarian and renal carcinomas. *Cancer Immunol Immunother* 1993; **36:** 191.

29. Finke JH, Tubbs R, Connelly B et al, Tumor-infiltrating lymphocytes in patients with renal cell carcinoma. *Ann NY Acad Sci* 1988; **532:** 387.

30. Bukowski R, Sharfman W, Murthy S et al, Clinical results and characterization of tumor-infiltrating lymphocytes with or without recombinant interleukin-2 in human metastatic renal cell cancer. *Cancer Res* 1991; **51:** 4199.

31. Pierce W, Belldegrun A, Figlin R, Cellular therapy: scientific rationale and clinical results in the treatment of metastatic renal cell carcinoma. *Semin Oncol* 1995; **22:** 74.

32. Figlin R, Pierce WC, Kaboo R et al, Treatment of metastatic renal cell carcinoma with nephrectomy, interleukin-2, and cytokine-primed or CD8(+) selected tumor infiltrating lymphocytes from primary tumor. *J Urol* 1997; **158:** 740.

33. Figlin RA, Thompson JA, Bukowski RM et al, Multicenter, randomized, phase III trial of CD8+ tumor-infiltrating lymphocytes in combination with recombinant interleukin-2 in metastatic renal cell carcinoma. *J Clin Oncol* 1999; **17:** 2521.

34. Osband ME, Lavin PT, Babayan RK et al, Effect of autolymphocytes therapy on survival and quality of life in patients with metastatic renal-cell carcinoma. *Lancet* 1990; **335:** 994.

35. Lavin PT, Maar R, Franklin M et al, Autolymphocyte therapy for metastatic renal cell carcinoma: initial clinical results from 335 patients treated in a multisite clinical practice. *Transplant Proc* 1992; **24:** 3059.

36. Graham S, Babayan RK, Lamm DL et al, The use of ex vivo-activated memory T cells (autolymphocyte therapy) in the treatment of metastatic renal cell carcinoma: final results from a randomized controlled multisite study. *Semin Urol* 1993; **11:** 27.

37. Gitlitz BJ, Belldegrun A, Figlin RA, Immunotherapy and gene therapy. *Semin Urol Oncol* 1996; **14:** 237.

38. Mulders P, Figlin RA, deKernion JB et al, Renal cell carcinoma: recent progress and future directions. *Cancer Res* 1997; **57:** 5189.

39. Chang AE, Aruga A, Cameron MJ et al, Adoptive immunotherapy with vaccine-primed lymph node cells secondarily activated with anti-CD3 and interleukin-2. *J Clin Oncol* 1997; **15:** 796.

40. Repmann R, Wagner S, Richter A, Adjuvant therapy of renal cell carcinoma with active-specific-immunotherapy (ASI) using autologous tumor vaccine. *Anticancer Res* 1997; **17:** 2879.

41. McCune CS, Schapira DV, Henshaw EC, Specific immunotherapy for advanced renal cell carcinoma: evidence for the polyclonality of metastases. *Cancer* 1981; **47:** 1984.

42. Galligioni E, Quaia M, Merlo A et al, Adjuvant immunotherapy treatment of renal cell carcinoma patients with autologous tumor cells and bacillus Calmette–Guérin. Five-year results of a prospective randomized study. *Cancer* 1996; **77:** 2560.

43. Fenton RG, Steis RG, Madara K et al, A phase I randomized study of subcutaneous IL-2 in combination with an autologous tumor vaccine in patients with advanced renal cell carcinoma. *J Immunother* 1996; **19:** 364.

44. Kirchner H, Anton P, Atzpodien J, Adjuvant treatment of locally advanced renal cancer with autologous virus-modified tumor vaccines. *World J Urol* 1995; **13:** 171.

45. Quesada JR, Swanson DA, Trindade A, Gutterman JU, Renal cell carcinoma: antitumor effects of leukocyte interferon. *Cancer Res* 1983; **43:** 940.

46. Lubeck MD, Steplewski Z, Baglia F et al, The interaction of murine IgG subclass proteins with human monocyte Fc receptors. *J Immunol* 1985; **135:** 1299.

47. Doveil GC, Fierno MT, Novelli M et al, Adjuvant therapy of stage IIIb melanoma with interferon alpha-2b: clinical and immunological relevance. *Dermatology* 1995; **191:** 234.

48. Krown SE, Interferon treatment of renal cell carcinoma. Current status and future prospects. *Cancer* 1986; **46:** 4315.

49. Ernstoff MS, Nair S, Bahnson RR et al, A phase Ia trial of sequential administration recombinant DNA-produced interferons: combination recombinant interferon gamma and recombinant interferon alpha in patients with metastatic renal cell carcinoma. *J Clin Oncol* 1990; **8:** 1637.

50. Gohji K, Fidler IJ, Tsan R et al, Human recombinant interferons-beta and -gamma decrease gelatinase production and invasion by human KG-2 renal cell carcinoma cells. *Int J Cancer* 1994; **58:** 380.

51. Ellerhorst JA, Kilbourn RG, Amato RJ et al, Phase II trial of low-dose γ-interferon in metastatic renal cell carcinoma. *J Urol* 1994; **152:** 841.

52. Small EJ, Weiss G, Dutcher J et al, Preliminary results from a multicenter open-label trial of active immune interferon γ-1 by injection (rIFN-γ) for the treatment of metastatic renal cell carcinoma: favorable safety profile. *Proc Am Soc Clin Oncol* 1996; **15:** 259.

53. Ernstoff MS, Gooding W, Nair S et al, Immunological effects of treatment with sequential administration of recombinant IFN-γ and α in patients with metastatic renal cell carcinoma during a phase I trial. *Cancer Res* 1992; **52:** 851.

54. Mulders P, Tso CL, Gitlitz B et al, Presentation of renal tumor antigens by human dendritic cells activates tumor-infiltrating lymphocytes against autologous tumor: implications for live kidney cancer vaccines. *Clin Cancer Res* 1999; **5:** 445.

55. Wirth MP, Immunotherapy for metastatic renal cell carcinoma. *Urol Clin North Am* 1993; **20:** 283.

56. Neidhart JA, Interferon therapy for the treatment of renal cancer. *Cancer* 1986; **57:** 1696.

57. Sarna G, Figlin R, deKernion J, Interferon in renal cell carcinoma. The UCLA experience. *Cancer* 1987; **59:** 610.

58. Muss HB, Costanzi JJ, Leavitt R et al, Recombinant α-interferon in renal cell carcinoma: a randomized trail of two routes of administration. *J Clin Oncol* 1987; **5:** 286.

59. Quesada JR, Rios A, Swanson D et al, Antitumor activity of recombinant-derived interferon alpha in metastatic renal cell carcinoma. *J Clin Oncol* 1985; **3:** 1522.

60. Medical Research Council Renal Cell Cancer Collaborators, Interferon-α and survival in metastatic renal carcinoma: early results of a randomised controlled trial. *Lancet* 1999; **353:** 14.

61. Pyrhönen S, Salminen E, Ruutu M et al, Prospective randomized trial of interferon alpha-2a plus vinblastine versus vinblastine alone in patients with advanced renal cell cancer. *J Clin Oncol* 1999; **17:** 2859.

62. Savage PD, Muss HB, Renal cell cancer. In: *Biologic Therapy of Cancer*, 2nd edn (DeVita VT, Hellman S, Rosenberg SA, eds). JB Lippincott: Philadelphia, 1995: 373.

63. Elias L, Blumenstein BA, Kish J et al, A phase II trial of interferon-α and 5-fluorouracil in patients with advanced renal cell carcinoma. *Cancer* 1996; **78:** 1085.

64. Gudas LJ, Retinoids, retinoid-responsive genes, cell differentiation, and cancer. *Cell Growth Differ* 1992; **3:** 655.

65. Smith MA, Parkinson DP, Cheson BD et al, Retinoids in cancer therapy. *J Clin Oncol* 1992; **10:** 839.

66. Dmitrovsky E, Bosl GJ, Active cancer therapy combining 13-*cis*-retinoic acid with interferon-alpha. *J Natl Cancer Inst* 1992; **84:** 218.

67. Motzer RJ, Murray-Law T, Schwartz L et al, Antitumor activity of interferon alfa-2 and 13-*cis*-retinoic acid in patients with advanced renal cell carcinoma. *Proc Am Soc Clin Oncol* 1994; **13**: 713.

68. Toma S, Monteghirfo S, Tasso P et al, Antiproliferative and synergistic effect of interferon alpha-2, retinoids and their association in established human cancer cell lines. *Cancer Lett* 1994; **82**: 209.

69. Buer J, Probst M, Ganser A, Atzpodien J, Response to 13-*cis*-retinoic acid plus interferon alfa-2a in two patients with therapy-refractory advanced renal cell carcinoma. *J Clin Oncol* 1995; **13**: 2679.

70. Lotze MT, Robb RJ, Sharrow SO et al, Systemic administration of interleukin-2 in humans. *J Biol Resp Mod* 1984; **3**: 475–82.

71. Rosenberg SA, Immunotherapy of patients with advanced cancer using interleukin-2 alone or in combination with lymphokine activated killer cells. In: *Important Advances in Oncology* (DeVita VT, Hellman S, Rosenberg SA, eds). Lippincott: New York, 1988: 217–57.

72. Fyfe G, Fisher RI, Rosenberg SA et al, Results of treatment of 255 patients with metastatic renal cell carcinoma who received high-dose recombinant interleukin-2 therapy. *J Clin Oncol* 1995; **13**: 688.

73. Fisher RI, Rosenberg SA, Sznol M et al, High-dose aldesleukin in renal cell carcinoma: longterm survival update. *Cancer J Sci Am* 1997; **3**: 70.

74. Rosenberg SA, Yang JC, Topalian SL et al, Treatment of 283 consecutive patients with metastatic melanoma or renal cell cancer using high-dose bolus interleukin-2. *JAMA* 1994; **271**: 907.

75. Fyfe G, Fisher R, Rosenberg S et al, Results of treatment in 225 patients with metastatic renal cell carcinoma who received high dose recombinant interleukin-2 therapy. *J Clin Oncol* 1995; **13**: 688.

76. Atkins MB, Dutcher JP, Renal cell carcinoma. *N Engl J Med* 1997; **336**: 809.

77. Yang J, Topalian S, Parkinson D et al, Randomised comparison of high-dose and low-dose interleukin-2 for the therapy of metastatic renal cell carcinoma: an interim report. *J Clin Oncol* 1994; **12**: 1572.

78. Kirchner GI, Franzke A, Buer J et al, Pharmacokinetics of recombinant human interleukin-2 in advanced renal cell carcinoma patients following subcutaneous application. *Br J Clin Pharmacol* 1998; **46**: 5.

79. Sherry RM, Rosenberg SA, Yang JC, Relapse after response to interleukin-2-based immunotherapy: patterns of progression and response to retreatment. *J Immunother* 1991; **10**: 371.

80. Escudier B, Farace F, Angevin E et al, Combination of interleukin-2 and gamma interferon in metastatic RCC. *Eur J Cancer* 1993; **29A**: 724.

81. Krigel RL, Padavic-Shaller KA, Rudolph AR et al, Renal cell carcinoma: treatment with recombinant interleukin-2 plus beta-interferon. *J Clin Oncol* 1990; **8**: 460.

82. Chikkala NF, Lewis I, Ulchaker J et al, Interactive effects of α-interferon A/D and interleukin-2 on murine lymphokine-activated killer activity: analysis at the effector and precursor level. *Cancer Res* 1990; **50**: 1176.

83. Brunda MJ, Tarnowski D, Davatelis V, Interaction of recombinant interferons with recombinant interleukin-2: differential effects on natural killer cell activity and interleukin-2-activated killer cells. *Int J Cancer* 1986; **37**: 787.

84. Iligo M, Sakurai M, Tamura T et al, In vivo antitumor activity of multiple injections of recombinant interleukin 2, alone and in combination with three different types of recombinant interferon, on various syngeneic murine tumors. *Cancer Res* 1988; **48**: 260.

85. Cameron RB, McIntosh JK, Rosenberg SA, Synergistic antitumor effects of combination immunotherapy with recombinant interleukin-2 and a recombinant hybrid alpha-interferon in the treatment of established murine hepatic metastases. *Cancer Res* 1988; **48**: 5810.

86. Sokoloff MH, deKernion JB, Figlin RA, Belldegrun A, Current management of renal cell carcinoma. *CA Cancer J Clin* 1996; **46**: 284.

87. Atkins MB, Sparano J, Fisher RI et al, Randomized phase II trial of high-dose interleukin-2 either alone or in combination with interferon-alfa-2b in advanced renal cell carcinoma. *J Clin Oncol* 1993; **11**: 661.

88. Philip T, Negrier S, Lasset C, Coronel B et al, Patients with metastatic RCC candidate for immunotherapy with cytokines. Analysis of a single institution study on 181 patients. *Br J Cancer* 1993; **68**: 1036.

89. Palmer PA, Atzpodien J, Philip T et al, A comparison of 2 modes of administration of recombinant interleukin-2: continuous intravenous infusion alone versus subcutaneous administra-

tion plus interferon alfa in patients with advanced RCC. *Cancer Biother* 1993; **8**: 123.

90. Negrier S, Escudier B, Lasset C et al, The FNCLCC Crecy trial: interleukin-2 (IL-2) + interferon (IFN) is the optimal treatment to induce responses in metastatic renal cell carcinoma (MRCC). *Proc Am Soc Clin Oncol* 1996; **15**: 248.

91. Lissoni P, Barni S, Ardizzoia A et al, A randomized study of low-dose interleukin-2 subcutaneous immunotherapy versus interleukin-2 plus interferon-alpha first line therapy for metastatic RCC. *Tumori* 1993; **79**: 397.

92. Bergmann L, Fenchel K, Weidmann E et al, Daily alternating administration of high-dose alpha-2b-interferon and interleukin-2 bolus infusion in metastatic renal cell cancer. A phase II study. *Cancer* 1993; **72**: 1733.

93. Spencer WF, Linehan WM, Walther MM et al, Immunotherapy with interleukin-2 and α-interferon in patients with metastatic renal cell cancer with in situ primary cancers: a pilot study. *J Urol* 1992; **147**: 24.

94. Rosenberg SA, Lotze MT, Yang JC et al, Combination therapy with interleukin-2 and alfa-interferon for the treatment of patients with advanced cancer. *J Clin Oncol* 1989; **7**: 1863.

95. Sznol M, Mier JW, Sparano J et al, A phase I study of high-dose interleukin-2 in combination with interferon-α2b. *J Biol Resp Mod* 1990; **9**: 529.

96. Figlin RA, Belldegrun A, Moldawer N et al, Concomitant administration of recombinant human interleukin-2 and recombinant interferon alfa-2a: an active outpatient regimen for metastatic RCC. *J Clin Oncol* 1992; **10**: 414.

97. Besana C, Borri A, Bucci E et al, Treatment of advanced renal cell cancer with sequential intravenous recombinant interleukin-2 and subcutaneous α-interferon. *Eur J Cancer* 1994; **9**: 1292.

98. Figlin RA, Citron M, Whitehead R et al, Low dose continuous infusion recombinant human interleukin-2 (rIL-2) and Roferon-A: an active outpatient regimen for metastatic RCC. *Proc Am Soc Clin Oncol* 1990; **9**: 142.

99. Dillman RO, Church C, Oldham RK et al, Inpatient continuous-infusion interleukin-2 in 788 patients with cancer. *Cancer* 1993; **71**: 2358.

100. Bukowski RM, McLain D, Olencki T et al, Interleukin-2: use in solid tumors. *Stem Cells* 1993; **11**: 26.

101. Fossa SD, Aune H, Baggerud E et al, Continuous intravenous interleukin-2 infusion and subcutaneous interferon-α in metastatic RCC. *Eur J Cancer* 1993; **29A**: 1313.

102. Raymond E, Boaziz C, Komarover H et al, Cancer du rein: variations des populations lymphocytaires sanguines sous traitement par interferon-2a et interleukine-2r. *Bull Cancer (Paris)* 1993; **80**: 299.

103. Lipton A, Harvey H, Givant E et al, A phase II trial of interleukin-2 and interferon alfa-2a in patients with advanced RCC. *J Clin Oncol* 1992; **10;** 1124.

104. Ilson DH, Mozter RJ, Kradin RI et al, A phase II trial of interleukin-2 and interferon alfa-2a in patients with advanced RCC. *J Clin Oncol* 1992; **10**: 1124.

105. Boaziz C, Breau JL, Morere JF et al, Interferon and interleukin-2 in metastatic cancer of the kidney: apropos of 18 cases. *Ann Urol (Paris)* 1991; **25**: 163.

106. Wersall JP, Masucci G, Hjelm AL et al, Low dose cyclophosphamide, alpha-interferon and continuous infusions of interleukin-2 in advanced renal cell carcinoma. *Med Oncol Tumor Pharmacother* 1993; **10**: 103.

107. Morant R, Richner J, Aapro M et al, Treatment of patients with metastatic RCC with subcutaneous recombinant interferon-alfa 2b and continuous infusion of recombinant interleukin-2: a phase II study. *Onkologie* 1994; **17**: 254.

108. Schiller JH, Hank J, Storer B et al, A direct comparison of immunological and clinical effects of interleukin-2 with and without interferon-α in humans. *Cancer Res* 1993; **53**: 1286.

109. Mittelmann A, Puccio C, Ahmed T et al, A phase II trial of interleukin-2 and interferon by intramuscular injection in patients with RCC. *Cancer* 1991; **68**: 1699.

110. Hirsh M, Lipton A, Harvey H et al, Phase I study of interleukin-2 and interferon-alfa2a as outpatient therapy for patients with advanced malignancy. *J Clin Oncol* 1990; **8**: 1657.

111. Atzpodien J, Korfer A, Franks CR et al, Home therapy with recombinant interleukin-2 and interferon-α2b in advanced human malignancies. *Lancet* 1990; **335**: 1509.

112. Thioun N, Mathiot C, Dorval T et al, Lack of efficacy of low dose subcutaneous recombinant interleukin-2 and interferon-α in the treatment of metastatic RCC. *Br J Urol* 1995; **75**: 586.

113. Atzpodien J, Lopez Hanninen E, Kirchner H et al, Multiinstitutional home therapy trial of recombinant human interleukin-2 and interferon alfa-2 in progressive metastatic RCC. *J Clin Oncol* 1995; **13**: 497.

114. Canobbio L, Rubagotti A, Miglietta L et al, Prognostic factors for survival in patients with advanced RCC treated with interleukin-2 and interferon-α. *J Cancer Res Clin Oncol* 1995; **121:** 753.

115. Schneekloth C, Korfer A, Hadam M et al, Low-dose interleukin-2 in combination with interferon-α effectively modulates biological response in vivo. *Acta Haematol* 1993; **89:** 13.

116. Vogelzang NJ, Lipton A, Figlin RA, Subcutaneous interleukin-2 plus interferon alfa-2a in metastatic renal cancer: an outpatient multicenter trial. *J Clin Oncol* 1993; **11:** 1809.

117. Funke I, Spath-Schwalbe E, Stohlmann G et al, Subcutaneous IL-2 and low-dose-IFN-α2a in the treatment of unselected patients with advanced renal cell cancer. *Onkologie* 1994; **17:** 263.

118. Vuoristo M, Jantumen J, Pyrhonen S et al, A combination of subcutaneous recombinant interleukin-2 and recombinant interferon-α in the treatment of advanced RCC or melanoma. *Eur J Cancer* 1994; **30A:** 530.

119. Ratain MJ, Priest ER, Janisch L, Vogelzang J, A phase I study of subcutaneous recombinant interleukin-2 and interferon alfa-2a. *Cancer* 1993; **71:** 2371.

120. Negrier S, Escudier B, Lasset C et al, Recombinant human interleukin-2, recombinant human interferon alfa-2a, or both in metastatic renal cell carcinoma. *N Engl J Med* 1998; **338:** 1272.

121. Lopez-Hanninen E, Kirchner H, Atzpodien J, Interleukin-2 based home therapy of metastatic renal cell carcinoma: risks and benefits in 215 consecutive single institution patients. *J Urol* 1996; **155:** 19.

122. Motzer RJ, Mazumdar M, Bacik J et al, Survival and prognostic stratification of 670 patients with advanced renal cell carcinoma. *J Clin Oncol* 1999; **17:** 2530.

123. Escudier B, Chevreau C, Lasset C et al, Cytokines in metastatic renal cell carcinoma: Is it useful to switch to interleukin-2 or interferon after failure of first treatment? *J Clin Oncol* 1999; **17:** 2039.

124. Stadler WM, Kuzel T, Dumas M, Vogelzang N, Multicenter phase II trial of interleukin-2, interferon-α, and 13-*cis*-retinoic acid in patients with metastatic renal-cell carcinoma. *J Clin Oncol* 1998; **16:** 1820.

125. Wigginton JM, Kuhns DB, Back TC et al, Interleukin-12 primes macrophages for nitric oxide production in vivo and restores depressed nitric oxide production by macrophages from tumor-bearing mice: implications for the antitumor activity of interleukin-12 and/or interleukin-2. *Cancer Res* 1996; **56:** 1131.

126. Figlin RA, deKernion JB, Maldazys J et al, Treatment of renal cell carcinoma with alpha (human leukocyte) interferon and vinblastine in combination: a phase I–II trial. *Cancer Treat Rep* 1987; **69:** 263.

127. Brunda M, Tarnowski D, Davatelis V, Interaction of recombinant interferons with recombinant interleukin-2: differential effects on natural killer cell activity and interleukin-2 activated killer cells. *Int J Cancer* 1986; **37:** 787.

128. Atzpodien J, Kichner H, Lopez-Hanninen E et al, Interleukin-2 in combination with alpha-interferon and 5-fluorouracil for metastatic renal cancer. *Eur J Cancer* 1993; **29:** 6.

129. Atzpodien J, Kirchner H, Franzke A et al, Results of a randomized clinical trial comparing sc interleukin-2, sc alpha-2a-interferon and iv bolus 5-fluorouracil against oral tamoxifen in progressive metastatic renal cell carcinoma patients. *Proc Am Soc Clin Oncol* 1997; **16:** 1164.

130. Joffe JK, Banks RE, Forbes MA et al, A phase II study of interferon-α, interleukin-2 and 5-fluorouracil in advanced renal carcinoma: clinical data and laboratory evidence of protease activation. *Br J Urol* 1996; **77:** 638.

131. Dutcher J, Logan T, Sosman J et al, 5FU + subcutaneous (sc) interleukin-2 (IL-2) plus sc intron (IFN) in metastatic renal cell cancer (RCC) patients (PTS). A CWG study. *Proc Am Soc Clin Oncol* 1996; **15:** 272.

132. Sella A, Kilbourn RG, Gray I et al, Phase I study of interleukin-2 combined with interferon-α and 5-fluorouracil in patients with metastatic renal cell cancer. *Cancer Biother* 1994; **9:** 103.

133. Sella A, Zukiwski A, Robinson E et al, Interleukin-2 (IL-2) with interferon-α (IFN-α) and 5-fluorouracil (5-FU) in patients (PTS) with metastatic renal cell cancer (RCC). *Proc Am Soc Clin Oncol* 1994; **13:** 237.

134. Lindenmann J, Klein P, Viral oncolysis: increased immunogenicity of host cell antigen associated with influenza virus. *J Exp Med* 1967; **126:** 93.

135. Jaffee EM, Pardoll DM, Gene therapy: its potential applications in the treatment of renal-cell carcinoma. *Semin Oncol* 1995; **22:** 81.

136. Jaffee EM, Marshall F, Weber C et al, Bioactivity of a human GM-CSF tumor vaccine for the

treatment of metastatic renal cell carcinoma. *Proc Am Soc Clin Oncol* 1996; **15**: 237.

137. Gansbacher B, Zier K, Daniels B et al, Interleukin-2 gene transfer into tumor cells abrogates tumorigenicity and induces protective immunity. *J Exp Med* 1990; **172**: 1217.

138. Gansbacher B, Bannerji R, Daniels B et al, Retroviral vector-mediated γ-interferon gene transfer into tumor cells generates potent and long lasting antitumor immunity. *Cancer Res* 1990; **50**: 7820.

139. Rosenberg SA, Aebersold P, Cornetta K et al, Gene transfer into humans – immunotherapy of patients with advanced melanoma, using tumor-infiltrating lymphocytes modified by retroviral gene transduction. *N Engl J Med* 1990; **323**: 570.

140. Fisher B, Packard BS, Read EJ et al, Tumor localization of adoptively transferred indium-111 labeled infiltrating lymphocytes in patients with metastatic melanoma. *J Clin Oncol* 1989; **7**: 250.

141. Griffith KD, Read EJ, Carrasquillo JA et al, In vivo distribution of adoptively transferred indium-111 labeled tumor infiltrating lymphocytes and peripheral blood lymphocytes in patients with metastatic melanoma. *J Natl Cancer Inst* 1989; **81**: 1709.

142. Kranenbourg MH, Boerman OC, Oosterwijk-Wakka JC et al, Development and characterization anti-renal cell carcinoma X antichelate bispecific monoclonal antibodies for two-phase targeting of renal cell carcinoma. *Cancer Res* 1995; **55**: 5864.

143. Valone FH, Kaufman PA, Guyre PM et al, Phase Ia/Ib trial of bispecific antibody MDX-210 in patients with advanced breast or ovarian cancer that overexpresses the proto-oncogene HER-2/neu. *J Clin Oncol* 1995; **13**: 2281.

144. Valone FH, Kaufman PA, Guyre PM et al, Clinical trials of bispecific antibody MDX-210 in women with advanced breast or ovarian cancer that overexpresses HER-2/neu. *J Hematother* 1995; **4**: 471.

145. Schwaab T, Schned AR, Heaney JA et al, In vivo characterization of dendritic cells in human renal cell carcinoma. *J Urol* 1999; **162**: 567.

146. Mulders P, Gitlitz B, Tso CL, Biological characterization of dendritic cells isolated from patients with advanced renal cell carcinoma (RCC) for potential use in adoptive immunotherapy. *Proc Am Soc Clin Oncol* 1997; **16**: 442A.

147. Gitlitz B, Mulders P, Tso CL, Specific anti-tumor response against human renal cell carcinoma by dendritic cells loaded with tumor antigens. *Proc Am Assoc Cancer Res* 1997; **38**: 345.

148. Hsu F, Benike C, Fagnoni F et al, Vaccination of patients with B-cell lymphoma using autologous antigen-pulsed dendritic cells. *Nature Med* 1996; **2**: 52.

149. Mukherji B, Chakraborty NG, Yamasaki S et al, Induction of antigen-specific cytolytic T cells in situ in human melanoma by immunization with synthetic peptide-pulsed autologous antigen-presenting cells. *Proc Natl Acad Sci USA* 1995; **92**: 8078.

150. Murphy G, Tjoa B, Ragde H et al, Phase I clinical trial: T-cell therapy for prostate cancer using autologous dendritic cells pulsed with HLA-A0201-specific peptides from prostate-specific membrane antigen. *Prostate* 1996; **29**: 371.

151. Holtl L, Rieser C, Papesh C et al, CD83+ blood dendritic cells as a vaccine for immunotherapy of metastatic renal-cell cancer. *Lancet* 1998; **352**: 1358.

152. Thurnher M, Rieser C, Holtl L et al, Dendritic cell-based immunotherapy of renal cell carcinoma. *Urol Int* 1998; **61**: 67.

153. Holtl L, Rieser C, Papesh C et al, Cellular and humoral immune responses in patients with metastatic renal cell carcinoma after vaccination with antigen pulsed dendritic cells. *J Urol* 1999; **161**: 777.

154. Vogelzang NJ, Lestingi TM, Sudakoff G, Kradjian SA, Phase I study of immunotherapy of metastatic renal cell carcinoma by direct gene transfer into metastatic lesions. *Hum Gene Ther* 1994; **5**: 1357.

155. Hofmockel G, Langer W, Theiss M et al, Immunotherapy for metastatic renal cell carcinoma using a regimen of interleukin-2, interferon-alpha and 5-fluorouracil. *J Urol* 1996; **156**: 18.

156. Kirchner H, Buer J, Probst-Kepper M et al, Risk and long-term outcome in metastatic renal cell carcinoma patients receiving sc interleukin-2, sc interferon-alfa2a and iv 5-fluorouracil. *Proc Am Soc Clin Oncol* 1998; **17**: 310a.

157. Samland D, Steinbach F, Reiher F et al, Results of immunochemotherapy with interleukin-2, interferon-alpha2 and 5-fluorouracil in the treatment of metastatic renal cancer. *Eur Urol* 1999; **35**: 204.

158. Elias L, Binder M, Mangalik A et al, Pilot trial of infusional 5-fluorouracil, interleukin-2, and subcutaneous interferon-alpha for advanced renal cell carcinoma. *Am J Clin Oncol* 1999; **22:** 156.

159. Subcutaneous interleukin-2, interferon alpha-2a, and continuous infusion of fluorouracil in metastatic renal cell carcinoma: a multicenter phase II trial. Groupe Français d'Immunotherapie. *J Clin Oncol* 1998; **16:** 2728.

160. Tourani JM, Pfister C, Berdah JF et al, Outpatient treatment with subcutaneous interleukin-2 and interferon alfa administration in combination with fluorouracil in patients with metastatic renal cell carcinoma: results of a sequential nonrandomized phase II study.

Subcutaneous administration propeukin program cooperative group. *J Clin Oncol* 1998; **16:** 2505.

161. Atzpodien J, Kirchner H, Duensing S et al, Biochemotherapy of advanced metastatic renal-cell carcinoma: results of the combination of interleukin-2, alpha-interferon, 5-fluorouracil, vinblastine, and 13-cis-retinoic acid. *World J Urol* 1995; **13:** 174.

162. Atzpodien J, Kirchner H, Bergmann L et al, 13 *cis*-retinoic acid, IFN-alpha, IL-2 and chemotherapy in advanced renal cell carcinoma: results of a prospectively randomized trial of the German cooperative renal carcinoma immunotherapy group (DGCIN). *Proc Am Soc Clin Oncol* 1999; **18:** 448a.

8

Adjuvant biological therapy of head and neck cancer

Julie G Izzo, Fadlo R Khuri, Waun Ki Hong

INTRODUCTION

Squamous cell carcinoma of the head and neck (HNSCC) has been proven to be a major public health problem worldwide, representing a significant cause of morbidity and mortality, with approximately 500 000 annual cases.[1] In the USA, HNSCC accounts annually for approximately 5% of all newly diagnosed cases of cancer and 2% of all cancer deaths. The National Cancer Institute has predicted 41 400 newly diagnosed cases of HNSCC (30 300 oral cavity and pharyngeal cancer, 11 000 laryngeal cancer) and 12 300 related deaths for 1998.[2] Over the past 50 years, the incidence rates of both oral and laryngeal cancer have substantially increased among all women and among men aged 45–65 years, while rate stabilization is now becoming evident among younger men.[3,4] Despite significant advances in early diagnosis and local management, the curability of this heterogeneous disease remains limited, with a five-year relative survival rate of 55% for Whites and 34% for Blacks.[5] Although in early-stage head and neck cancers a high cure rate can be achieved with surgery and/or radiotherapy, more than 60% of patients present with

stage III/IV locally advanced disease. The probability of cure of advanced disease is only marginal, with loco-regional recurrences occurring in 40–60% of the cases and distant metastases in 30% of the cases, and with an overall five-year survival of less than 30%.[6–11]

Even in early-stage HNSCC, treatment advances have been undermined by the significant number of patients initially presumed cured who subsequently develop second primary tumors (SPTs).[12–14] SPTs in head and neck patients are not treatment-related, and their high incidence and particular distribution within the upper aerodigestive tract (UADT) and lungs are believed to result from the same continuous carcinogenic exposure occurring in the 'field' and responsible for the initial primaries. SPTs, whether synchronous or metachronous, represent the major impediment to long-term survival after successful primary therapy, and occur at a constant rate of 4–7% per year in patients previously treated for stage I/II disease.[15–18] Data from the Radiation Therapy Oncology Group (RTOG) and the Memorial Sloan-Kettering Cancer Center have shown that the rate of SPTs increases continuously with long-term survival, regardless of the initial tumor stage, with an estimated risk of 10% within three years, 15% within five years and 24% within eight years of the initial radiotherapy.[12,17] The incidence of metachronous SPTs varies by primary site from 10% in the glottic larynx to 40% in the oropharynx.[16,18–22] Approximately one-half of the SPTs associated with oral cavity primaries occur in the overlapping oropharyngeal region, one-third in the lung and one-fifth in the esophagus. In contrast, over 40% of SPTs associated with laryngeal primaries develop in the lung.[18,20,21,23] While the control rate for early-stage laryngeal cancer is excellent after primary surgery and/or radiotherapy, with a five-year survival rate of 60–90%, the prognosis for patients with SPTs, especially of the lung, is extremely poor, with a median survival of 5–10 months and a two-year survival rate of less than 10%.[19,20,23–26]

Given these grim statistics, the recent concept of interventional preventive strategies has been developed as an innovative approach to circumvent the high overall failure rates of the classic therapies. The term 'chemoprevention' was coined by Sporn in 1976, and can be defined as the use of specific natural and synthetic chemical agents to reverse, suppress or prevent premalignancy from progressing to invasive cancer.[27] Advances in the understanding of the processes driving tumorigenesis in the UADT represent a crucial aspect of the successful development of chemopreventive strategies. In particular, the basic concepts of diffuse field carcinogenesis and multistep carcinogenesis, and the identification of individuals at particularly increased risk, along with retinoid-based intervention in the reversal of premalignancy, have been extensively developed to support the role of chemoprevention in UADT epithelial cancers.

In this chapter, we shall focus on issues regarding the biology of aerodigestive carcinogenesis, retinoid biology and its impact in HNSCC, clinical chemopreventive interventions, and cytokine-based therapy, as well as the role of new biological therapeutic approaches.

BIOLOGY OF AERODIGESTIVE CARCINOGENESIS

A critical point in the development of efficient primary and secondary adjuvant therapies is the understanding of the biological mechanisms underlying the tumorigenic process and the identification of specific biomarkers for this process. These biomarkers can be subsequently utilized both for risk assessment of malignant transformation and for evidence of the ongoing carcinogenic process, and may eventually prove useful to monitor the response to chemopreventive intervention.

Field carcinogenesis

Proposed by Slaughter et al in 1953, the concept of field cancerization hypothesizes that the entire aerodigestive epithelial lining is exposed to carcinogenic injury, usually through tobacco smoke, and therefore remains at increased risk for tumor development at multiple sites, which may simultaneously exhibit different stages of the process.[28] The clinical projection of field carcinogenesis is the development of SPTs, which occur at different rates depending upon the primary tumor and various environmental and genetic risk factors.

Extensive clinical, histological and cytogenetic evidence exists to support this concept. In the UADT, for example, the use of tobacco, along with the extent and duration of the exposure, greatly increase tumor risk throughout the entire exposed epithelium. The concomitant exposure to other potential carcinogenic agents, such as alcohol, increases the risk within the exposed field. Furthermore, premalignant lesions and multiple primary tumors occur at increased frequency throughout the whole field.

Histologically, in the late 1950s Auerbach et al, demonstrated that pathological changes (e.g. loss of cilia, hyperplasia, dysplasia) were present throughout the lung epithelial field of light and heavy smokers. Moreover, the degree of histological change noted in the carcinogen-exposed field correlated strongly with the extent of tobacco exposure.[29]

Substantial data exist to support the hypothesis that cellular genetic instability is associated with continuous carcinogen exposure and is an ongoing process detectable in the field.[30,31] Studies of epithelial UADT cancers have demonstrated the existence of common genetic changes between the tumor and adjacent tissue appearing histologically normal, supporting a possible clonal origin. However, in some cases, distinct cytogenetic changes were noted in the normal epithelia, suggesting a continuous accumulation of genetic damage that might lead to the development of multiple primaries.[32–35]

New insights into the process of field cancerization have been enhanced by the characterization of molecular events occurring in the carcinogenic field. An increasing number of specific genetic changes involving oncogenes and tumor suppressor genes have been identified in aerodigestive tract tumors.[36–38] Of all the specific molecular abnormalities identified to date in premalignant lesions and head and neck cancers, alterations (e.g. point mutations, deletions, insertions) of the *p53* gene are among the most frequently observed. Brennan et al analyzed the pattern of *p53* mutations in a large number of patients, and demonstrated a strong correlation between *p53* mutations and cigarette smoking alone (33%) or in combination with alcohol use (58%).[39] In particular, they found a prevalence of smoking-associated mutations at endogenous sites, thus implicating tobacco in the molecular progression of HNSCC. Several investigators have shown *p53* inactivation in head and neck tumors, while others have demonstrated that this inactivation is an early clonal event in premalignant lesions, and is less frequent in normal epithelium adjacent to head and neck tumors.[40–46] The use of the *p53* mutation status as a clonality marker has provided further proof for a multifocal, polyclonal field cancerization process with the finding of distinct *p53* mutations in different tumor-distant epithelia of head and neck patients.[47] This has lent further support to the theory of the independent origin of SPTs, and has enhanced the differentiation between SPT and primary tumor recurrence.[48–50]

The study of *p53* alterations as a marker of the carcinogenic process can have wide clinical research implications, especially in the adjuvant therapy setting. Lately, Sidransky's group at the Johns Hopkins Cancer Center has demonstrated the feasibility of molecular staging in head and neck cancer by showing that *p53* mutations specific for the primary tumor were present in the histologically negative margins in 56% of completely resected HNSCC. In addition, these mutations were also strongly predictive of local recurrence.[39] Shin et al conducted a study in patients who had surgical resection or biopsy of a head and neck tumor in an attempt to correlate clinical outcome with p53 immunoreactivity. Although the cases were matched for clinical characteristics and therapeutic intervention, the rates of overall survival and event-free survival were significantly shorter in the p53-positive group. Moreover, p53 accumulation in the primary tumor was significantly associated with earlier recurrence and earlier relapse, as well as an increased frequency of SPT.[51]

Support for field cancerization also come from studies of allelic losses at 9p and 3p chromosomal loci that have been observed not only in HNSCC but also in premalignant head and neck lesions.[52–54] Several groups have reported high rates (50–74%) of loss of constitutional heterozygosity at single or multiple areas on the short arm of chromosome 3 in oral premalignant lesions and invasive head and neck cancers.[55–58] Mao and co-workers have detected a focal clonal expansion in the form of loss of heterozygosity (LOH) at 9p21 in 32% and at 3p14 in 35% of oral leukoplakia samples obtained from patients enrolled in a clinical chemoprevention trial with 13-*cis*-retinoic acid.[59] With a median follow-up of 63 months, the LOH status of the patients was significantly correlated with an earlier and greater risk for the development of cancer, often away from the biopsy site, further supporting the observation that tumorigenesis is an ongoing process throughout the entire tissue field.[54]

Califano et al, attempting to define a progression model for head and neck carcinogenesis, performed a polymerase chain reaction (PCR)-based microsatellite analysis at 10 critical, frequently altered loci in lesions of the head and neck, including preinvasive lesions and benign lesions associated with carcinogen exposure. They observed a high frequency of alterations at 9p, 3p, 17p and 11q. They additionally observed that the accumulation of genetic events was correlated with histological progression from hyperplasia to dysplasia, to carcinoma in situ, and finally to invasive cancer. The authors proposed that the findings of shared genetic alterations between abnormal epithelia surrounding preinvasive and microinvasive lesions support the field cancerization theory, in the sense of migration of common altered progenitors followed by their clonal expansion.[60]

In a recent study, Bedi et al analyzed X-chromosome inactivation and allelic losses at 9p and 3p chromosomal loci as molecular clonal markers in multiple primary head and neck tumors. Their findings suggested that, at least in a proportion of patients, multiple cancers share a common clonal origin.[61]

Multistep carcinogenesis

The carcinogenic process in epithelial tumors involves complex interactions between several factors, both exogenous (such as the degree of continuous carcinogen exposure) and endogenous (e.g. genetic, hormonal, enzymatic or immunological), and is most consistent with a multistep process occurring over several years.[62–65] The transition from normal to malignant phenotype involves a multistep process whereby the sequential and progressive accumulation of genetic changes results in dysregulated proliferation with loss of cellular differentiation and disruption of apoptotic mechanisms. From a clinical point of view, this concept is illustrated in the aerodigestive tract by the frequent presence of abnormal lesions in the carcinogen-damaged field, such as oral leukoplakia/erythroplakia, bronchial metaplasia/dysplasia or Barrett's esophagus. While these lesions often precede tumor development, they do not necessarily progress to frank neoplasms; however, their presence indicates a high tumor risk in the field.[66–68] For example,

individuals with oral leukoplakia/erythroplakia with histologic evidence of dysplasia have a 30–40% long-term risk of developing head and neck cancers.[69] This concept of multistep carcinogenesis has been supported over the past years by compelling cellular and molecular evidence demonstrating that in multiple organ sites, including head and neck, bladder, esophagus, breast, and colon, the premalignant lesions frequently share specific genetic abnormalities with the tumor.[61,64,70,71] These genetic changes are thought to result in dysfunctional cellular processes, with dysregulation of proliferation and differentiation. These can be manifested by phenotypic changes that are histologically apparent as a progression from hyperplasia to dysplasia and finally to cancer, with invasive and metastatic potential.

While several groups have examined some of the events characterizing the multistep process, focusing on those factors that might be constituents in the dysregulation of growth (e.g. inappropriate expression of epidermal growth factor receptors as well as of cyclin D1), or elements that might serve as markers of dysregulated cell proliferation (e.g. proliferating cell nuclear antigen expression), other groups have searched for evidence of ongoing genetic instability (e.g. polysomy, *p53*).[72–83]

The concept of multistep carcinogenesis has developed along with the development of clinical chemoprevention trials, whose goal is to use specific compounds to block and/or reverse the progression to invasive cancer at various points of the tumorigenesis process. Furthermore, the enhanced understanding of the cellular and molecular changes accompanying the multistep pathway has allowed the identification of biomarkers that might be useful in assessing tumor risk and monitoring responses subsequent to specific chemopreventive interventions.

Biomarkers

The concept of biomarkers as intermediate endpoints for risk assessment and for monitoring the efficacy of intervention has developed over the past decade. This process has been tightly linked to the design and development of clinical intervention trials. While the identification of biomarkers could substantially alleviate the problems encountered by current primary chemopreventive phase III trials (e.g. duration, size, cost), it may play an equally important role in the development of more appropriate and efficient secondary interventions.[84–87]

The identification of specific phenotypic and genotypic events occurring during the multistep process might lead to the development of strategies targeting the particular dysfunction. Additionally, the development of markers that can represent the ongoing tumorigenic process in randomly biopsied material from the field is fundamental to the identification of individual cancer risk in carcinogen-exposed subjects.

In addition to the specific influences of exposure to carcinogenic compounds, in particular tobacco and alcohol, it has been suggested that the development of cancers may depend on an individual intrinsic cancer susceptibility. Therefore another important aspect is the development of biomarkers that can assess the genetic predisposition of exposed individuals to a defined dose of carcinogen. Several studies have demonstrated the value of in vitro analysis of chromosomal sensitivity to genotoxic stress as a potential marker of cancer risk.[85,86] Hsu and co-workers developed a mutagen sensitivity assay, based on bleomycin-induced chromatid breaks in cultured lymphocytes, to measure human risk for environmentally caused cancers.[85] The same investigators reported in a case-control analysis that in vitro bleomycin-induced mutagen sensitivity was an independent risk factor for head and neck cancers. In addition, head and neck cancer patients appeared to have a higher inherent mutagen sensitivity compared with noncancer controls.[87] Furthermore, individuals developing second primary tumors showed the highest degree of mutagen sensitivity at relative 'hot spots' for chromosome breakage, preferentially at chromosomes 3 and 7.[88,89] A recent multicenter, interdisciplinary meta-analysis of head and neck cancers has combined previously published data and new data, and has confirmed these findings. In particular, this study has emphasized the concept of genetic predisposition and has substantiated the value of mutagen sensitivity as a biomarker of susceptibility to head and neck cancer.[90] In a recent study conducted in several lymphoblastoid cell lines, Wei et al reported that increased mutagen-induced chromatid breaks were significantly correlated with an overall reduced cellular DNA repair capacity.[91]

These findings raise the hypothesis that carcinogen-exposed individuals, because of an inherent predisposition for instability at relevant genetic loci, may have a different susceptibility to genetic injury, thereby accounting for a different cancer risk. This concept has been recently supported by Gadzar et al, who showed an allele-specific loss in different regions of the tumor-associated field, despite the apparent development of these lesions through genetically different pathways.[92]

Although over the past years substantial progress has been accomplished in the identification of molecular events in the initiation and progression of HNSCC, the continuation of an intensive and exhaustive investigation of these events is critical to our understanding of the disease. Nevertheless, the integration of translational research concepts, such as diffuse field injury, multistep carcinogenesis, and intermediate biomarkers in the setting of adjuvant chemopreventive trials, represents a unique tool for progress in the appropriate treatment of those individuals at greatest risk.

RETINOIDS

Retinoids include the naturally occurring and synthetic derivatives of vitamin A.[93,94] Several natural and synthetic retinoids have been investigated in clinical trials, including vitamin A (retinol), β-all-*trans*-retinoic acid (ATRA) and its two isoforms, 9-*cis*-retinoic acid (9-*c*RA) and 13-*cis*-retinoic acid (13-*c*RA or isotretinoin), retinyl palmitate, etretinate, and the two synthetic retinamides 4-HPR (4-*N*-(4-hydroxyphenyl)retinamide) and 4-HCR (4-(hydroxycarbophenyl)retinamide). Figure 8.1 illustrates the structure of retinoids currently used in

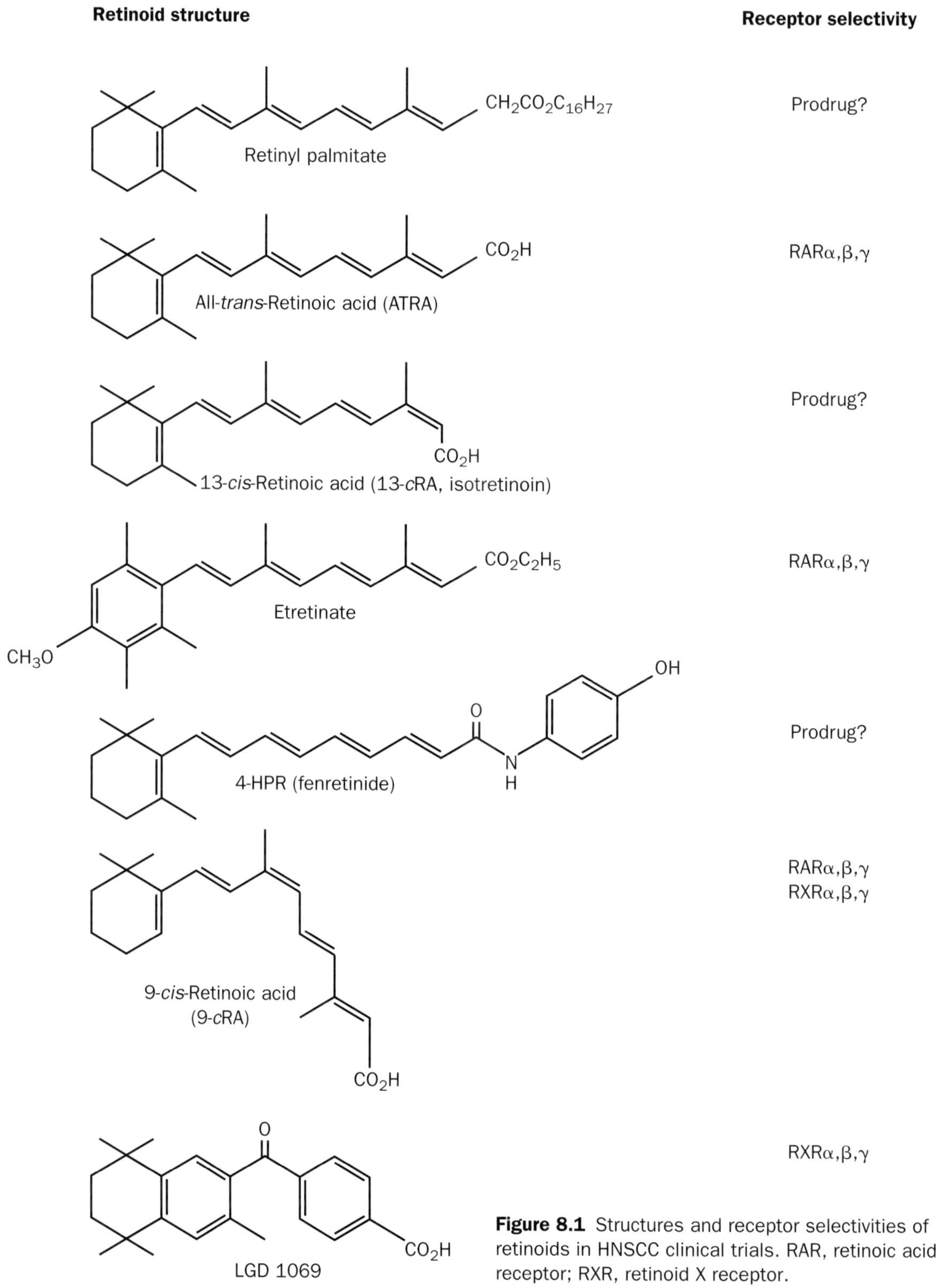
Retinoid structure
Receptor selectivity
CH2CO2C16H27
Retinyl palmitate
Prodrug?
CO2H
All-trans-Retinoic acid (ATRA)
RARα,β,γ
CO2H
13-cis-Retinoic acid (13-cRA, isotretinoin)
Prodrug?
CO2C2H5
Etretinate
CH3O
RARα,β,γ
OH
O
N
H
4-HPR (fenretinide)
Prodrug?
9-cis-Retinoic acid
(9-cRA)
CO2H
RARα,β,γ
RXRα,β,γ
O
CO2H
LGD 1069
RXRα,β,γ

Figure 8.1 Structures and receptor selectivities of retinoids in HNSCC clinical trials. RAR, retinoic acid receptor; RXR, retinoid X receptor.

clinical trials and their receptor-selectivity characteristics.

Retinoids have been extensively studied in preclinical animal models, where they have been shown to suppress carcinogenesis in various tissues, including skin, bladder, oral cavity, lung, breast, cervix and prostate.[95–98] Vitamin A-deficient animals often exhibit a high incidence of tumors; in these animals, the exogenous administration of retinol in the diet has been shown to reverse premalignant lesions and to play a role as adjuvant therapy after resection of the initial tumor.[99,100] In other models, such as the two-stage mouse skin carcinogenesis model, the topical application of retinoids exerted inhibitory effects on tumor promotion but had no impact on tumor initiation.[101] Several investigators have conducted animal studies demonstrating the efficacy of retinoids in the reversal of tumorigenesis and in reduction of the size and number of squamous cell oropharyngeal carcinomas.[102–106]

Cellular biological activities of retinoids

Although the mechanisms underlying their anti-tumorigenic activity have not been entirely elucidated, retinoids appear to be implicated in various physiological, developmental and morphogenic processes, particularly in the regulatory control of proliferation and differentiation of normal, premalignant and malignant cells.[107]

Exposure to retinoids induces a decrease in the cell growth rate of many tumor cell types, including carcinomas of the head and neck, lung, skin and cervix.[108–110] Furthermore, the maintenance of this inhibition requires the continuous presence of retinoids.[110] This growth-inhibitory activity appears to be mediated by the restoration of cellular anchorage dependence, which is often lost by cells undergoing malignant transformation in vitro.[108,110] Interestingly, the same phenomenon has been observed in vivo with fresh tumor cells dissociated from biopsies and exposed to different retinoids.[111]

An aspect of retinoid function receiving increased interest is the ability of retinoids to induce apoptosis during the normal develop-

ment of a wide variety of tissues (e.g. mesenchymal, neuroectodermal, hematopoietic and epithelial).[112,113] Cultured untransformed tumor cells demonstrate an apoptotic pathway after retinoid exposure, but the mechanisms involved appear to differ, depending upon the cell type. Whereas in HL60 myeloid leukemia cells the apoptosis induced by ATRA follows cellular differentiation, in neuroblastoma cell lines the apoptosis appears to be temporally independent from cellular differentiation.[114]

A major physiological function of vitamin A is the prevention of squamous differentiation of epithelial cells in nonkeratinizing tissues.[115] While retinoids have been demonstrated to restore in vitro the differentiation of HL60 myeloid leukemia cells and other malignant cells (e.g. melanoma, neuroblastoma), in cultured keratinocytes and squamous cell carcinomas they inhibit squamous differentiation.[110,115] This effect appears to be mediated by the recovery of cellular responses to growth control mechanisms, such as suppression of oncogene expression and increase in gap-junctional communication.[116,117] Based on these particular differentiating properties of retinoids, a number of clinical trials have been successfully conducted in acute promyelocytic leukemia, using ATRA.[118]

The effects of retinoids on cellular growth, apoptosis and differentiation have significant clinical implications that constitute the rationale for their use in the chemopreventive setting. This ability to modulate cellular differentiation was seen as a promising mechanism whereby the reversal of aberrant differentiation states of preneoplastic cells, particularly squamous cells, could be achieved. Therefore the recovery of growth control and the induction of appropriate apoptosis may serve to reverse the carcinogenic process.

The retinoid signaling pathway

The regulatory properties of retinoids on cellular growth and differentiation appear to result from a signal transduction cascade in which these compounds bind to and activate specific nuclear receptors, which ultimately modulate

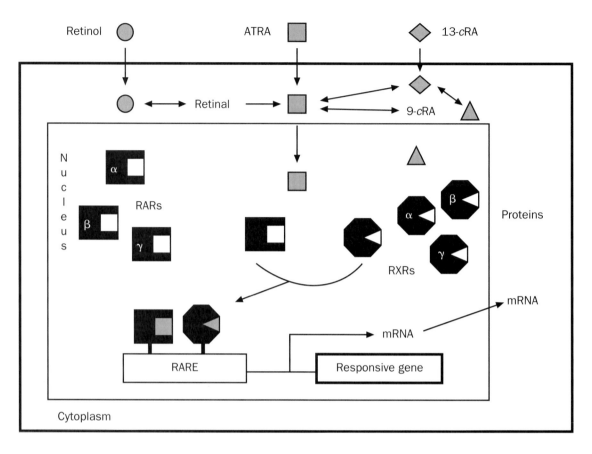

Figure 8.2 A schematic view of the retinoid signal transduction pathways. After cellular uptake of retinol and retinoic acids, and metabolism of retinol to retinoic acid via retinal, there follows isomerization among retinoic acids, diffusion of the retinoic acids into the nucleus, binding to retinoic acid receptors (RARs) and retinoid X receptors (RXRs), activation of these receptors to bind retinoic-acid-responsive elements (RARE) and finally induction of the transduction of retinoid-responsive genes.

gene expression. A number of nuclear retinoid receptors have been identified and cloned to date; they are considered to be members of the steroid/vitamin D_3/thyroid hormone family. Two subfamilies of retinoid receptors have been identified: the retinoic acid receptors (RARs) and the retinoid X receptors (RXRs). Each of the subfamilies harbor different subtypes designated as RARα, -β, -γ and RXRα, -β, -γ, which are divided further into a large number of isoforms produced through differential promoter usage and alternative splicing of receptor transcripts.[119–121] Both RARs and RXRs

form heterodimers, while RXRs can form both homodimers and heterodimers before binding to specific DNA sequences, and both RARs and RXRs control a series of overlapping and unique target genes.[121,122] However, the determination of differential patterns of tissue distribution, the identification of RXR-specific target genes, and also the differences in transactivated domains and in ligand affinity have suggested that there may be two distinct retinoid receptor pathways.[119] These observations have led to the development of strategies designed to identify compounds that selectively bind specific receptor subtypes, thereby allowing a more receptor-specific intervention with potentially fewer side-effects. For example, the development of 9-*c*RA, a pan-agonist that binds both RAR:RXR heterodimers and RXR:RXR homodimers, was initiated by the observation that RXR receptors were unable to bind ATRA with high affinity.[123,124] Figure 8.2 schematically represents the retinoid signal transduction pathway.

Retinoid receptors and head and neck cancer

Recent insights into the molecular identification of retinoid receptors, as well as increasing knowledge of the distinct retinoid signaling pathways, have promoted the assumption that changes in receptor expression and function may be important in carcinogenesis. In the framework of the design and development of chemopreventive strategies, Hong and colleagues have focused on the possible relationships between retinoid receptors and aerodigestive tract carcinogenesis. Studies conducted in several HNSCC and lung carcinoma cell lines have demonstrated the absence of RARβ nuclear receptor expression, therefore supporting the hypothesis that RARβ loss may be linked to tumorigenesis.[125,126] Lotan and co-workers have further expanded the study of RARβ expression by using in situ hybridization with antisense RAR and RXR riboprobes in histological specimens obtained from HNSCC patients and normal volunteers. They observed a progressive decrease in the expression of RARβ in adjacent normal tissues, hyperplasia, dysplasia and finally carcinoma, which displayed expression in only 35% of the cases. In contrast, all specimens from normal volunteers expressed RARβ.[127] These observations were further extended in a study of RARα, -β, and -γ expression in premalignant oral lesions in patients without cancer; RARβ was detected in only 40% of the oral leukoplakia specimens analyzed, while RARα and RARγ were expressed in 88% and 94% of the specimens respectively. Treatment with 13-*c*RA restored RARβ expression in 90% of these lesions, with a correlated clinical response.[128] These observations strongly implicate RARβ in oral squamous carcinogenesis, and suggest that its upregulation may be an important and potentially useful intermediate biomarker of retinoid responsiveness.

An additional relevant aspect is the potential link between retinoids and *p53*. When evaluated through in vitro systems, retinoids have been shown to modulate *p53* transcription and p53 protein levels associated with carcinogenesis.[129] Moreover, in specimens from 40 cancer-free patients with oral premalignant lesions, Lippman et al demonstrated that the increasing accumulation of p53 protein was directly correlated with histological grade and lack of modulation by isotretinoin, with a strong correlation between retinoid resistance and the level of p53 protein accumulation.[130] This retinoid resistance may be related to the lack of an apoptotic pathway as a result of the loss of wild-type p53. Therefore it appears that premalignant and malignant lesions that have lost functional p53 protein will not benefit from retinoid-based intervention, and will require the development of entirely different strategies, which potentially target the p53 abnormality, such as gene therapy.[131]

These findings have strongly implicated retinoids both in the development of the tumorigenic process and in its potential reversal, and have lent support to the extensive exploration of clinical retinoid activity in the UADT, particularly in the setting of reversal of oral premalignant lesions and adjuvant chemoprevention of SPT.

The chemoprevention of oral premalignancy

Oral leukoplakia and erythroplakia, clearly associated with the development of oral cancer, have been the object of chemopreventive studies since the late 1950s. These oral premalignant lesions histologically may harbor multiple lesions of hyperplasia and/or dysplasia, and are strongly associated with exposure to carcinogens such as tobacco, alcohol and betel nut.[132,133] Despite a spontaneous regression rate of 10–20% in these lesions, their natural history demonstrates a significant rate of malignant transformation – from 18% to 36% for some dysplastic lesions at seven years.[69] Oral premalignant lesions therefore provide a unique model to determine the impact of chemopreventive interventions on the control of UADT epithelial cancers. Several agents have been used in the chemoprevention trials of oral premalignancy, including selenium, β-carotene, α-tocopherol and retinoids. Stich et al have reported a pioneering series of trials with β-carotene in high-risk groups (snuff or betel-nut users), being the first to introduce an early intermediate endpoint as a marker of activity with the study of micronuclei.[132,133] The same group conducted a three-arm study (placebo, β-carotene, β-carotene plus retinol) involving 130 patients, and observed that the combination of β-carotene plus retinol was twice as active as β-carotene alone in the reversal of established leukoplakia lesions.[134] At six months, the leukoplakia in the control group showed improvement in 15% of the cases and worsened in 15%, while in the combined-treatment group, 28% of the patients had improvement, with development of new lesions in only 8% of the cases. The single-arm trials that followed these studies using β-carotene reported an unexplained inverse relationship between escalating doses and decreasing response rates. While all of these studies confirmed the minimal toxicity of β-carotene, none of them were randomized, and the histological responses reported were not documented with biopsies.[135–137]

Benner et al conducted a single-arm phase II study of α-tocopherol in patients with oral leukoplakia. Forty-three patients completed 24 weeks of therapy, 20 (46%) having clinical responses and 9 (21%) having histological responses. Interestingly, responses were observed in some retinoid-resistant lesions.[138]

While the use of chemoprevention is not yet considered a standard practice, Hong et al at the MD Anderson Cancer Center have conducted a series of randomized trials since 1984 to explore the chemopreventive potential of retinoids. Five randomized studies involving natural or synthetic retinoids have been reported in oral premalignancy. Table 8.1 summarizes the currently completed chemopreventive randomized trials conducted in head and neck cancer. The ongoing studies are summarized in Table 8.2.

Hong et al conducted a three-month placebo-controlled trial of high-dose 13-cRA given at 2 mg/kg/day, with an additional follow-up of six months in patients with oral leukoplakia. The endpoints of the trial were clinical and histological response (reversal of cytological abnormalities). The complete and partial response rates achieved in 44 evaluable patients were 67% in the retinoid arm and 10% in the placebo arm ($p = 0.0002$). The impact of the retinoid intervention was also significantly higher in the histological improvement rate (54% versus 10%; $p = 0.01$). However, the toxic effects reported in the retinoid arm were significant and unacceptable for this relatively low-risk patient setting. Additionally, owing to a short-term intervention, over 50% of the responders recurred subsequently or presented with new lesions within the three-month interval after the completion of the treatment.[139]

Based on these findings, a subsequent randomized maintenance trial was designed.[59] All patients received an induction course of 13-cRA (1.5 mg/kg/day) for three months. Participants who responded or demonstrated stable lesions were randomized to receive maintenance therapy for nine months with a low dose of 13-cRA (0.5 mg/kg/day) or β-carotene (30 mg/day). This was the first randomized maintenance trial with relapse rate as the primary endpoint. The low-dose 13-cRA arm was chosen in an effort to maintain the good clinical responses obtained with the higher induction dose while minimizing the toxicity; the β-carotene arm was based on epidemiological evidence and previous positive uncontrolled studies. The study confirmed that high-dose 13-cRA induction is active in these premalignant lesions, with 55% of 66 patients achieving a clinical response. The maintenance therapy also demonstrated that low-dose 13-cRA was more effective than β-carotene, with 8% of the maintenance retinoid patients progressing versus 55% of the β-carotene patients ($p < 0.001$). Maintenance

Table 8.1 Completed randomized head and neck chemoprevention trials

Author (year)	Setting	Phase	Number of patients	Agent (dose)	Outcome
Hong[139] (1986)	Oral leukoplakia	IIb	44	Isotretinoin 1–2 mg/kg/day (13-cRa)	Positive
Stich[143] (1988)	Oral leukoplakia	IIb	65	Vitamin A 200 000 U/week	Positive
Han[144] (1990)	Oral leukoplakia	IIb	61	4-HCR 40 mg/day	Positive
Lippman[59] (1993)	Oral leukoplakia	IIb[a]	70	Isotretinoin 0.5 mg/kg/day (13-cRA)	Positive
Costa[145,146] (1992/1994)	Oral leukoplakia	IIb[a]	153	Fenretinide 200 mg/day (4-HPR)	Positive
Hong[150] (1990/1994)	Prior SCC	III	103	Isotretinoin 50–100 mg/m^2/day (13-cRA)	Positive
Bolla[154] (1994)	Prior SCC	III	316	Etretinate 50–25 mg/day	Negative

[a] Maintenance.

therapy was well tolerated, with no dropouts related to toxicity. An update of this study with a median follow-up of 66 months revealed a similar rate of malignant transformation between the two arms (23% in the 13-cRA arm versus 27% in the β-carotene arm), thus confirming the high rate of head and neck cancer SPTs and reinforcing the necessity of a more prolonged intervention.[140] The conclusions of this trial were the basis for the design of an ongoing long-term randomized trial comparing low-dose 13-cRA (0.5 mg/kg/day for one year followed by 0.25 mg/kg/day for the second and third years), versus combined retinyl palmitate and β-carotene for three years. However, because of the findings of the ATBC and CARET studies, demonstrating an increased risk of lung cancer in current smokers receiving β-carotene, the β-carotene treatment

was discontinued from the retinyl palmitate arm of this study.[141,142]

The efficacy of retinoids in the reversal of oral premalignancy has been supported by three subsequent randomized trials. Stich et al compared natural vitamin A (200 000 IU/week orally for six months) with placebo in tobacco or betel nut users who had developed oral leukoplakia. They observed a significantly higher rate of complete remission in the vitamin A arm (57.1%) compared with the placebo arm (3%), and additionally a significant reduction in the rate of progression in the vitamin A arm.[143]

Two randomized trials of synthetic retinamides (4-HPR, or fenretinide, and 4-HCR) also have been conducted in oral premalignancy. Han et al conducted a four-month placebo-controlled study randomizing 61

Table 8.2 Ongoing randomized head and neck chemoprevention trials

Trial[a]	Setting[b]	Agents	Sample size	Primary endpoint[c]
UTMDACC	Oral leukoplakia	Isotretinoin (13-cRA) versus retinyl palmitate	154	Reversal leukoplakia, intermediate biomarkers
RTOG 91-15	Stage I–II HNSCC	Isotretinoin (13-cRA), low-dose	1302	SPT
EUROSCAN (EORTC)	Stage I–II HNSCC or NSCLC	Retinyl palmitate N-acetylcysteine	>2500	SPT
ECOG	Stage I–II HNSCC	Isotretinoin (13-cRA)	525	SPT
Yale	Stage I–II HNSCC	β-Carotene	560	SPT, local recurrence
Australia	Stage I–II HNSCC	Isotretinoin (13-cRA), low-dose	600	SPT

[a] UTMDA, University of Texas MD Anderson Cancer Center; RTOG, Radiation Therapy Oncology Group; EORTC, European Organization for the Research and Treatment of Cancer; ECOG, Eastern Cooperative Oncology Group.
[b] HNSCC, squamous cell carcinoma of the head and neck; NSCLC, non-small cell lung cancer.
[c] SPT, second primary tumor.

patients to either 4-HCR (40 mg/day) or placebo, in which the retinamide arm achieved significant activity in reversing oral premalignant lesions.[144] A maintenance trial comparing 12 months of 4-HPR with no treatment following complete laser resection of oral premalignant lesions began in Italy in 1988. One-hundred and thirty-seven patients have been randomized to receive either 4-HPR (200 mg/day for 52 weeks) or no intervention, with a three-day drug holiday in the fenretinide arm to minimize side-effects. The results reported have confirmed the protective effect of retinoid treatment, with an 8% relapse rate in the 4-HPR arm versus 29% in the nontreatment arm.[145,146]

Second primary tumors: adjuvant chemoprevention

SPTs represent a major cause of death following surgical cure of HNSCC, with a lifetime risk of between 20% and 40% for patients successfully treated for initial disease.[14,23,147] While the risk of recurrence declines sharply over time, the risk of SPT development for early-stage patients remains constant for at least eight years, and constitutes the leading cause of death.[12,14,20,23,148] Despite the increasing emphasis on smoking cessation programs, to date their impact as primary or secondary prevention remains unclear.[149]

These elements, along with the recognized activity of retinoids in oral premalignancy, have provided the rationale for the development of adjuvant chemoprevention trials in head and neck cancer. Several extensive randomized studies of adjuvant retinoids have been completed or are ongoing, as can be seen in Tables 8.1 and 8.2.

In the first phase III randomized adjuvant trial of high-dose 13-cRA, reported by Hong et al, a significant reduction in the rate of SPTs was achieved.[150] Following definitive local surgical and/or radiotherapeutic treatment for stage III–IV HNSCC, 103 head and neck cancer patients were randomized to 12 months of 13-cRA ($50–100 \, mg/m^2/day$) or placebo. The two main endpoints of the study were primary disease recurrence and SPT development. At the first median follow-up of 32 months, no significant differences were observed between the two arms in either the rate of recurrence or in overall survival. Fifteen (31%) of the retinoid-treated group and 17 (33%) of the placebo-treated patients developed local, regional or distant recurrences. However, there was a marked reduction in the development of SPTs in the retinoid arm when compared with the control group. Only 2 (4%) patients of the 13-cRA treated group developed SPTs, compared with 12 (24%) of the placebo patients ($p = 0.005$). Significant toxic effects were associated with the retinoid arm, and the dose of 13-cRA was decreased to $50 \, mg/m^2/day$ during the course of the trial, owing to intolerable toxicity in 13 of the 44 patients receiving the initial high-dose retinoid. The side-effects included cheilitis (25%), conjunctivitis (19%), hypertriglyceridemia (27%) and skin dryness (63%). Only one-third of the retinoid-treated patients were able to complete the 12-month therapy without a dose reduction.[151]

The updated analysis of this trial with a median follow-up of 55 months demonstrated that the retinoid group continued to have fewer SPTs than the placebo arm (14% versus 31%; $p = 0.04$).[152] Furthermore, when evaluating only tobacco-related SPTs (located in the aerodigestive tract) the retinoid intervention was revealed to be strikingly effective in terms of SPT reduction (7% versus 33% for the placebo group; $p = 0.008$) and in terms of a longer delay prior to SPT development. Furthermore, consistent with field carcinogenesis, approximately 80% of the SPTs developed in the carcinogen-exposed field of the head and neck, esophagus and lung; in addition, four patients, all within the placebo-treated group, developed more than one SPT. The overall outcome of this trial suggests that, despite the relatively short-term intervention and the reduced doses, the retinoid chemoprevention was effective, with some prolonged protection from SPTs maintained after the 12-month intervention. Moreover, while 13-cRA had no impact on primary disease recurrence or survival, the reduction in SPTs suggests that retinoids are active against premalignant lesions but are unable to eradicate frankly neoplastic tumor foci. Finally, through the close follow-up and accurate diagnostic criteria applied, this study reported a twofold higher rate of SPTs compared with those reported in retrospective data, suggesting that perhaps the reported incidence of SPT might be underestimated.[147]

Based on the encouraging positive results and toxicity data of this high-dose adjuvant trial, a large-scale multicentric phase III NCI trial, evaluating low-dose 13-cRA as adjuvant chemoprevention in stage I and II HNSCC, was initiated through the intergroup mechanism. After an eight-week run-in period, the patients enrolled in this randomized, double-blind, placebo-controlled study will be treated for three years with $30 \, mg/day$ of 13-cRA versus placebo and subsequently followed for an additional four years. Patients treated up to three years previously for an initial head and neck cancer are eligible for this study. The development of SPTs as defined by Warren and Gates will be the study endpoint.[153] This pivotal clinical trial is complemented by laboratory-based investigations that will assess the mechanism of retinoid action and the expression and validation of potential intermediate biomarkers, as well as the development of an individual risk assessment model for head and neck squamous cell cancer. An interim report on this ongoing trial demonstrated a reasonable tolerance to low-dose 13-cRA, confirming the toxicity data from the previous low-dose trial in oral premalignancy reported by Lippman et al.[59] After its completion, this trial should define the role of

13-*c*RA in preventing SPTs in patients with prior HNSCC.

Bolla et al have recently completed a randomized adjuvant chemoprevention trial using low doses of the synthetic retinoid etretinate for the prevention of SPTs after definitive therapy of early-stage oropharyngeal squamous cell carcinomas.[154] This trial has enrolled 316 patients, who were randomized to receive placebo or etretinate given at doses of 50 mg/day for the first month, followed by 25 mg/day for two years. While this study confirmed the absence of impact of retinoids on primary disease recurrence and overall survival, it also demonstrated no significant differences in the rate of SPTs between the etretinate and placebo arms. However, the data reported have confirmed the high incidence of head and neck cancer-associated SPTs: after a median follow-up of 41 months, 24% of the placebo patients developed SPTs, 80% of which arose in the carcinogen-exposed field, including the head and neck, lungs, or esophagus. Since data on patient compliance and the diagnostic criteria for SPTs have not been reported, it is difficult to extract definitive conclusions.

Another ongoing trial has been initiated through the Northern California Oncology Group (NCOG) and the Eastern Cooperative Oncology Group (ECOG), also evaluating the impact of 13-*c*RA on the prevention of second primary tumors. Shortly after the completion of primary definitive therapy, patients with stage I or II head and neck cancer are randomized to receive placebo versus low-dose (0.15 mg/kg/day) 13-*c*RA. This low-dose 13-*c*RA therapy has yet to demonstrate a reversal of premalignant lesions; moreover, in a negative multicentric clinical trial, a comparable dose, 10 mg/day of 13-*c*RA, was found to be inactive in the prevention of basal cell carcinoma.[155]

An additional placebo-controlled, double-blind trial is currently ongoing at Yale to evaluate the activity of β-carotene (50 mg/day) in the reduction of local recurrences and SPT in head and neck cancers.[156]

A large European randomized chemoprevention study, called Euroscan, is being conducted through the European Organization for the

Research and Treatment of Cancer (EORTC). The design of this ongoing study has been supported by the favorable outcome of a previous trial conducted by Pastorino et al, comparing retinyl palmitate (300 000 IU/day) treatment for 12 months versus observation among patients previously treated for stage I non-small cell lung cancer (NSCLC). Eighteen patients in the retinyl palmitate group developed SPTs, compared with 29 patients in the control arm. A significant reduction in tobacco-related SPTs occurred in the retinoid arm, with 13 SPTs versus 25 in the control arm. A statistically significant difference ($p = 0.045$) in time to development of SPTs within the carcinogen-exposed field was found in favor of the retinoid-treated group.[157]

The Euroscan trial uses a 2×2 factorial design in an attempt to prevent SPTs in two high-risk populations: patients with completely resected NSCLC and HNSCC after curative treatment. The interventions used are retinyl palmitate (300 000 IU/day for one year and 150 000 IU/day for the second and third years) versus *N*-acetylcysteine (600 mg/day for two years). *N*-acetylcysteine is a potent antioxidant used to prevent hepatotoxicity following acetaminophen (paracetamol) overdose.[158] Patients are randomized to receive either one of these agents alone, both agents, or placebo. The projected endpoints for this trial include the development of SPTs, loco-regional recurrence, development of distant metastases and long-term survival. A recent update indicates that accrual is progressing well and that both regimens appear to be well tolerated. Most of the reported side-effects, including headache, dyspepsia and skin changes, have been associated with the retinyl palmitate.

Finally, a large randomized study in Australia is currently comparing the efficacy of low-dose versus high-dose 13-*c*RA in early-stage head and neck cancer patients.

Bio-chemoprevention

In human hematological and solid tumor model systems, various combinations of retinoids and biological response modifiers, such as the interferon (IFN) family, have demonstrated synergistic antiproliferative, antiangiogenic and differentiating activities. Although further studies are needed to understand better the mechanisms underlying the retinoid–IFN interaction, the synergistic activity has been correlated with an increased antiproliferative activity of IFN, a higher level of IFN-induced genes, and an enhancement of the activity of IFN by the differentiation properties of retinoic acid.[159–164] The combination of retinoids and interferons has demonstrated efficacy in vitro and in clinical trials. Lippman et al have conducted several clinical trials with combined 13-cRA and IFN-α to explore the clinical potential of this regimen in advanced skin and cervical cancer.[165,166] The encouraging results of these trials led to the design of studies of the retinoid–IFN-α combination in UADT chemoprevention. Retinoids and IFN-α are individually active in vitro against cells transformed with human papillomavirus and in vivo against HPV-induced diseases, such as recurrent respiratory papillomatosis and cervical dysplasia.[167–169]

Voravud et al reported a phase II trial of 13-cRA (1 mg/kg/day) and IFN-α (3 MUI/m^2/day s.c.) in 28 head and neck cancer patients with recurrent disease. Of the 21 evaluable patients, none developed a complete response, one had a partial response, and two had minor responses. In terms of side-effects, grade 3 toxicities were seen in five patients, all of whom required dose reduction. The median survival duration was 25.5 weeks. Because of the low activity and substantial toxicity, this particular regimen does not appear to be suitable as second-line therapy in head and neck cancer.[170]

Despite these disappointing results, the potential activity of this regimen in advanced oral premalignancy is currently being investigated.[170,171] Based on their previous experience with retinoids in oral premalignancy and the demonstrated usefulness of α-tocopherol as a modulator of retinoid toxicity with potential additional chemopreventive activity, Hong and colleagues have recently begun a biochemopreventive phase II trial combining 13-cRA, α-tocopherol and IFN-α for advanced premalignant lesions of the oral cavity and larynx.[172,173] These premalignant lesions, including moderate to severe dysplasia or carcinoma in situ, are very unlikely to reverse in response to either antioxidant or single-agent retinoid therapies, and are frequently destined to develop into invasive squamous carcinoma. This pilot trial combines, after an initial biopsy, 13-cRA (100 mg/m^2/day), α-tocopherol (1200 IU/day) and IFN-α2b (3.0 MU/m^2/day) twice a week for six months, followed by six more months of treatment if there is evidence of disease stabilization or clinical response. To assess both tumor development and the effectiveness of the therapeutic intervention, an evaluation of several biomarkers of tumorigenesis has been integrated in this protocol. The aim of the present study is to establish the role of biological response modifiers, differentiating agents and antioxidants as combination biochemopreventive therapy in prognostically unfavorable advanced premalignant lesions. This trial is still in the early stages, but preliminary results appear very promising.

Other combination therapies

Further interest has focused on the combination of retinoids with chemotherapeutic agents. Preclinical studies demonstrate promising activity for retinoids in combination with cytotoxic agents, including etoposide, 1,3-bis-(2-chloroethyl)-1-nitrosourea, 5-fluorouracil (5-FU) and cisplatin.[174] In the early 1970s, a series of innovative nonrandomized clinical trials were conducted in Japan to investigate the efficacy of the combination of 5-FU, vitamin A and radiation (FAR) in UADT cancers. The basic regimen, reported by Komiyama et al, was given alone or with surgical resection and incorporated 5-FU (250 mg) and vitamin A (50 000 IU), given one and six hours before each 200 cGy fraction of radiation, which was given five times per week.[175,176] Two-hundred and seventy patients were treated from 1972 to 1977; of note, the five-year survival rates of radiotherapy-treated laryngeal cancer patients treated with ($n = 53$) or without ($n = 138$) FAR therapy were 83% and 65% respectively. Similar results were achieved in hypopharyngeal cancer, with five-year survivals of 38% with FAR and 24% without. Another Japanese group substituted etretinate for vitamin A in the FAR regimen, and achieved promising pilot-study results in 16 patients.[177]

In another pilot study, Thatcher et al reported a chemotherapeutic regimen combining natural vitamin A with doxorubicin (Adriamycin), bleomycin, 5-FU and methotrexate in 25 advanced recurrent HNSCC patients. This regimen produced an acceptable response rate of 40% (3 complete and 7 partial responses), and suggested that vitamin A may ameliorate treatment-related oral mucositis.[178] A similar pilot study using β-carotene arrived at the same conclusions.[179]

More recently, Shalinsky et al have explored the potential synergistic effect of cisplatin in combination with 9-cRA in a human oral xenograft model. Mice bearing HNSCC xenografts received 9-cRA (5 days/week) and/or cisplatin (twice weekly). The combination of the two agents synergistically inhibited tumor growth by up to 86%, without subsequently increased toxicities associated with either cisplatin or 9-cRA. Interestingly, in combination, the predominant morphological changes were those induced by 9-cRA, such as suppression of squamous cell differentiation with an increased number of basal cells, suggesting a possible basis for the enhancement of cisplatin sensitivity in tumors exposed to both agents.[180]

Future directions

Since the initial discovery by Petkovic and Giguere of the human 'orphan' retinoic acid receptors in 1987, followed by the identification of different receptor subtypes, the retinoid research domain has been greatly expanded, with particular emphasis on the development of new compounds with unique pharmacological properties.[181–183] New natural and synthetic agents, selectively binding to distinct receptor types or to 'unknown' receptors, have been generated and are undergoing clinical investigation in humans.

4-HPR, which does not bind to RXRs or RARs, has received considerable interest as a potential chemopreventive agent, and has been used in 4- and 12-month placebo-controlled studies conducted in oral premalignancy. With a 12-month follow-up, these results have confirmed a lower relapse rate in the retinoid arm (8% versus 29% for the placebo), with minimal toxicity, prompting further clinical applications for this promising agent.[144–146]

LGD 1069, currently under experimental investigation in advanced HNSCC, is a bicyclic retinoid derivative with specific RXR agonist activity, a possibly improved therapeutic index, a unique biological activity and a reduced toxicity profile.[184] Hawkins and co-workers are currently conducting a phase I study of oral LGD 1069 (Targretin) in patients with advanced solid tumors. In a preliminary report, 42 patients were treated with escalating doses from 5 to $500 \, mg/m^2$, without the occurrence of any major toxicity except an asymptomatic hypertriglyceridemia. One out of four patients with advanced HNSCC who had progressed on prior chemotherapy developed a prolonged disease stabilization with subsequent improvement of quality of life; prolonged disease stability was also observed in 3 out of 11 patients with metastatic lung cancer.[185]

Finally, two groups have recently completed encouraging phase I studies in solid tumors of 9-cRA, a pan-agonist stereoisomer of all-trans-retinoic acid that binds both RXR:RXR homodimers and RAR:RXR heterodimers. Kurie et al and Miller et al conducted phase I trials of 9-cRA in 23 and 28 patients respectively with advanced or recurrent tumors. In both trials, 9-cRA was generally well tolerated, with headaches and diarrhea as dose-limiting toxicities; other toxicities included mild myalgia, hypertriglyceridemia, hypercalcemia, facial flushing and fatigue. Pharmacokinetic studies were also conducted, and demonstrated a reduction in the peak of the 9-cRA plasma level occurring with chronic administration. No major antitumor responses were observed at the doses administered; however, preclinical data on this compound, as well as the previous results obtained with other retinoids, suggest that it should be tested further both as a single agent and also in combination with other agents.[186,187]

Retinoids have thus far demonstrated promising activity in primary and secondary interventions in head and neck cancers. Through the continuous expansion of translational investigations, allowing an increasing understanding of the mechanisms of retinoid activity along with better knowledge of the process of aerodigestive tract cancerization, physicians and scientists hope to further explore the role of retinoid chemoprevention in the neoadjuvant and adjuvant standard therapy of HNSCC.

CYTOKINE-BASED THERAPY

Over the past decade, cytokines have represented an active area of research, and they have entered the clinical arena as important effectors of the immune and hematological systems. Furthermore, through the development of new techniques, a growing list of recombinant cytokines has become available, including the interleukins (ILs), the interferons (IFNs), the colony-stimulating factors (CSFs), and tumor necrosis factors (TNF)-α and -β.

The use of IFNs as single agents or in combination with chemotherapy for HNSCC patients has been reported by several groups. In four small pilot studies conducted with human leukocyte IFN, complete and partial responses were noted in 11 out of the 35 treated patients.[188–191] The largest trial using IFN-α (high-dose versus low-dose) in HNSCC was conducted by the Eastern Cooperative Oncology Group (ECOG).[192] A total of 71 patients with recurrent or metastatic HNSCC were entered into a phase II noncomparative randomized trial of IFN-α at two dose schedules: low- and high-dose IFN-α. Median survivals of patients receiving six or more weeks of IFN-α were 10 and 12 months for low- and high-dose IFN-α respectively. Among 35

patients who received six or more weeks of therapy, high baseline natural killer (NK) activity was a significant predictor of the duration of survival both in univariate ($p = 0.04$) and multivariate ($p = 0.005$) analysis. Survival of patients with median baseline NK activity of 192 lytic units was more than 24 months versus 6–12 months for patients with median NK activity of 67. This study concluded that elevated baseline NK activity was associated with increased survival in patients receiving IFN-α for more than six weeks. The efficacy of IFN-α combined with chemotherapeutic agents has also been investigated by several groups. In a phase I/II study of combined IFN-α, cisplatin and 5-FU, Huber et al reported a 30% response rate and an encouraging median survival duration of 48 weeks in patients with recurrent HNSCC.[193] Vokes et al conducted a phase I/II study of combined IFN-α, cisplatin, 5-FU and leucovorin in 34 patients with stage III/IV HNSCC. Nineteen of the 34 patients treated at the maximum tolerated dose (cisplatin 100 mg/m², 5-FU 640 mg/m²/day × 5, leucovorin 100 mg orally and IFN-α 2 MU/m²/day) achieved a complete response.[194] More recently, the ECOG group has reported their phase II noncomparative randomized trial of recombinant IFN-α with 5-FU or cisplatin conducted in 62 patients with recurrent or metastatic HNSCC. Significant toxic effects were reported for both arms, with six treatment-related deaths related to septicemia, acute renal failure, hemorrhage and sepsis. While the IFN-α–5-FU arm was suspended owing to a low response rate (2 partial responses out 19 patients), in the IFN-α–cisplatin arm a 23.6% response rate was reported (1 complete and 8 partial responses). The median overall survivals were 5.3 and 5.4 months for the IFN-α–5-FU and the IFN-α–cisplatin arms respectively.[195] These studies have not addressed the individual contribution of IFN-α in such chemotherapy regimens; neither have they demonstrated the role of IFN-α in potentiating the effects of cytotoxic compounds such as platinum or fluorouracil. However, IFN-α appears to have important biological activity in patients with HNSCC, and several currently ongoing studies are exploring its potential impact in the treatment of HNSCC.

IL-2 has emerged in a relatively short time as a prototypical biological response modifier with a significant antitumor activity in vitro as well as in vivo against selected neoplasms.[196] IL-2 is a glycoprotein secreted predominantly by T-helper cells whose major role appears to be the activation and proliferation of T-cell subpopulations and NK cells. Additionally, through the secretion of secondary cytokines (IL-4, IL-5 and IL-6), IL-2 may induce B-cell growth, antibody production, and the release of other cytokines such as IFN-γ, granulocyte–macrophage (GM)-CSF and TNF.

Earlier studies have consistently demonstrated that patients with advanced HNSCC often present with impaired cell-mediated immunity, and that the quantitation of such deficiency (e.g. NK-cell function and count of CD8$^+$ cytotoxic lymphocytes) may provide information about survival and patterns of disease recurrence.[197–201] In vitro studies conducted in head and neck cancer have shown the potential effect of IL-2 in terms of modulation of the susceptibility to immune effector cells as well as direct growth inhibition of HNSCC tumors. Several investigators have demonstrated that the immunodeficiency of HNSCC patients may be reversed by the addition of IL-2, and, moreover, that the combination of IL-2 and IFN-α may result in lymphokine-activated killer (LAK) cell generation and increased cytotoxic effects.[202,203] Further, these results have been confirmed in vivo in a nude mice xenograft model of HNSCC in which IL-2, as well as IFN-γ and supernatant of A-NK cells, have been shown to induce control of tumor growth and regression of established tumors.[204,205] Based on these preclinical data, several investigators have evaluated the use of IL-2, administered directly into the tumor and/or into draining lymph nodes in HNSCC patients. Forni et al reported four objective responses among seven patients with inoperable recurrent HNSCC treated with low-dose natural IL-2, which was injected into the regional draining lymph nodes.[206] Subsequently, the same Italian group has reported several phase I trials of loco-regional injection of natural (n) or recombinant (r) IL-2 in

advanced recurrent HNSCC patients. Although the overall response rates varied from 13% with rIL-2 to 65% with nIL-2, the responses reported were always transient and refractory to further injection of IL-2.[207,208] Local preoperative therapy with low-dose nIL-2 was assayed by Musiani et al in four patients with advanced primary tumors, with a documented clinical and histological decrease or total disappearance of some neoplastic lesions.[209] ECOG conducted a dose-escalating phase I trial of rIL-2 in 36 untreated unresectable patients. For this study, rIL-2 was injected among the four quadrants of the tumor and bilateral upper jugular nodes, followed by standard chemotherapy or radiotherapy. Two objective responses and 21 cases of stable disease were observed.[210] This clinical study was complemented by an extensive immunological laboratory investigation which demonstrated the ability of IL-2 local therapy to activate local as well as systemic antitumor effector cells. One other trial combining perilymphatic IL-2 administration with peritumoral injection of LAK cells reported three partial and three minor responses in patients with a minimal tumor burden (<20 cm^2).

Several studies have combined systemic IL-2 with IFN-α or chemotherapy. Urba et al and Schantz et al reported on the combination of IL-2 (3 MU/m^2/day) and IFN-α (5 MU/m^2/day) administered during two four-week courses in patients with locally recurrent, metastatic or previously untreated bulky stage IV HNSCC.[211,212] Side-effects were significant, with fatigue, oliguria, hypotension and gastrointestinal distress, allowing only 12% of the patients to complete two cycles of therapy. Among 25 patients, four (16%) achieved a partial response and four (16%) had stable disease; no complete responses were seen. Although no statistically significant correlations existed, the immunological laboratory evaluation suggested a correlation between tumor response, tumor differentiation and improved lymphocyte-mediated immunity (increase in number of CD56$^+$ lymphocytes and NK cell activity).[213]

Several investigations of the feasibility and activity of regimens combining rIL-2 and conventional chemotherapy have been carried out.

Valone et al treated 12 HNSCC and 22 NSCLC patients with a $12\,MU/m^2$ five-day infusion of IL-2 in the middle of a monthly cycle of high-dose cisplatin and 5-FU. A 55% response rate, including two complete and four partial responses, was reported in the HNSCC group. Interestingly, two responding patients had failed prior therapy with cisplatin/5-FU alone.[214] Dimery et al conducted a phase I trial of cisplatin, 5-FU and escalating doses of rIL-2 (from 0.5 up to $6\,MU/m^2$ by bolus injection over four days, twice in a 28-day cycle) in 25 patients with advanced head and neck cancer. A 35% response rate (one complete and six partial responses) was observed, and the rIL-2 maximum tolerable dose in combination with cisplatin and 5-FU was determined to be $4\,MU/m^2$.[215]

Despite the acceptable tolerance, as well as the response rate reported with the combination of rIL-2 and chemotherapy, it appears difficult to evaluate the individual contribution of IL-2, since similar activities have been shown to be achieved with cisplatin and 5-FU alone. Convincing evidence has demonstrated the ability of loco-regional IL-2 therapy to activate the local and systemic immune effector cells in HNSCC patients, and has also demonstrated the feasibility and safety of such an approach. However, the clinical outcome has been disappointing, perhaps compromised by the limited time of IL-2 administration and the advanced stage of the patients treated. Future strategies for the use of IL-2 will require the selection of patients with minimal residual disease or early limited disease, as well as optimization of the modalities of IL-2 administration, eventually in combination with other biological or differentiating agents.

NEW TREATMENT STRATEGIES

As knowledge of the mechanisms of carcinogenesis continue to grow, along with advances in molecular biology, immunology and genetic engineering, the ability to consider novel strategies for tumor management is becoming a reality.

Gene therapy in head and neck cancer

The advent of polymerase chain reaction (PCR) technology has led to the discovery of oncogenes and tumor suppressor genes implicated in tumorigenesis – an important step in biotechnology. These developments have laid the conceptual and technical foundations for gene therapy, which is one of the most heralded novel therapeutic approaches to emerge in the past decade.

Gene therapy involves the introduction of novel genes into somatic cells to produce a desired therapeutic effect. The potential selectivity of the treatment is the most important expected property of the gene therapy approach. Gene transfer can be done either directly in vivo or ex vivo into explanted cells that are subsequently reimplanted to the patients via recombinant viruses or through one of several physical methods, such as transfection, lipofection or receptor-mediated delivery.[216,217] Four major strategies are currently being tested in most experimental or clinical investigations of cancer gene therapy:[218–221]

- protection of normal tissues, which are principal targets of the cytotoxic effects of both radiotherapy and chemotherapy;
- improvement of host antitumor responses either by modifying the tumor cells in order to render them more immunogenic or by increasing the antitumor activity of the immunological effectors infiltrating the tumor;
- direct killing of tumor cells by cytotoxic or drug-activating genes;
- reversal of the malignant phenotype either by downregulation of oncogene expression or by insertion of normal tumor suppressor genes.

Among these different approaches, the last two have been pursued to date in preclinical as well as clinical investigations in HNSCC. Based on the rationale of introducing 'suicide genes', O'Malley et al have performed studies using an adenovirus-mediated gene transfer of the herpes simplex virus thymidine kinase in human squamous cell cancer implanted in a nude mouse model.[222] The importance of herpes thymidine kinase gene transfer is its ability to render cells sensitive to the nucleoside analogue ganciclovir. Upon viral transduction, the thymidine kinase gene selectively kills dividing cells by converting ganciclovir into a phosphorylated compound that is critical in DNA synthesis. This property may be valuable for the treatment of rapidly growing tumors that invade normal surrounding non-proliferating tissues. However, this strategy requires further investigation, particularly because of its potential toxicity to normal dividing cells.

The second approach has mainly focused on the reintroduction of *p53* tumor suppressor gene function. Liu et al studied this approach in vitro and demonstrated that transfected wild-type *p53* may induce growth suppression of human head and neck squamous carcinoma cells.[223,224] Clayman et al demonstrated the in vivo efficacy of such an approach in a xenograft animal model with microscopic residual disease, mimicking the postsurgical environment of head and neck patients with advanced disease. In this model, the establishment of tumors was prevented by transiently introducing exogenous wild-type *p53*.[225]

The rationale underlying the use of wild-type *p53* is based on the observation that the wild type appears to be dominant over its mutant gene, preferentially affecting proliferating cells when transduced into cells containing the mutant gene. This suppression of cell growth appears to be mediated by two distinct pathways: one transient pathway in which the p53 protein exerts its cell cycle checkpoint function, and one permanent pathway with the induction of programmed cell death or apoptosis.[226–228] Furthermore, the transient overexpression of wild-type *p53* does not affect the growth of nonmalignant cells with an endogenous wild-type *p53*, thus allowing the protection of normal cells from adverse effects. Standard dose-escalation phase I trials are currently ongoing in several institutions, enrolling patients with clinical evidence of advanced local or regional disease that is unresectable, or for which no surgically negative margins will be attainable. Clayman et al recently reported

on a phase I study enrolling 33 patients who were injected intratumorally with adenoviral vector delivering the wild-type *p53* (Ad–*p53*). Interestingly, this trial showed several encouraging outcomes:

- objective antitumor activity was detected in several patients;
- the infectious Ad–*p53* in body fluids was asymptomatic.

These results suggest that systemic or regional treatment may be tolerable, and provide encouragement for further investigation of Ad–*p53* as a therapeutic agent for patients with HNSCC.[229]

An alternative approach targeting *p53* abnormal function is the use of the human adenovirus Onyx-015, which lacks the E1B genetic region, and therefore selectively replicates in and lyses tumor cells that are deficient in *p53* function. In preclinical models of cancer, this adenovirus has shown dramatic activity and is now undergoing clinical trials in refractory recurrent head and neck patients.[230,231] The preliminary results of the phase II study have shown encouraging results, with a good tolerance and an objective antitumor activity (of the 13 evaluable patients, 2 achieved partial response and 2 achieved complete response) and subjective clinical benefit.[232] However, the selective action of the Onyx-015 is currently disputed and further studies are necessary to assess the real selectivity of this approach.[233,234]

Another tumor suppressor gene, *p16*[INK4A], located at the 9p21 chromosomal locus, appears to show further promise for gene therapy. The *p16* gene is an attractive candidate because of its important function in the cell cycle as a negative regulator of the G_1–S phase transition, as well as the high frequency of its homozygous deletion in premalignant lesions and tumors of the head and neck.[52,54,235,236] Preliminary in vitro studies have shown growth suppression of human HNSCC lines, mediated by G_1 phase growth arrest. In vivo animal studies are currently underway to further assess this approach.

Another area of development is the application of topical gene constructs for the treatment of oral cancer. Several therapeutic approaches have been investigated, including the use of antisense molecules directed toward transforming papillomavirus genes as well as the transfer of a toxic phenotype to the oral mucosa. This approach appears to be very attractive, since the topical application of agents to oral mucosa is extremely simple. However, several attempts to induce topical transduction in mouse, hamster and human (ex vivo) oral epithelia have yet to be successful.

The preliminary results of gene therapy in HNSCC are encouraging. Moreover, this approach is feasible and potentially may be integrated in the setting of adjuvant multimodality therapy, targeting patients with residual disease harboring specific molecular abnormalities.

Monoclonal antibodies and receptor-based therapy in head and neck tumors

A second important achievement has been the development of recombinant technology utilizing the hybridoma technique, which requires the fusing of an immortal cell with an antibody-producing cell, yielding monoclonal antibodies (MoAbs) specifically directed at a desired tumor target. These MoAbs have found wide applications in diagnostic testing, and continue to be explored for therapeutic purpose in conjugates, such as immunotoxins, and in other new chimeric forms. Among the multiple classical applications of MoAbs in cancer therapy, a new alternative approach is to use them to block the physiological activity of a receptor by blocking the function of the receptor itself or its ligand. The growth factor receptors implicated in cell proliferation, such as the epidermal growth factor (EGF) receptor (EGFR), are an appealing target for this approach, and are currently under investigation at the Memorial Sloan-Kettering Cancer Center and the MD Anderson Cancer Center.

Premalignant lesions and tumors of the head and neck frequently harbor high expression levels of EGFR and of its ligand, transforming growth factor alpha (TGF-α).[72-75] Increased

EGFR expression has been correlated with poor clinical outcome in several malignancies.[237-240] Furthermore, increased expression of EGFR has also been observed in premalignant lesions of HNSCC, suggesting a potential role for this receptor in the carcinogenic process.[75]

Since the initial description of MoAbs against EGFR by Schlessinger et al, a large panel of MoAbs that block EGF- and TGF-α-induced stimulation of cell growth have been produced.[241,242] The blockade of the increased proliferation rate induced by exogenous EGF/TGF-α by the antireceptor MoAb has been demonstrated in tumor cell lines and in vivo against human tumor xenografts in athymic mice.[242,243] Mendelsohn and co-workers conducted a series of phase I trials with gradually increasing doses of the human chimeric MoAb C225 in patients with diverse tumor types, including head and neck cancer patients. They demonstrated that this approach is safe, feasible and potentially fruitful.[244,245] Perez-Soler et al conducted a phase I trial of the anti-EGFR murine MoAb RG83852 in patients with non-small cell lung cancer and HNSCC, examining the modulation of EGFR tyrosine kinase activity, tumor EGFR saturation and toxicity. RG83852 was well tolerated, and induced a high degree of EGFR saturation in the tumor. Post-therapy, a three- to fourfold upregulation of EGFR tyrosine kinase activity was observed in two patients, while a moderate upregulation of EGFR itself was observed in four patients.[246]

Since high EGFR expression in tumors has been associated with increased sensitivity to cytotoxic chemotherapy, the suggestion of antibody-mediated upregulation of EGFR may be useful in enhancing chemotherapeutic efficacy.[247-249] Pursuing this rationale, Perez-Soler's group has also recently reported a phase I trial combination of the humanized anti-EGFR MoAb C225 with cisplatin in recurrent head and neck cancer.[250] Although the results are still preliminary, this study appears promising. Two of the five patients treated at the first dose level have shown transient minor responses, and biologically the post-therapy samples have demonstrated a complete functional inhibition of the tumor EGFR.

These observations may suggest a potential future role for anti-EGFR MoAbs as part of a chemopreventive adjuvant strategy for premalignant lesions, perhaps eventually combined with differentiating agents and/or chemoradiotherapeutic modalities.

SUMMARY

In the past two decades, despite treatment advances, the mortality rates of HNSCC have decreased only marginally. Nevertheless, encouraging advances are being made in our understanding of tumor biology, particularly multistep and field carcinogenesis, and molecular biology. These advances in biotechnology, as well as in the understanding of the genetic regulation of cellular differentiation, the cell cycle and tumor progression, are rapidly changing the concepts of solid malignancy management. Since chemoprevention was initially conceived in the 1970s, it has become apparent that this approach is no longer speculative, demonstrating important achievements through the completion of rigorous, randomized clinical trials. However, challenges still exist in identifying the best agents, the optimal duration of intervention, and the individuals at highest risk in whom these interventions should be initiated. Potential application of monoclonal antibodies, as well as gene therapy, are just beginning to be explored: while it is premature to predict the direction of those therapies, the preliminary results appear promising.

Appropriate basic, translational and clinical research trials are necessary to further advance the exploration of novel approaches such as gene therapy, and to further define the role of retinoid chemoprevention and biochemoprevention in the realm of standard clinical practice for the management of head and neck cancer.

ACKNOWLEDGEMENTS

We are very grateful to Arianne Morgan for critical editorial review and assistance in preparing the manuscript.

REFERENCES

1. Parkin DM, Pisani P, Ferlay J, Estimates of the worldwide incidence of eighteen major cancers in 1995. *Int J Cancer* 1995; **54:** 594–606.
2. Landis SH, Murray T, Bolden S, Wingo PA, Cancer statistics, 1998. *CA Cancer J Clin* 1998; **48:** 6–29.
3. Devesa SS, Silverman DT, Young JL et al, Cancer incidence and mortality trends among whites in the United States, 1947–84. *J Natl Cancer Inst* 1987; **79:** 701–7.
4. Blot WJ, Devesa SS, McLaughlin JK, Fraumeni JF Jr, Oral and pharyngeal cancers. *Cancer Surv* 1994; **20:** 23–42.
5. Wingo PA, Tong T, Bolden S, Cancer Statistics 1995. *CA Cancer J Clin* 1995; **45:** 8–30.
6. Cvitkovic E, Neoadjuvant chemotherapy (NACT) with epirubicin (EPI), cisplatin (CDDP), bleomycin (BLEO) (BEC) in undifferentiated nasopharyngeal cancer (UCNT): preliminary results of an international (Int) phase (PH) III trial. *Proc Am Soc Clin Oncol* 1994; **14:** 283 (abst).
7. Kotwall C, Sako K, Razack MS et al, Metastatic pattern in squamous cell cancer of the head and neck. *Am J Surg* 1987; **154:** 439–42.
8. Zbären P, Lehmann W, Frequency and sites of distant metastases in head and neck squamous cell carcinoma. *Arch Otolaryngol Head Neck Surg* 1987; **113:** 762–4.
9. Vokes EE, Head and neck cancer. In: *Chemotherapy Source Book* (Perry MC, ed). Williams and Wilkins: Baltimore, 1992: 918–31.
10. Vokes EE, Weichselbaum RR, Lippman S et al, Head and neck cancer. *N Engl J Med* 1993; **328:** 184–94.
11. Vokes EE, Weichselbaum RR, Chemoradiotherapy for head and neck cancers. *Prin Prac Oncol Updates* 1993; **7:** 1–8.
12. Vikram B, Changing pattern of failure in advanced head and neck cancer. *Arch*

Otolaryngol 1984; **110**: 564–5.

13. Lippman SM, Hong WK, Second malignant tumors in head and neck squamous cell carcinoma: the overshadowing threat for patients with early-stage disease. *Int J Radiat Oncol Biol Phys* 1989; **17**: 691–4.

14. Lippman SM, Hong WK, Chemotherapy and chemoprevention. In: *Cancer of the Head and Neck*, 3rd edn (Myers EN, Suen JY, eds). WS Saunders: Philadelphia, 1995: 782–804.

15. Batsakis JG, Synchronous and metachronous carcinomas in patients with head and neck cancer. *Int J Radiat Oncol Biol Phys* 1984; **10**: 2163–4.

16. Boice ZD, Fraumeni ZF, Second cancer following cancer of the respiratory system in Connecticut, 1935–1982. *Natl Cancer Inst Monogr* 1985; **68**: 83–98.

17. Cooper JS, Pajak TF, Rubin P et al, Second malignancies in patients who have head and neck cancers. Incidence, effect on survival and implications for chemoprevention based on the RTOG experience. *Int J Radiat Oncol Biol Phys* 1989; **17**: 449–56.

18. Gluckman J, Crissman JD, Survival in 548 patients with multiple neoplasms of the upper aerodigestive tract. *Laryngoscope* 1983; **93**: 71–4.

19. Jesse RH, Sugarbaker EV, Squamous cell carcinoma of the esopharynx: why we fail. *Am J Surg* 1976; **132**: 435–8.

20. Licciardello JTW, Spitz MR, Hong WK, Multiple primary cancer in patients with cancers of the head and neck: second cancer of the head and neck, esophagus and lung. *Int J Radiat Oncol Biol Phys* 1988; **17**: 467–76.

21. Schottenfeld D, Gantt RC, Wynder EL, The role of alcohol and tobacco in multiple primary cancers of the upper digestive system, larynx and lung: a prospective study. *Prev Med* 1974; **3**: 277–93.

22. Horoligk GH, DeJong JMA, Synchronous and metachronous tumors in patients with head and neck cancers. *J Laryngol* 1983; **93**: 71–4.

23. McDonald S, Haie C, Rubin P et al, Second primary tumors of laryngeal carcinoma: diagnosis, treatment and prevention. *Int J Radiat Oncol Biol Phys* 1989; **17**: 457–65.

24. McGuirt WF, Matthews B, Koufman JA, Multiple simultaneous tumors in patients with head and neck cancer: a prospective, sequential panendoscopic study. *Cancer* 1982; **50**: 1195–9.

25. Hong WK, Multiple primary squamous cell carcinoma of the head and neck. *Am J Clin Oncol* 1987; **10**: 182–3.

26. Olsen JH, Second cancer following cancer of the respiratory system in Denmark 1943–1980. *Natl Cancer Inst Monogr* 1985; **68**: 309–12.

27. Sporn MB, Lippman SM, Chemoprevention of cancer. In: *Cancer Medicine*, 4th edn (Holland JF, Frei E, Bast RC et al, eds). Lea and Febiger: Philadelphia, 1997: 495–508.

28. Slaughter DP, Southwick HW, Smejkal W, 'Field cancerization' in oral stratified squamous epithelium: clinical implications of multicentric origin. *Cancer* 1953; **6**: 963–8.

29. Auerbach O, Stout AP, Hammond EC, Changes in bronchial epithelium in relation to cigarette smoking and in relation to lung cancer. *N Engl J Med* 1961; **265**: 253–67.

30. Lippman SM, Lee JS, Lotan R et al, Biomarkers as intermediate endpoints in chemoprevention trials. *J Natl Cancer Inst* 1990; **82**: 555–60.

31. Benner SE, Lippman SM, Wargovich MJ et al, Micronuclei, a biomarker for chemoprevention trials: results of a randomized study in oral premalignancy. *Int J Cancer* 1994; **59**: 457–9.

32. Stich HF, Micronucleated exfoliated cells as indicators for genotoxic damage and as markers in chemoprevention trials. *J Nutr Growth Cancer* 1987; **4**: 9–18.

33. Stich HF, Rosin MP, Vallejera MO, Reduction with vitamin A and beta-carotene administration of the proportion of micronucleated buccal mucosal cells in Asian betel nut and tobacco chewers. *Lancet* 1984; **i**: 1204–6.

34. Hittelman WN, Premature chromosome condensation in the diagnosis of malignancies. In: *PCC: Applications in Basic and Clinical Research* (Johnson R, Rao PN, Sperling K, eds). Academic Press: New York, 1982: 309–58.

35. Kim SY, Lee JS, Ro JY et al, Interphase cytogenetics in paraffin sections of lung tumors by non-isotopic in situ hybridization. Mapping genotype/phenotype heterogeneity. *Am J Pathol* 1993; **142**: 307–17.

36. Speicher MR, Howe C, Crotty P et al, Comparative genomic hybridization detects novel deletions and amplifications in head and neck squamous cell carcinomas. *Cancer Res* 1995; **55**: 1010–13.

37. Brzoska PM, Levin NA, Fu KK et al, Frequent novel DNA copy number increase in squamous cell head and neck tumors. *Cancer Res* 1995; **55**: 3055–9.

38. Papadimitrakopoulou VA, Shin DM, Hong WK, Molecular and cellular biomarkers for field can-

cerization and multistep process in head and neck tumorigenesis. *Cancer Metas Rev* 1996; **15:** 53–76.

39. Brennan JA, Mao L, Hruban RH et al, Molecular assessment of histopathological staging in squamous-cell carcinoma of the head and neck. *N Engl J Med* 1995; **332:** 429–35.

40. Field JK, Spandidos SA, Malliri A et al, Elevated p53 expression correlates with a history of heavy smoking in squamous cell carcinomas of the head and neck. *Br J Cancer* 1991; **64:** 573–7.

41. Maestro R, Dolcetti R, Gasparotto D et al, High frequency of p53 alterations associated with protein over-expression in human squamous-cell carcinoma of the larynx. *Oncogene* 1992; **7:** 1159–66.

42. Somers KD, Merrick MA, Lopez ME et al, Frequent p53 mutations in head and neck cancer. *Cancer Res* 1992; **52:** 5997–6000.

43. Gusterson BA, Anbazhagan R, Warren W et al, Expression of p53 in premalignant and malignant squamous epithelium. *Oncogene* 1991; **6:** 1785–9.

44. Boyle JO, Koch W, Hruban RH et al, The incidence of p53 mutations increases with progression of head and neck cancer. *Cancer Res* 1993; **53:** 4477–80.

45. El-Naggar A, Lai S, Luna MA et al, Sequential p53 mutation analysis of pre-invasive and invasive head and neck squamous cell carcinoma. *Int J Cancer* 1995; **64:** 196–201.

46. Shin DM, Kim J, Ro JY et al, Activation of p53 gene expression in premalignant lesions during head and neck tumorigenesis. *Cancer Res* 1994; **54:** 321–6.

47. Nees M, Homann N, Disher H et al, Expression of mutated p53 occurs in tumor-distant epithelia of head and neck cancer patients: a possible molecular basis for the development of multiple tumors. *Cancer Res* 1993; **53:** 4189–96.

48. Chung KY, Mukhopadhyay T, Kim J et al, Discordant p53 gene mutations in primary head and neck cancers and corresponding second primary cancers of the upper aerodigestive tract. *Cancer Res* 1993; **53:** 1676–83.

49. Zariwala M, Schmid S, Pfaltz M et al, p53 mutations in oropharyngeal carcinomas: a comparison of solitary and multiple primary tumors and lymph-node metastases. *Int J Cancer* 1994; **56:** 807–11.

50. Gasparotto D, Maestro R, Barzan L et al, Recurrences and second primary tumors in the head and neck region: differentiation by p53 mutation analysis. *Ann Oncol* 1995; **6:** 933–9.

51. Shin DM, Lee JS, Lippman SM et al, p53 expression: predicting recurrence and second primary tumors in head and neck squamous cell carcinoma. *J Natl Cancer Inst* 1996; **88:** 519–29.

52. Van der Riet P, Nawroz H, Hruban RH et al, Frequent loss of chromosome 9p21–22 early in head and neck cancer progression. *Cancer Res* 1994; **54:** 1156–8.

53. Nawroz H, van der Riet P, Hruban RH et al, Allelotype of head and neck squamous cell carcinoma. *Cancer Res* 1994; **54:** 1152–5.

54. Mao L, Lee JS, Fan YH et al, Frequent microsatellite alterations at chromosome 9p21 and 3p14 in oral premalignant lesions and their value in cancer risk assessment. *Nature Med* 1996; **2:** 682–5.

55. Roz L, Wu CL, Porter S et al, Allelic imbalance on chromosome 3p in oral dysplastic lesions: an early event in oral carcinogenesis. *Cancer Res* 1996; **56:** 1228–31.

56. Latif F, Fivosh M, Glenn G et al, Chromosome 3p deletions in head and neck carcinomas: statistical ascertainment of allelic losses. *Cancer Res* 1992; **52:** 1451–6.

57. Maestro R, Gasparotto D, Vuksavljevic T et al, Three discrete regions of deletions in head and neck cancers. *Cancer Res* 1993; **53:** 5775–9.

58. El-Naggar AK, Lee MS, Wang G et al, Polymerase chain reaction-based restriction fragment length polymorphism analysis of the short arm of chromosome 3 in primary head and neck squamous carcinomas. *Cancer* 1993; **72:** 881–6.

59. Lippman SM, Batsakis JG, Toth BB et al, Comparison of low-dose 13cRA with beta carotene to prevent oral carcinogenesis. *N Engl J Med* 1993; **328:** 15s–19s.

60. Califano J, van der Riet P, Westra W et al, Genetic progression model for head and neck cancer: implications for field cancerization, *Cancer Res* 1996; **56:** 2488–92.

61. Bedi GC, Westra WH, Gabrielson E et al, Multiple head and neck tumors: evidence for a common clonal origin. *Cancer Res* 1996; **56:** 2484–7.

62. Auerbach O, Stout AP, Hammond EC et al, Changes in bronchial epithelium in relation to cigarette smoking and in relation to lung cancer. *N Engl J Med* 1961; **265:** 253–67.

63. Farber E. The multistep nature of cancer development. *Cancer Res* 1984; **44:** 4217–23.

64. Vogelstein B, Fearon ER, Hamilton SR, Genetic

alterations during colorectal tumoral development. *N Engl J Med* 1988; **319:** 525–32.

65. Boone C, Kelloff GJ, Steele VE, Natural history of intraepithelial neoplasia in humans with implications for cancer chemoprevention strategy. *Cancer Res* 1992; **52:** 1651–9.

66. Einhorn J, Wersall J, Incidence of oral carcinoma in patients with leukoplakia of the oral mucosa. *Cancer* 1967; **20:** 2189–93.

67. Mashberg AL, Erythroplasia vs leukoplakia in the diagnosis of early asymptomatic oral squamous carcinoma. *N Engl J Med* 1977; **297:** 109–10.

68. Sklar G, Oral leukoplakia. *N Engl J Med* 1986; **315:** 1544–6.

69. Silverman S Jr, Gorsky M, Lozada F, Oral leukoplakia and malignant transformation: a follow-up study of 257 patients. *Cancer* 1984; **53:** 563–8.

70. Simoneau AR, Mikkelsen T, Schwechheimer K et al, Bladder cancer: the molecular progression to invasive disease. *World J Urol* 1994; **12:** 89–95.

71. Boland CR, Sato J, Appelman HD et al, Microallelotyping defines the sequence and tempo of allelic losses at tumor suppressor gene loci during colorectal cancer progression. *Nature Med* 1995; **1:** 902–9.

72. Eisbruch A, Blick M, Lee JS et al, Analysis of epidermal growth factor receptor gene in fresh human head and neck tumors. *Cancer Res* 1987; **47:** 3603–5.

73. Santini J, Formento JL, Francoval M et al, Characterization, quantitation and potential clinical value of the epidermal growth factor receptor in head and neck squamous cell carcinomas. *Head Neck* 1991; **13:** 132–9.

74. Grandis JR, Tweardy DJ, Elevated levels of transforming growth factor alpha and epidermal growth factor receptor messanger RNA are early markers of carcinogenesis in head and neck cancer. *Cancer Res* 1993; **53:** 3579–84.

75. Shin DM, Ro YJ, Hong WK et al, Dysregulation of epidermal growth factor receptor expression in premalignant lesions during head and neck tumorigenesis. *Cancer Res* 1994; **54:** 3153–9.

76. Izzo J, Papadimitrakopoulou VA, Li XQ et al, Dysregulated cyclin D1 expression early in head and neck tumorigenesis: in vivo evidence for an association with subsequent gene amplification. *Oncogene* 1998; **17:** 2313–22.

77. Arber N, Lightdale C, Rotterdam H et al, Increased expression of the cyclin D1 gene in Barrett's esophagus. *Cancer Epidemiol Biomarkers Prev* 1996; **5:** 457–9.

78. Shin DM, Voravud N, Ro YJ et al, Sequential upregulation of proliferating cell nuclear antigen in head and neck tumorigenesis: a potential biomarker. *J Natl Cancer Inst* 1993; **85:** 971–8.

79. Huang WY, Coltrera M, Schubert M et al, Histopathologic evaluation of proliferating cell nuclear antigen (PCNA) in oral epithelial hyperplasias and premalignant lesions. *Oral Surg Oral Med Oral Pathol* 1994; **78:** 748–54.

80. Girod SC, Pape HD, Krueger GR, *p53* and PCNA expression in carcinogenesis of the oropharyngeal mucosa. *Eur J Cancer B Oral Oncol* 1994; **30b:** 419–23.

81. Shin DM, Ro YJ, Shah T et al, *p53* expression and genetic instability in head and neck multistep tumorigenesis. *Proc Am Assoc Cancer Res* 1994; **35:** 944 (abst).

82. Lee JS, Kim SY, Hong WK et al, Detection of chromosomal polysomy in oral eukoplakia, a premalignant lesion. *J Natl Cancer Inst* 1993; **85:** 1951–4.

83. Voravud N, Shin DM, Ro YJ et al, Increased polysomies of chromosomes 7 and 17 during head and neck multistage tumorigenesis. *Cancer Res* 1993; **53:** 2874–83.

84. Schatzin A, Freedman LS, Schiffman MN et al, Validation of intermediate endpoint in cancer research. *J Natl Cancer Inst* 1990; **82:** 1746–52.

85. Stockman MS, Gupta PK, Pressman NJ et al, Considerations in bringing a cancer biomarker to clinical application. *Cancer Res* 1992; **52**(Suppl): 2711–18.

86. Lippman SM, Lee JS, Lotan R et al, Biomarkers as intermediate endpoints in chemoprevention trials. *J Natl Cancer Inst* 1990; **82:** 555–60.

87. Shin DM, Hittelman WN, Hong WK, Biomarkers in upper aerodigestive tract tumorigenesis. *Cancer Epidemiol Biomarkers Prev* 1994; **3:** 697–709.

85. Hsu TC, Cherry LM, Samaan NA, Differential mutagen susceptibility in cultured lymphocytes of normal individuals and cancer patients. *Cancer Genet Cytogenet* 1985; **17:** 307–13.

86. Hagmar L, Brogger A, Hansteen IL et al, Cancer risk in humans predicted by increased levels of chromosomal aberrations in lymphocytes: Nordic study group on the health risk of chromosome damage. *Cancer Res* 1994; **54:** 2919–22.

87. Spitz MR, Fueger JJ, Beddingfield NA et al, Chromosome sensitivity to bleomycin-induced mutagenesis, an independent risk factor for

upper aerodigestive tract cancers. *Cancer Res* 1989; **49:** 4626–8.

88. Spitz MR, Hoque A, Hong WK et al, Mutagen sensitivity as a risk factor for second malignant tumors following upper aerodigestive tract malignacies. *J Natl Cancer Inst* 1994; **86:** 1681–4.

89. Dave BH, Hsu TC, Hong WK et al, Nonrandom distribution of mutagen-induced chromosome breaks in lymphocytes of patients with different malignancies. *Int J Oncol* 1994; **5:** 733–40.

90. Cloos J, Spitz MR, Schantz SP et al, Genetic susceptibility to head and neck squamous cell carcinoma. *J Natl Cancer Inst* 1996; **88:** 530–5.

91. Wei Q, Spitz MR, Gu J et al, DNA repair capacity correlates with mutagen sensitivity in lymphoblastoid cell lines. *Cancer Epidemiol Biomarkers Prev* 1996; **5:** 199–204.

92. Gadzar AF, Molecular changes preceding the onset of invasive lung cancers. *Lung Cancer* 1994; **11:** 16–17.

93. Lippman SM, Kessler JF, Meyskens FL, Retinoids as preventive and therapeutic anticancer agents (Part I). *Cancer Treat Rep* 1987; **71:** 391–405.

94. Smith MA, Parkinson DR, Cheson BD et al, Retinoids in cancer therapy. *J Clin Oncol* 1992; **10:** 839–64.

95. Jetten AM, Multistep process of squamous differentiation of tracheobronchial epithelial cells: role of retinoids. *Dermatologica* 1987; **175:** 37–44.

96. Lippman SM, Kessler JF, Meyskens F Jr et al, Retinoids as preventive and therapeutic anticancer agents. Parts I and II. *Cancer Treat Rep* 1987; **71:** 391–405 and 493–515.

97. Moon RC, Mehta RG, Retinoid inhibition of experimental carcinogenesis. In: *Chemistry and Biology of Synthetic Retinoids* (Dawson MI, Okamura WH, eds). CRC Press: Boca Raton, FL, 1990: 501–19.

98. Lippman SM, Heyman RA, Kurie JM et al, Retinoids and chemoprevention: clinical and basic studies. *J Cell Biochem* 1995; **22** (Suppl): 1–10.

99. Harris CC, Kaufman DG, Sporn MB et al, Histogenesis of squamous metaplasia and squamous cell carcinoma of the respiratory epithelium in an animal model. *Cancer Chemother Rep* 1973; **2**(3): 43–54.

100. Mehta RG, Rao KVN, Detrisac CJ et al, Inhibition of diethylnitrosamine-induced lung carcinogenesis by retinoids. *Proc Am Assoc Cancer Res* 1988; **29:** 129 (abst).

101. Klein-Szanto AJ, Ruggeri B, Bianchi A et al, Cellular and molecular changes during mouse skin tumor progression. *Rec Res Cancer Res* 1993; **128:** 193–204.

102. Shklar G, Marefat P, Korhauser A et al, Retinoid inhibition of lingual carcinogenesis. *Oral Surg Oral Med Oral Pathol* 1980; **49:** 325–32.

103. Shklar G, Schwartz J, Grau D et al, Inhibition of hamster buccal pouch carcinogenesis by 13-*cis*-retinoic acid. *Oral Surg* 1980; **50:** 45–52.

104. Goodwin WJ, Bordash GD, Huijing F et al, Inhibition of hamster tongue carcinogenesis by selenium and retinoic acid. *Ann Otol Rhinol Laryngol* 1986; **95:** 162–6.

105. Huang CC, Effects of retinoids on the growth of squamous cell carcinoma of the palate in rats. *Am J Otolaryngol* 1987; **7:** 55–7.

106. Slaga TJ, Gimenez-Conti IB, An animal model for oral cancer. *Natl Cancer Inst Monogr* 1992; **13:** 55–60.

107. Leroy P, Krust A, Kastner P et al, Retinoic acid receptors. In: *Retinoids in Normal Development and Teratogenesis* (Morriss-Kay G, ed). Oxford University Press: New York, 1992: 7–25.

108. Amos B, Lotan R, Retinoid sensitive cells and cell lines. *Meth Enzymol* 1991; **190:** 217–25.

109. Lotan R, Clifford JL, Nuclear receptors for retinoids: mediators of retinoids effects on normal and malignant cells. *Biomed Pharmacother* 1990; **45:** 145–56.

110. Gudas LJ, Sporn MB, Roberts AB, Cellular biology and biochemistry of the retinoids. In: *The Retinoids* (Sporn MB, Roberts AB, Goodman DS, eds). Raven Press: New York, 1994: 443–520.

111. Hong WK, Lippman SC, Hittelman WN et al, Retinoid chemoprevention of aerodigestive cancer: from basic research to the clinic. *Clin Cancer Res* 1995; **1:** 667–86.

112. Delia D, Aiello A, Lombardi L et al, *N*-(4-hydroxyphenyl)retinamide induces apoptosis of malignant hematopoietic cell lines including those unresponsive to retinoic acid. *Cancer Res* 1993; **53:** 6036–41.

113. Davies PJ, Stein JP, Chiocca EA et al, Retinoid-regulated expression of transglutaminases: links to the biochemistry of programmed cell death. In: *Retinoids in Normal Development and Teratogenesis* (Morriss-Kay G, ed). Oxford University Press: New York, 1992: 249–63.

114. Roberts AB, Sporn MD, Mechanistic interrelationships between two superfamilies: the steroid/retinoid receptors and transforming growth factor-β. *Cancer Surv* 1992; **14:** 204–20.

115. Lotan R, Retinoids and squamous differentia-

tion. In: *Retinoids in Oncology* (Hong WK, Lotan R, eds). Marcel Dekker: New York, 1993: 43–72.

116. Thiele C, Deutsch LA, Israel MA, The expression of multiple protooncogenes is differentially regulated during retinoic acid induced maturation of human neuroblastoma cell line. *Oncogene* 1988; **3**: 281–8.

117. Bertram JS, Role of gap junctional cell/cell communication in the control of proliferation and neoplastic transformation. *Radiat Res* 1990; **123**: 252–6.

118. Huang M, Ye Y, Chen S, Use of all-*trans*-retinoic acid in the treatment of acute promyelocytic leukemia. *Blood* 1988; **72**: 567–72.

119. Mangelsdorf DJ, Umesono K, Evans RM, The retinoid receptors. In: *The Retinoids* (Sporn MB, Roberts AB, Goodman DS, eds). Raven Press: New York, 1994: 319–49.

120. DeLuca LM, Retinoids and their receptors in differentiation, embryogenesis and neoplasia. *FASEB J* 1991; **5**: 2924–33.

121. Chambon P, The retinoid signalling pathway: molecular and genetic analyses. *Semin Cell Biol* 1994; **5**: 115–25.

122. Pfahl M, Vertebrate receptors: molecular biology, dimerization and response elements. *Semin Cell Biol* 1994; **5**: 95–103.

123. Heyman RA, Mangelsdorf DJ, Dyck JA et al, 9-*cis*-retinoic acid is a high affinity ligand for the retinoid X receptor. *Cell* 1992; **68**: 397–406.

124. Levin AA, Sturzenbecker LJ, Kazmer S et al, 9-*cis* retinoic acid stereoisomer binds and activates the nuclear receptor of RXRα. *Nature* 1992; **355**: 359–61.

125. Gebert JF, Moghal N, Frangioni JV et al, High frequency of retinoic acid receptor beta abnormalities in human lung cancer. *Oncogene* 1991; **6**: 1859–68.

126. Hu L, Crowe DL, Rheinwald JG et al, Abnormal expression of retinoic acid receptors and keratin 19 by human oral and epidermal squamous cell carcinoma cell lines. *Cancer Res* 1991; **51**: 3972–81.

127. Xu XC, Ro YJ, Lee JS et al, Differential expression of nuclear retinoic acid receptors in normal, premalignant and malignant head and neck tissues. *Cancer Res* 1994; **54**: 3580–7.

128. Lotan R, Xu XC, Lippman SM et al, Suppression of retinoic acid receptor β in premalignant oral lesions and its upregulation by isotretinoin. *N Engl J Med* 1995; **332**: 1405–10.

129. Maxwell SA, Mukhopadhyay T, Transient stabilization of p53 in non-small cell lung carcinoma

cultures arrested for growth by retinoic acid. *Exp Cell Res* 1994; **214**: 67–74.

130. Lippman SM, Shin DM, Lee JS et al, p53 and retinoid chemoprevention in oral carcinogenesis. *Cancer Res* 1993; **53**: 4817–22.

131. Clayman GL, El-Naggar AK, Roth JA et al, In vivo therapy with p53 adenovirus for microscopic residual head and neck squamous carcinoma. *Cancer Res* 1995; **55**: 1–6.

132. WHO Collaborating Center for Oral Precancerous lesions, Definition of leukoplakia and related lesions: an aid to studies on precancer. *Oral Surg Oral Med Oral Pathol* 1978; **46**: 517–39.

133. Silverman S, Shillitoe EJ, Etiology and predisposing factors. In: *Oral Cancer* (Silverman S, ed). American Cancer Society: Atlanta, GA, 1988: 7–39.

134. Stich HF, Rosin MP, Hornby AP, Remission of oral leukoplakias and micronuclei in tobacco/betel quid chewers treated with beta-carotene and vitamin A. *Int J Cancer* 1988; **42**: 195–9.

135. Garewal HS, Meyskens FL, Kilen D et al, Response of oral leukoplakia to beta-carotene. *J Clin Oncol* 1990; **8**: 1715–20.

136. Malaker K, Anderson BJ, Beecroft WA et al, Management of oral mucosal dysplasia with β-carotene retinoic acid: a pilot cross-over study. *Cancer Detect Prev* 1991; **15**: 335–40.

137. Toma S, Coialbu T, Collecchi P et al, Treatment of oral leukoplakia with beta-carotene. *Oncology* 1992; **42**: 77–81.

138. Benner SE, Winn RJ, Lippman SM et al, Regression of oral leukoplakia with α-tocopherol: a Community Clinical Oncology Program (CCOP) chemoprevention study. *J Natl Cancer Inst* 1993; **85**: 44–7.

139. Hong WK, Endicott J, Itri LM, 13-*cis*-Retinoic acid in the treatment of oral leukoplakia. *N Engl J Med* 1986; **315**: 1501–5.

140. Papadimitrakopoulou V, Lippman SM, Lee JS et al, Long term follow-up of low-dose isotretinoin (13cRA) versus beta-carotene to prevent oral carcinogenesis. *Proc Am Soc Clin Oncol* 1996; **15**: 340 (abst).

141. The Alpha-Tocopherol, Beta-Carotene Prevention Study Group, The effect of vitamin E and beta-carotene on the incidence of lung cancer and other cancers in male smokers. *N Engl J Med* 1994; **330**: 1029–35.

142. Omenn GS, Goodman GE, Thornquist MD et al, Effects of beta-carotene and vitamin A on lung

cancer. *N Engl J Med* 1996; **334**: 1150.

143. Stich HF, Hornby AP, Mathew B et al, Response of oral leukoplakias to the administration of vitamin A. *Cancer Lett* 1988; **40**: 93–101.

144. Han J, Jiao L, Lu L et al, Evaluation of *N*-4(hydroxycarbophenyl)retinamide as a cancer prevention agent and as a cancer chemotherapeutic agent. *In Vivo* 1990; **4**: 153–60.

145. Chiesa F, Tradati N, Marazza M et al, 4HPR in chemoprevention of oral leukoplakia. *J Cell Biochem Suppl* 1993; **17F**: 255–61.

146. Costa A, Formelli F, Chiesa F et al, Prospects of chemoprevention of human cancers with the synthetic retinoid fenretinamide. *Cancer Res* 1994; **54**: 2032s–7s.

147. Lippman SM, Hong WK, Not yet standard: retinoids versus second primary tumors. *J Clin Oncol* 1993; **11**: 1204–7.

148. Tepperman BS, Fitzpatrick PJ, Second respiratory and upper digestive tract cancers after oral cancer. *Lancet* 1981; **ii**: 547–9.

149. Dan GL, Blot WJ, Shore RE et al, Second cancers following oral and pharyngeal cancers: role of tobacco and alcohol. *J Natl Cancer Inst* 1994; **86**: 131–7.

150. Hong WK, Lippman SM, Itri LM et al, Prevention of secondary primary tumors with isotretinoin in squamous-cell carcinoma of the head and neck. *N Engl J Med* 1990; **323**: 795–801.

151. Benner SE, Pajak TF, Stetz J et al, Toxicity of isotretinoin in a chemoprevention trial to prevent second primary tumors following head and neck cancer. *J Natl Cancer Inst* 1994; **86**: 1799–801.

152. Benner SE, Pajak TF, Lippman SM et al, Prevention of second primary tumors with isotretinoin in squamous cell carcinoma of the head and neck: long term follow-up. *J Natl Cancer Inst* 1994; **86**: 140–1.

153. Warren S, Gates O, Multiple primary malignant tumors: a survey of the literature and statistical study. *Am J Cancer* 1932; **51**: 1358–403.

154. Bolla M, Lefur R, Ton Van J et al, Prevention of second primary tumors with etretinate in squamous cell carcinoma of the oral cavity and oropharynx. Results of a multicentric double-blind randomized study. *Eur J Cancer* 1994; **30A**: 767–72.

155. Tangrea JA, Edwards BK, Taylor PR et al, Long term therapy with low-dose isotretinoin for prevention of basal cell carcinoma: a multicenter clinical trial. *J Natl Cancer Inst* 1992; **84**: 328–32.

156. Mayne ST, Tongzhang Z, Janerich DT et al, A population based trial of β-carotene chemoprevention of the head and neck. *Oncology* 1992; **6**: 61–6.

157. Pastorino U, Ifante M, Maioli M et al, Adjuvant treatment of stage I lung cancer with high-dose vitamin A. *J Clin Oncol* 1993; **11**: 1216–22.

158. van Zanwijk N, *N*-Acetylcystein (NAC) in chemoprevention. In: *Chemoimmuno Prevention of Cancer* (Pastorino U, Hong WK, eds). Thieme Medical Publishers: New York, 1991: 147–59.

159. Marth C, Daxenbichler G, Dapunt O, Synergistic antiproliferative effect of human recombinant interferons and retinoic acid in cultured breast cancer cells. *J Natl Cancer Inst* 1986; **77**: 1197–202.

160. Marth C, Kirchebner P, Daxenbichler G, The role of polyamines in interferon and retinoic acid mediated synergistic antiproliferative action. *Cancer Lett* 1989; **44**: 55–9.

161. Hemmi H, Breitman TR, Combination human interferon and retinoic acid synergistically induced differentiation of the human promyelocytic leukemia cell line HL60. *Blood* 1987; **69**: 501–7.

162. Wadler S, Schwartz EL, Antineoplastic activity of the combination of interferon and cytotoxic agents against experimental and human malignancies: a review. *Cancer Res* 1990; **50**: 3473–86.

163. Peck R, Bollag W, Potentiation of retinoid-induced differentiation of HL-60 and U937 cell lines by cytokines. *Eur J Cancer* 1991; **27**: 53–7.

164. Frey JR, Peck R, Bollag W, Antiproliferative activity of retinoids, interferon-α and combination in five human transformed cell lines. *Cancer Lett* 1991; **57**: 223–7.

165. Lippman SM, Kavanagh JJ, Paredees-Espinoza M et al, 13-cRA plus interferon α-2a: highly active systemic therapy for squamous cell carcinoma of the cervix. *J Natl Cancer Inst* 1992; **84**: 241–6.

166. Lippman SM, Parkinson DR, Itri LM et al, 13-*cis*-retinoic acid and interferon α-2a: effective combination therapy for advanced squamous cell carcinoma of the skin. *J Natl Cancer Inst* 1992; **84**: 235–41.

167. Lippman SM, Donovan DT, Frankenthaler RA et al, 13-*cis*-retinoic acid and interferon α-2a in recurrent respiratory papillomatosis. *J Natl Cancer Inst* 1992; **84**: 859–61.

168. Healy GB, Gelber RD, Trowbridge AL et al, Treatment of recurrent respiratory papillomatosis with human leucocyte interferon. Results of a multicenter randomized clinical trial. *N Engl J*

Med 1988; **319**: 401–47.

169. Toma S, Palumbo R, Gustavino C et al, Efficacy of the association of 13-*cis*-retinoic acid (13cRA) and interferon α2a (IFN α2a) in cervical intraepithelial neoplasia (CIN II-III): a pilot study. *Proc Am Soc Clin Oncol* 1994; **13**: 258 (abst).

170. Voravud N, Lippman SM, Weber RS et al, Phase II trial of 13-*cis*-retinoic acid plus interferon-α in recurrent head and neck cancer. *Invest New Drugs* 1993; **11**: 57–60.

171. Toma S, Palumbo R, Vincenti M et al, Efficacy of recombinant alpha-interferon 2a and 13-*cis*-retinoic acid in the treatment of squamous cell carcinoma. *Ann Oncol* 1994; **5**: 463–5.

172. Besa EC, Abraham JL, Bartholomew MJ et al, Treatment with 13-*cis*-retinoic acid in transfusion-dependent patients with myelodysplastic syndrome and decreased toxicity with addition of alpha-tocopherol. *Am J Med* 1990; **89**: 739–47.

173. Dimery I, Shirinian M, Heyne K et al, Reduction in toxicity of high dose 13-*cis*-retinoic acid (13-cRA) with alpha-tocopherol (AT). *Proc Am Soc Clin Oncol* 1992; **11**: 145 (abst).

174. Sacks PJ, Harris D, Chou TC, Modulation of growth and proliferation in squamous cell carcinoma by retinoic acid: a rationale for combination chemotherapy with chemotherapeutic agents. *Int J Cancer* 1995; **61**: 1–7.

175. Takaku F, Clinical trials and cancer risk in Japan. *J Natl Cancer Inst* 1984; **73**: 1483–5.

176. Komiyama S, Kudoh S, Yanagita T et al, Synergistic combination therapy of 5-fluorouracil, vitamin A and cobalt-60 radiation for head and neck tumors: antitumor combination therapy with vitamin A. *Auris Nasus Larynx* 1985; **12**: 5239–43.

177. Edamatsu H, Chikuda K, Hasegawa M, Vitamin A: disorder of otorhinolaryngology. *Otorhinolaryngology* 1982; **54**: 941–3.

178. Thatcher N, Blackledge G, Crowther D, Advanced recurrent squamous cell carcinoma of the head and neck. Results of a chemotherapeutic regimen with Adriamycin, bleomycin, 5-fluorouracil, methotrexate, and vitamin A. *Cancer* 1980; **46**: 1324–8.

179. Millis EED, The modifying effect of beta-carotene on radiation and chemotherapy induced oral mucositis. *Br J Cancer* 1988; **57**: 416–17.

180. Shalinsky DR, Bischoff ED, Gregory ML, Enhanced antitumor efficacy of cisplatin in combination with ALRT 1057 (9-*cis* retinoic acid) in human oral squamous carcinoma xenografts in nude mice. *Clin Cancer Res* 1996; **2**: 511–20.

181. Petkovic M, Brand NJ, Krust A et al, A human retinoic acid receptor which belongs to the family of nuclear receptors. *Nature* 1987; **330**: 444–50.

182. Giguere V, Ong ES, Segui P et al, Identification of a receptor for the morphogen retinoic acid. *Nature* 1987; **330**: 624–9.

183. Brand N, Petkovic M, Krust A et al, Identification of a second human retinoic acid receptor. *Nature* 1988; **332**: 850–3.

184. Boehm M, McClurg M, Pathirana C et al, Synthesis of high specific activity [^{3}H]-9-*cis*-retinoic acid and application for identifying retinoids with unusual binding properties. *J Med Chem* 1994; **37**: 2930–41.

185. Rizvi NA, Marschall JL, Loewen GR et al, A phase I study of Targretin, an RXR-selective retinoid agonist. *Proc Am Assoc Cancer Res* 1996; **37**: 1135 (abst).

186. Kurie JM, Lee JS, Griffin T et al, Phase I trial of 9-*cis* retinoic acid in adults with solid tumors. *Clin Cancer Res* 1996; **2**: 287–93.

187. Miller VA, Rigas JR, Benedetti FM, Initial clinical trial of the retinoid receptor pan agonist 9-*cis* retinoic acid. *Clin Cancer Res* 1996; **2**: 471–5.

188. Healy GB, Gelber RD, Trowbridge AL et al, Treatment of recurrent respiratory papillomatosis with human leukocyte interferon. Results of a multicenter randomized clinical trial. *N Engl J Med* 1988; **319**: 401–7.

189. Fierro R, Johnson J, Myers E et al, Phase II trial of non-recombinant interferon alpha (IFN) in recurrent squamous cell carcinomas of the head and neck (SCCHN). *Proc Am Soc Clin Oncol* 1988; **7**: 156 (abst).

190. Argarwala S, Vlock D, Johnson J et al, Phase II of interferon alpha (IFN-α) in locally recurrent or metastatic head and neck cancer. Results of ECOG trial. *Proc Am Soc Clin Oncol* 1991; **10**: 205 (abst).

191. Ikic D, Padovan I, Pipic N et al, Interferon therapy for basal cell carcinoma and squamous cell carcinoma. *Int J Clin Pharmacol Ther Toxicol* 1991; **29**: 342–6.

192. Vlock D, Anderson J, Whiteside T et al, Immunologic correlated in patients with head and neck cancer treated with interferon alpha: association between natural killer cell activity and prolonged survival. *Proc Am Soc Clin Oncol* 1994; **13**: 280 (abst).

193. Huber MH, Shirinian M, Lippman SM et al, Phase I/II study of cisplatin, 5-fluorouracil and α-interferon for recurrent carcinoma of the head and neck. *Invest New Drugs* 1994; **12**: 223–9.

194. Vokes EE, Ratain MJ, Mick R et al, Cisplatin, fluorouracil and leucovorin augmented by interferon alpha-2b in head and neck cancer: a clinical and pharmacologic analysis. *J Clin Oncol* 1993; **11**: 360–8.

195. Vlock D, Leong T, Wonson W et al, Phase II trial of interferon alpha (IFN) and chemotherapy in locally recurrent or metastatic head and neck cancer (SCCHN). *Proc Am Soc Clin Oncol* 1995; **14**: 303 (abst).

196. Lotze MT, Interleukin-2: basic principles. In: *Biologic Therapy of Cancer*, 2nd edn (De Vita VT Jr, Hellman S, Rosenberg SA, eds). JB Lippincott: Philadelphia, 1995: 207–34.

197. Wanebo HJ, Jun MY, Strong EW et al, T-cell deficiency in patients with squamous cell cancer of the head and neck. *Am J Surg* 1975; **130**: 445–51.

198. Berlinger NT, Hilal EY, Oettgen H, Deficient cell-mediated immunity in head and neck cancer patients secondary to autologous suppressive immune cells. *Laryngoscope* 1978; **88**: 470–81.

199. Schantz SP, Ordonez NG, Quantitation of natural killer cell function and risk of metastatic poorly differentiated head and neck cancer. *Nat Immun Cell Growth Regul* 1991; **10**: 278–88.

200. Schantz SP, Brown BW, Lira E et al, Evidence for the role of natural immunity in the control of metastatic spread of head and neck cancer. *Cancer Immunol Immunother* 1987; **25**: 141–8.

201. Wolf GT, Schmaltz S, Hudson J et al, Alterations in T-lymphocytes subpopulations in patients with head and neck cancer. *Arch Otolaryngol Head Neck Surg* 1987; **113**: 1200–6.

202. Wanebo HJ, Jones T, Pace R et al, Immune restoration with interleukin-2 in patients with squamous cell carcinoma of the head and neck. *Am J Surg* 1989; **158**: 356–60.

203. Wang MB, Lichtenstein A, Michel RA, Hierarchical immunosuppression of regional lymph nodes in patients with head and neck squamous cell carcinoma. *Arch Otolaryngol Head Neck Surg* 1991; **105**: 517–27.

204. Sacchi M, Snyderman CH, Heo DS et al, Local adoptive immunotherapy of human head and neck cancer xenograft in nude mice with lymphokine-activated killer cells and interleukin 2. *Cancer Res* 1990; **50**: 3113–18.

205. Sacchi M, Kaplan I, Johnson JT et al, Antiproliferative effects of cytokines on squamous cell carcinoma. *Arch Otolaryngol Head Neck Surg* 1991; **177**: 321–6.

206. Forni G, Cavallo GP, Giovarelli M et al, Tumor immunotherapy by local injection of interleukin 2 and non-reactive lymphocytes. *Prog Exp Tumor Res* 1988; **32**: 187–212.

207. Cortesina G, De Stefani A, Giovarelli M et al, Treatment of recurrent squamous cell carcinoma of the head and neck with low-dose of interleukin 2 (IL-2) injected perilymphatically. *Cancer* 1988; **62**: 2482–7.

208. Cortesina G, De Stefani A, Galeazzi E et al, Interleukin-2 injected around tumor-draining lymph nodes in head and neck cancer. *Head Neck* 1991; **13**: 125–31.

209. Musiani P, De Campora P, Valitutti S et al, Effect of low-doses of interleukin-2 injected perilymphatically and perotumorally in patients with advanced primary head and neck squamous cell carcinoma. *J Biol Response Mod* 1989; **8**: 571–8.

210. Whiteside TL, Letessier E, Hirabayashi H et al, Evidence for local and systemic activation of immune cells by peritumoral injections of interleukin 2 in patients with advanced squamous cell carcinoma of the head and neck. *Cancer Res* 1993; **53**: 5654–62.

211. Urba S, Forastiere A, Wolf G et al, Intensive recombinant interleukin-2 and alpha-interferon therapy in patients with advanced head and neck squamous carcinoma. *Cancer* 1993; **71**: 2326–31.

212. Schantz SP, Dimery I, Lippman SM et al, A phase II study of interleukin-2 and interferon-alpha in head and neck cancer. *Invest New Drugs* 1992; **10**: 217–23.

213. Schantz SP, Clayman G, Racz T et al, The in vivo biologic effect of interleukin 2 and interferon alpha on natural immunity in patients with head and neck cancer. *Arch Otolaryngol Head Neck Surg* 1990; **116**: 1302–8.

214. Valone FH, Gandara DR, Deisseroth AB et al, Interleukin-2, cisplatin, and 5-fluorouracil for patients with non-small cell lung cancer and head/neck carcinoma. *J Immunother* 1991; **10**: 207–13.

215. Dimery I, Martin T, Bradley E et al, Phase I trial of interleukin-2 (rIL-2) plus cisplatin (CDDP) and 5-fluorouracil (5-FU) in recurrent or advanced squamous cell carcinoma of the head and neck. *Proc Am Soc Clin Oncol* 1989; **8**: 170 (abst 660).

216. Morgan RA, Anderson WF, Human gene therapy. *Annu Rev Biochem* 1993; **62**: 191–217.

217. Vile R, Russel S, Gene therapy technologies for the gene therapy of cancer. *Gene Ther* 1994; **1**: 88–98.

218. Tepper RI, Mule JJ, Experimental and clinical studies of cytokines modified tumor cells. *Hum Gene Ther* 1994; **5**: 153–64.

219. Pardoll DM, Cancer vaccines. *Immunol Today* 1993; **14**: 310–16.

220. Rosenberg SA, The immunotherapy and gene therapy of cancer. *J Clin Oncol* 1992; **10**: 180–99.

221. Russel SJ, Lymphokines gene therapy for cancer. *Immunol Today* 1990; **11**: 196–9.

222. O'Malley BW Jr, Chen SH, Schwartz MR et al, Adenovirus-mediated gene therapy for human head and neck squamous cell cancer in a nude mouse model. *Cancer Res* 1995; **55**: 1080–5.

223. Liu TJ, Zhang WW, Taylor DL, Growth suppression of human head and neck cancer cells by the introduction of a wild-type p53 gene via a recombinant adenovirus. *Cancer Res* 1994; **54**: 3662–7.

224. Liu TJ, El-Naggar AK, McDonnell TJ, Apoptosis induction mediated by wild-type p53 adenoviral gene transfer in squamous cell carcinoma of the head and neck. *Cancer Res* 1995; **55**: 3117–22.

225. Clayman GL, El-Naggar AK, Roth JA. In vivo molecular therapy with p53 adenovirus for microscopic residual head and neck squamous carcinoma. *Cancer Res* 1995; **55**: 1–6.

226. Martinez J, Georgoff I, Martinez J et al, Cellular localization and cell cycle regulation by a temperature-sensitive p53 protein. *Genes Dev* 1991; **5**: 151–9.

227. Diller L, Kassell J, Nelson CE et al, p53 functions as a cell cycle control protein in osteosarcoma. *Mol Cell Biol* 1990; **10**: 5772–81.

228. Kamb A, Gruis NA, Weaver-Feldhaus J et al, A cell cycle regulator potentially involved in genesis of many tumor types. *Science* 1994; **264**: 436–40.

229. Clayman GL, El-Naggar AK, Lippman SM et al, Adenovirus mediated p53 gene transfer in patients with advanced recurrent head and neck squamous cell carcinoma. *J Clin Oncol* 1998; **16**: 2221–32.

230. Bischoff JR, Kirn DH, Williams A et al, An adenovirus mutant that replicates selectively in p53-deficient tumor cells. *Science* 1996; **274**: 373–6.

231. Heise C, Sampson-Johannes A, Williams A et al, Onyx-015, an E1B gene-attenuated adenovirus causes tumor-specific cytolysis and antitumoral efficacy that can be augmented by standard chemotherapeutic agents. *Nature Med* 1997; **6**: 639–45.

232. Kirn D, Nemunaitis J, Ganly I et al, A phase II trial of intratumoral injection with an E1B-deleted adenovirus, Onyx-015, in patients with recurrent, refractory head and neck cancer. *Proc Am Soc Clin Oncol* 1998; **17**: 391 (abst).

233. Plant DP, Killing tumor cells with viruses – a question of specificity. *Nature Med* 1998; **4**: 1012–13.

234. Hall AR, Dix BR, O'Carrol SJ et al, p53-dependent cell death/apoptosis is required for a productive adenovirus infection. *Nature Med* 1998; **4**: 1068–72.

235. Nobori T, Miura K, Wu DJ et al, Deletions of the cyclin-dependent kinase-4 inhibitor gene in multiple human cancers. *Nature* 1994; **370**: 753–6.

236. Cairns P, Mao L, Merlo A et al, Rate of p16 (MTS1) mutations in primary tumors with 9p loss. *Science* 1994; **265**: 415–16.

237. Derynck R, Goeddel D, Ullrich A et al, Synthesis of messenger RNAs for transforming growth factors α and β and the epidermal growth factor receptor by human tumors. *Cancer Res* 1987; **47**: 707–12.

238. Harris AL, Nicholson S, Sainsbury JRC et al, Epidermal growth factor receptors: a marker of early relapse in breast cancer and tumor stage progression in bladder cancer; interaction with neu. In: *The Molecular Diagnostics of Human Cancer* (Furth M, Greaves M, eds). Cold Spring Harbor Laboratory Press: New York, 1989: 353–7.

239. Sainsbury JRC, Malcom AJ, Appleton DR et al, Presence of epidermal growth factor receptor as an indicator of poor prognosis in patients with breast cancer. *J Clin Pathol* 1985; **38**: 1225–8.

240. Hendler FJ, Shum-Siu A, Nanu L et al, Increased EGF receptors and the absence of an alveolar differentiation marker predict a poor survival in lung cancer. *Proc Am Soc Clin Oncol* 1989; **8**: 223 (abst).

241. Schlessinger J, Schreiber AB, Levi A et al, Regulation of cell proliferation by epidermal growth factor. *CRC Crit Rev Biochem* 1983; **14**: 92–111.

242. Mendelsohn J, Baselga J, Interaction of biological agents with chemotherapy. In: *Biologic Therapy of Cancer*, 2nd edn (De Vita VT Jr, Hellman S, Rosenberg SA, eds). JB Lippincott:

Philadelphia, 1995: 607–23.

243. Masui H, Kawamoto T, Sato JD et al, Growth inhibition of human tumor cells in athymic mice by anti-EGF receptor monoclonal antibodies. *Cancer Res* 1984; **44**: 1002–7.

244. Divgi CR, Welt C, Kris M et al, Phase I and imaging trial of indium-111 labeled anti-EGF receptor monoclonal antibody 225 in patients with squamous cell lung carcinoma. *J Natl Cancer Inst* 1991; **83**: 97–104.

245. Bos M, Mendelsohn J, Bowden C et al, Phase I studies of anti-epidermal growth factor receptor (EGFR) chimeric monoclonal antibody C225 in patients with EGFR overexpressing tumors. *Proc Am Soc Clin Oncol* 1996; **15**: 443.

246. Perez-Soler R, Donato NJ, Shin DM et al, tumor epidermal growth factor receptor studies in patients with non small cell lung cancer or head and neck cancer treated with monoclonal antibody RG 83852. *J Clin Oncol* 1994; **12**: 730–9.

247. Baselga J, Norton L, Masui H et al, Antitumor effects of doxorubicin in combination with anti-epidermal growth factor receptor monoclonal antibodies. *J Natl Cancer Inst* 1993; **85**: 1327–32.

248. Fan Z, Baselga J, Masui H et al, Anti-tumor effect of anti-EGF receptor monoclonal antibodies plus cis-diamminedichloroplatinum (cis-DDP) on well established A431 cell xenografts. *Cancer Res* 1993; **53**: 4637–42.

249. Baselga J, Norton L, Coplan K et al, Antitumor activity of paclitaxel in combination with anti-growth factor receptor monoclonal antibodies in breast cancer xenografts. *Proc Am Assoc Cancer Res* 1996; **35**: 380 (abst).

250. Perez-Soler R, Shin DM, Donato N et al, Tumor studies in patients with head and neck cancer treated with humanized anti-epidermal growth factor (EGFR) monoclonal antibody C225 in combination with cisplatin. *Proc Am Soc Clin Oncol* 1998; **17**: 393a (abst).

9

Adjuvant therapies for non-small cell lung cancer

Karin V Mattson

INTRODUCTION

Adjuvant therapies were originally defined as those systemic treatments given after successful primary local therapy, surgery or radical radiotherapy in the case of non-small cell lung cancer (NSCLC). Surgery is the primary treatment for the early stages of NSCLC, but only 75% of cases of stage I NSCLC will be cured by a complete resection of the primary tumour. Extrathoracic recurrence is the main reason for failure in both autopsy and clinical trials, even in patients with very early disease.[1,2] In the more advanced and inoperable stages of the disease, radiotherapy is the main local therapy, but the five-year survival rate is at best 39% and at worst 5%.[3]

The case for adjuvant therapy as part of the routine local management of non-disseminated NSCLC would therefore seem rather obvious. However, it remains controversial because randomized controlled trials evaluating *post*operative adjuvant chemotherapy, radiotherapy and biological therapies over the last 30 years have not produced convincing evidence that any postoperative treatments significantly prolong the lives of patients with NSCLC.[3-6] However,

the advent of new more active drugs, better clinical management of toxicity, and improvements in patient selection by more accurate staging are encouraging a great deal of clinical research into neoadjuvant (induction) cytoreductive therapies prior to definitive locoregional treatment. The goal is to improve control of both macroscopic local disease and distant microscopic metastatic disease as early as possible, in order to improve survival. Newly available data from adjuvant therapy trials in patients with both stage IIIa and IIIb disease are most promising.[7-11] The initial encouraging results have already been confirmed by one long-term analysis.[12]

This chapter will concentrate on adjuvant therapies for NSCLC, which accounts for 75% of all cases of lung cancer. There is an increasing understanding that NSCLC is a disseminated disease, so that chemotherapy is becoming a main component of the treatment for all stages.[13] Current adjuvant trials tend to use chemotherapy before *and* after surgery, or before and concurrently with radiotherapy, and for a minimum number of three cycles.[14-16] Postoperative adjuvant studies provide the historical background to this development.

Alternative adjuvant therapies for lung cancer include immunotherapy (including the use of monoclonal antibodies), chemoprevention, gene therapy, and therapies using anti-angiogenesis factors.

In the earliest trials, the chemotherapy was not platinum-based, and subsequent trials with this agent did not use effective doses of platinum-based chemotherapy because of toxicity. Not surprisingly, most randomized postoperative chemotherapy trials recorded only modest survival benefits.[3] A number of newer agents, including vinorelbine, gemcitabine, paclitaxel and docetaxel, are now showing activity as single agents in more than 25% of patients, achieving one-year survival rates of 35%.[17] All of these active new drugs have been tested in platinum-based combinations, with convincing results. Response rates have repeatedly been greater than 45%, median survival more than 10 months and one-year survival rates close to 40% or more. The first phase III studies of platinum–new-drug combinations are now maturing.[17–23] The optimistic preliminary results indicate that the new drugs together with new strategies for administering the chemotherapy early in the treatment schedule are achieving the long-awaited step forward in the treatment of NSCLC.

It is now realized that the revised AJCC/UICC 1988 TNM classification of lung tumours has limitations.[24] Retrospective and prospective reviews have recognized that the stage categories for NSCLC are heterogeneous with respect to T and N categories, and have identified a number of subsets within the stages with important prognostic differences.[16,25] Minor modifications in TNM definitions and the reallocation of subsets to different stages are assuming greater importance as new multi-modality treatment strategies are being developed. In the early trials, patients who would now be recognized as having very different prognoses were grouped together, and it is hardly surprising that the results were inconclusive and controversial. Staging, and therefore patient selection, need to be very precise so that the results of the trials of different treatments, including adjuvant therapies, can be accurately interpreted.[26,27]

Locally advanced NSCLC presents particular problems of staging. Tumours classified as stage III form a very heterogeneous group, comprising any T3 tumour and any N2 tumour. A T3N0 tumour has a very much better prognosis at five years (39%) than does a T1N2 tumour (15%).[16,24] Ginsberg's analysis of prognoses within stage III illustrates the variation: for T2–3N0M0 tumours, the five-year survival rate is 57%, for T3N0–1M0 tumours it is 33–39%, for T1–2N2M0 it is 15%, and for T4 and N3 tumours it is 5–8% (Table 9.1). The differences are based on the possibility of performing a complete resection, on the extent of possible microscopic metastatic dissemination (which increases with nodal involvement), and on invasive tumour growth. Within the node categories are subcategories relating to resectability and to the numbers and sites of the nodes.[28] Accurate detailed staging, of the mediastinum in particular, is needed before decisions on treatment strategies, especially adjuvant therapies, can be made.[26,27] Neoadjuvant chemotherapy or chemo-radiotherapy can increase the success of resection, as well as attacking microscopic metastases earlier.[29–31]

In a review of the literature, Buccheri and Ferringo[32] found that performance status and disease stage were thought to be the only prognostic factors for NSCLC. In the early stages (I and II), molecular biology and cytogenetics have revealed other prognostic factors.[33–35] The fact that only 75% of patients with stage I (T1N0M0) NSCLC can be cured following a complete resection implies that there must be other factors that have prognostic significance. Flow cytometry and DNA studies have shown that a high fraction of S-phase cells in the tumour confers a worse prognosis, as does DNA aneuploidy.[36] Cytogenetic studies have shown that mutations in the *p53* tumour suppressor gene, the retinoblastoma susceptibility gene (*Rb*) and the *ras* genes all worsen the prognosis of patients with NSCLC.[37,38] The *p53* gene is mutated in 50% of NSCLC tumours, and these patients have less chance of survival than those who have similar tumours with no *p53* mutations.[33,39,40] In a study of 271 patients with stage I NSCLC, the five-year survival for

Table 9.1 Survival according to clinical and surgical/pathological stage of NSCLC (revised AJCC Lung Cancer Staging System[24]). Adapted from Bunn et al[102]

Clinical stage	Five-year survival (%)	Surgical/pathological stage	Five-year survival (%)
c IA	61	p IA	67
c IB	38	p IB	57
c IIA	34	p IIA	55
c IIB	24	p IIB	39
c IIIA	13	p IIIA	23
c IIIB	5		
c IV	1		

patients showing mutated *p53* was 53%, compared with 68% for those showing no mutated *p53* (*p* < 0.01). Similarly, Xu et al[41] found that median survival in stage I and II NSCLC was 18 months for patients with mutations in the retinoblastoma gene product (pRb), compared with 32 months for those having no mutated pRb (*p* < 0.05). The difference in prognosis was more pronounced for stage II patients. A number of studies have found a significant difference in prognosis for patients with any stage of adenocarcinoma and K-*ras* mutations.[42,43]

There is therefore potential for neoadjuvant chemotherapy to provide a significant improvement in outcome for patients with locally advanced NSCLC. Patients with N2T3 disease or N3T4 disease need systemic treatment, because micrometastases cause relapse in the majority of cases that are treated only locally, by surgery or radiotherapy respectively. The new drugs that are now available offer the possibility of effective and economical chemotherapy, as well as being less toxic than the earlier chemotherapeutic regimes.

OPERABLE NSCLC, STAGES I, II AND IIIA (T3)

The treatment of choice for the early stages of NSCLC is surgical resection, with five-year survival rates following complete resection of 70% and 60% for stage I and II disease respectively.[13] Nevertheless, less than half of the patients who have undergone complete resection are cured. Eighty percent of relapses occur at distant sites.[1,2]

Postoperative adjuvant therapy

The last IASLC workshop on staging and combined modality treatment in 1993 concluded that stage I (T1N0) patients should not be given postoperative adjuvant chemotherapy. However, the biological prognostic factors that have now been identified suggest that certain subsets of stage I patients could benefit from adjuvant chemotherapy, even at such an early stage in the disease. Clinical trials are currently being performed to test this new concept in a neoadjuvant setting.[31]

Routine postoperative radiotherapy is not recommended if the surgical margins are negative, and a recent meta-analysis has demonstrated that such treatment actually reduces survival.[44] However, for patients with positive surgical margins, there is some evidence that chemotherapy and radiotherapy may benefit patients more than radiotherapy alone.[45] Previously there was little proof that either radiotherapy or chemotherapy given postoperatively increased survival,[46,47] although there were benefits in terms of local tumour control.[48] A recent randomized trial involving a total of 728 patients who had been completely resected of stage I, II or III NSCLC has reported a significant *decrease* in survival for those patients who received postoperative radiotherapy.[44,48] The five-year survival rate was 41% for the control group and 29% for the treatment group ($p < 0.005$). Mortality during the trial period was also significantly higher in the radiotherapy group, at 25% compared with 8% in the control group ($p < 0.0001$). Although there were a number of stage I and II patients who were not expected to suffer local recurrence, no survival benefit was seen for the patients with stage III disease either.

Neoadjuvant therapy

More recent trials have concentrated on induction or 'neoadjuvant' chemotherapy or chemoradiotherapy.[7,8,10,12,49] Thirty percent of patients with stage IIIA (T3) survive for five years, whereas only 15% of patients with stage IIIA (N2) disease survive for five years, but an improvement to 15–39% can be demonstrated if complete resection of all tumour tissue can be carried out.[50] Patients who respond to preoperative therapy should have a better chance of complete resection.

The largest published phase II trial of neoadjuvant chemotherapy for NSCLC took place at the Memorial Sloan–Kettering Cancer Center, where 136 patients suffering from inoperable stage IIIA NSCLC received two or three cycles of mitomycin, vinblastine or vincristine, and cisplatin (MVP) before exploratory surgery.[51] Seventy-eight of the patients responded to the neoadjuvant chemotherapy, and 68% of all the patients underwent complete resection of all tumour tissue. No viable tumour cells were found in specimens from 19 patients. The median survival of all patients was 19 months, with one-year, three-year and five-year rates of 72%, 28% and 17% respectively. However, for the patients who had a complete resection, the figures were 27 months, 83%, 41% and 26% respectively. To offset these encouraging results, there were significant pulmonary complications associated with mitomycin administration: all patients received mitomycin at a dose of $24\,mg/m^2$, and 5% died of treatment-related complications. Burkes et al[52] reported similar results in a trial involving 39 patients in Toronto, who had received two preoperative and two postoperative courses of MVP chemotherapy. There were seven treatment-related deaths (18%), and 18 patients (46%) underwent complete resection of all tumour tissue. The overall survival of the completely resected patients was 29.7 months, with one-year, two-year and three-year survival rates of 73%, 55% and 40% respectively. Both studies demonstrated an improvement in long-term survival over historical controls. Only a few patients achieved a complete response to the induction chemotherapy, but their survival record was impressive: 61–66% at five years. This would suggest that future strategies should concentrate on improving the response rate in the induction phase, by using the newer more-active agents now available.[9,53]

A number of phase II studies conducted along similar lines using various cisplatin-based chemotherapy regimes have pointed towards improved survival for those patients able to undergo a complete resection.[54–56] Overall, the phase II studies suggest that preoperative chemotherapy can achieve response rates of 60–70% for stage IIIA patients, leading to a complete resection rate of 50–60%. The two-year and five-year survival rates also showed an improvement over historical controls (Table 9.2).

There have been two phase III studies comparing preoperative chemotherapy plus surgery with surgery alone in stage IIIA (mixed N2 or T3 lesions) NSCLC. Rosell et al[8] reported

Table 9.2 Non-randomized trials of induction chemotherapy before surgery in stage IIIA NSCLC. Adapted from Cameron and Ginsberg[49]

Ref	Number of patients	CT[a]	Responses[b]		Complete resections[c]	MST[d] (months)	Survival estimates (%)		
			PR	CR			1-yr	2-yr	3-yr
51	136	MVP	92 (68%)	13 (10%)	89 (65%)	19.0	72	28	17
52	39	MVP	22 (56%)	3 (8%)	22 (56%)	18.6	63	26	NS
54	44	Multi	NS	NS	66%	17.5	NS	NS	16
55	27	EVP	13 (48%)	0	4 (15%)	8.0	33	4	NS
56	35	FEP	22 (63%)	2 (6%)	26 (74%)	19.0	77	40	37

[a] Chemotherapy regimes: M, mitomycin; V, vindesine; P, cisplatin; E, etoposide; F, 5-fluorouracil; Multi, multiple chemotherapeutic regimes.
[b] PR, partial response; CR, complete response.
[c] The complete resection rate is calculated as the number of patients undergoing a complete resection with negative pathological margins divided by the number of patients in the study, and expressed as a percentage.
[d] Median survival time.
NS, not specified.

a phase III study in which three cycles of preoperative chemotherapy (mitomycin 6 mg/m^2, ifosfamide 3 g/m^2 with mesna 1 g/m^2, and cisplatin 50/mg/m^2 every three weeks: MIP) followed by surgery was compared with surgery alone in 60 patients with stage IIIA NSCLC. Postoperative radiation therapy (59 Gy in 1.8–2.0 GY/fraction, 5 fractions/week) was administered to both groups.

However, the eligibility criteria were different from other studies in that patients with stage IIIA (T3) disease without N2 status (T3N0–1M0) accounted for 27% (16 of 60) of all patients. The results support the role of preoperative chemotherapy. The therapy outcomes included a resection rate of 77% (23 of 30) versus 90% (27 of 30) and a median survival time (MST) of 26 months versus 8 months for the chemotherapy-plus-surgery group versus the surgery-alone group. The risk of death in the surgery-alone group was five times that in the preoperative chemotherapy-plus-surgery

group. Local–regional recurrence accounted for 54% of all relapses in the chemotherapy-plus-surgery group, whereas distant failure accounted for 55% of all recurrences in the surgery-alone group.

Roth et al[7] also reported a phase III study in which perioperative chemotherapy plus surgery was compared with surgery alone in stage IIIA NSCLC. Patients with stage IIIA (T3) disease, T3N0–1M0 status, accounted for 27% (16 of 60) of all patients in this study as well. The chemotherapy consisted of three cycles of cyclophosphamide 500 mg/m^2 intravenously (i.v.) on day 1, etoposide 100 mg/m^2 i.v. on days 1–3, and cisplatin 100 mg/m^2 i.v. on day 1 every 28 days (CEP regimen) before and after surgery. The complete resection rate with negative margins was low at 39% (11 of 28), compared with 31% (10 of 32) of the control group. The MST and two- and three-year survival rates were 64 months and 60% and 56% respectively for preoperative chemotherapy plus surgery versus 11 months and 25% and 15% respectively for surgery alone ($p = 0.018$). The long-term results of this study confirm that an increase in survival is conferred by perioperative chemotherapy.[12]

The data from these two randomized studies support the role of preoperative cisplatin-based chemotherapy in improving survival over surgery alone in stage IIIA NSCLC. However, the magnitude of the treatment benefit remains unresolved because of the small sample size in both studies. There was no difference in complete resection rate between the two groups in either study, and local–regional recurrence accounted for 54% of all relapses in the chemotherapy-plus-surgery group in the Rosell study. Therefore the survival benefit achieved by the preoperative chemotherapy seems most likely to be attributable to an improved control of distant microscopic disease.

Large international multicentre randomized studies are currently ongoing to test the usefulness of neoadjuvant chemotherapy with new drugs before surgery or radiotherapy.[9]

Neoadjuvant chemotherapy or chemo-radiotherapy, with or without postoperative radiotherapy

The results of five representative phase II studies on this subject are shown in Table 9.3. The chemotherapy comprised two to four cycles of intensive cisplatin-containing regimes. The complete resection rate ranged from 54% to 88%. Tumour downstaging and complete resection were correlated with a better therapeutic outcome.

Fleck et al[57] conducted a phase III randomized clinical trial in which preoperative concurrent chemo-radiotherapy was compared with preoperative chemotherapy alone in patients with stage IIIA (N2) and stage IIIB (T4) NSCLC. Surgery was performed 12 weeks after the initiation of the treatment. The results of this study supported chemo-radiotherapy over chemotherapy alone for this group of patients. The objective response rates were 67% (32 of 48) and 44% (21 of 48) for the chemo-radiotherapy

group and the chemotherapy group respectively ($p = 0.02$). The resection rates were 52% (25 of 48) and 31% (15 of 48) respectively ($p = 0.03$); and the rates of freedom from progression were 40% (19 of 48) and 21% (10 of 48) respectively ($p = 0.04$).

The above summary of trials using concurrent chemo-QD-radiotherapy (i.e. daily radiotherapy, as opposed to twice daily for hyperfractionated radiotherapy) as preoperative therapy is instructional for exploring the potential for synergy between chemo- and radiotherapy.[58–62] Cisplatin-containing chemotherapy regimes were used, and the total radiation doses varied from 30 Gy in 15 fractions given over three weeks to 60 Gy in 30 fractions over six weeks. The therapeutic outcome for patients with stage IIIB disease was also found to be similar to that for patients with stage IIIA disease in some of the studies. The three-year survival rate, ranging from 20% to 40% for both stage IIIA and IIIB after preoperative concurrent chemo-QD-radiotherapy, is very encouraging. However, the optimum radiation dose schedule in such chemo-radiotherapy regimes for stage IIIA and IIIB NSCLC remains to be determined. Schedules should be designed to provide an adequate total dose and dose intensity for the desired level of tumour response. The current level of chemo-radiation interaction needs to be improved by using new drugs such as paclitaxel, docetaxel, gemcitabine and vinorelbine.[63–65]

The role of surgery after induction chemo-radiotherapy for stage IIIA (N2) NSCLC is being evaluated in several large randomized studies.[66] Significant progress in imaging will further improve patient selection for a number of different treatments.

All of these trials, which used a variety of older chemotherapy regimes, indicate that neoadjuvant chemo-radiotherapy improves resectability and survival for stage III patients. Phase III studies are currently underway to compare these neoadjuvant strategies with standard therapy, surgery or radiotherapy, and to assess the best chemotherapy to use.[9]

Table 9.3 Non-randomized trials of induction chemo-radiotherapy before surgery in stage III NSCLC. Adapted from Cameron and Ginsberg[49]

| Ref | Number of patients and stage | CT[a] | RT[b] | Responses[b] | | Complete resections[d] | MST[e] (months) | Survival estimates (%) | | |
				PR	CR			1-yr	3-yr	5-yr
58	85 IIIA	FP 2/0	30 Gy C/–	46 (54%)	2 (2%)	29 (54%)	13.0	53	20	NS
59	41 IIIA	FVP 2/1	30 Gy C/30 Gy	21 (51%)	0	24 (59%)	15.5	58	29	22
60	41 IIIA/B	CAP 2/4	30 Gy S/27 Gy	12 (29%)	2 (5%)	36 (88%)	32.3	75	66[f]	31
61	83 IIIA/B	FP ± E 4/0	40 Gy C/–	84%	0	60 (72%)	NS	NS	40	NS
62	75 IIIA/B	EP 2/0	45 Gy C/–	51 (68%)	1 (1%)	55 (73%)	17.0	NS	40[f]	NS

[a] Preoperative/postoperative chemotherapy regimes: F, 5-fluorouracil; P, cisplatin; V, vinblastine; C, cyclophosphamide; A, doxorubicin; E, etoposide.
[b] Preoperative/postoperative radiation therapy: C, given concurrently with CT; S, given sequentially with CT.
[c] PR, partial response; CR, complete response.
[d] The complete resection rate is calculated as the number of patients undergoing complete resection with negative pathological margins divided by the number of patients in the study.
[e] Median survival time.
[f] Two-year survival data.
NS, not specified.

INOPERABLE LOCALLY ADVANCED NSCLC STAGES IIIA (N2) AND IIIB

Chemotherapy before radiotherapy

The standard treatment for inoperable stage IIIA (N2) tumours, and for all stage IIIB tumours, is radical radiotherapy. However, a meta-analysis of 22 randomized trials comparing chemotherapy plus radiotherapy versus radiotherapy alone for locally advanced unresectable NSCLC concluded that the addition of chemotherapy confers a small improvement in survival.[67] Recent phase III trials of chemo-radiotherapy have concentrated on stage IIIA (N2) and IIIB disease, using neoadjuvant chemotherapy and/or concurrent chemotherapy with radiotherapy, sometimes followed by surgery. A summary of trials is shown in Table 9.4.

Dillman et al[10] randomly assigned patients with stage III (T3 or N2) NSCLC to high-dose radiotherapy alone, or to radiotherapy preceded by induction chemotherapy using vinblastine and cisplatin. The median survival for the patients who received induction chemotherapy

Table 9.4 Summary of positive trials of sequential or concurrent chemotherapy and radiotherapy in unresectable NSCLC

Ref	Phase	Number of patients	Schedule	CT[a]	RT[b] or CT + RT	Response rate (%)	Survival MS[e] (months)	2-yr (%)
10	III	155	CT → RT	PV × 2	60 Gy/6 wk		13.8	30
			RT[d]				9.7	13
11	III	308	CT + RT	P daily[e]	30 Gy/2 wk +		13	26
			RT[d]		25 Gy/2 wk		12	13
68	III	452	CT → RT	PV × 2	60 Gy/6 wk		13.8	30
			RT[d]				11.4	19
71	I/II	9	CT → CT + RT	TP × 2	60 Gy/6 wk + TP × 2	89	Too early	
72	I/II	14	CT → CT + RT	TCb × 2	60 Gy/6 wk + TCb × 2	88	Too early	
73	II	33	CT → CT + RT	TP(E) × 2	60 Gy/6 wk + TP(E) × 2	67	>12	NS
63	II	7	CT → CT + RT	TCb × 3	56 Gy/5.5 wk + TP × 2	71	Too early	
74	II	33	CT + RT	T weekly × 6	60 Gy/6 wk	86	1-yr survival = 73%	

[a] Chemotherapy regimes: P, cisplatin; V, vinblastine; T, paclitaxel; Cb, carboplatin. Etoposide (E) was only given at the beginning of the Hainsworth study.[73]
[b] Radiotherapy.
[c] Median survival.
[d] Control arm of phase III study: the same RT given without CT.
[e] Cisplatin (P) was given on each treatment day before RT.
NS, not specified.

was longer (13.8 months) than for those who received only radiotherapy (9.7 months; $p = 0.0066$). Long-term survival also improved, with 23% of the induction chemotherapy patients surviving three years, compared with 11% of the radiotherapy patients. However, a majority of patients still died within three years, which strongly suggests that both the systemic and local treatments need further improvement.

Schaake-Koning et al[11] treated 331 patients suffering from inoperable NSCLC with radiotherapy alone (30 Gy over two weeks, followed by three weeks rest, followed by 25 Gy over two weeks); with the same radiotherapy plus weekly cisplatin (30 mg/m^2/week); or with the same radiotherapy plus daily cisplatin (6 mg/m^2/day). The survival rate for the group receiving radiotherapy plus daily cisplatin was 16% at three years, compared with 2% at three years for the group receiving radiotherapy alone ($p = 0.009$). The improvement in survival was a function of better control of local disease: 59% of the patients receiving radiotherapy plus daily cisplatin survived one year without recurrence. Comparable figures for the group receiving radiotherapy plus weekly cisplatin were 42% and 30%, and for the radiotherapy-only group 41% and 19%. However, substantial side-effects were experienced.

Sause et al[68] have recently compared the results obtained from standard radiotherapy with those from adjuvant chemotherapy followed by standard radiotherapy, and with those from hyperfractionated radiotherapy. In this study, 452 patients with inoperable NSCLC were eligible for assessment, of whom 95% had stage IIIA or B disease. The patients who received induction cisplatin and vinblastine, followed by standard radiotherapy, did significantly better (one-year survival 60%; median survival 13.8 months) than the standard radiotherapy group (46%; 11.4 months) or the hyperfractionated radiotherapy group (51%; 12.3 months) (log-rank $p = 0.03$).

These multimodality schemes for treating locally advanced NSCLC seem to provide an improvement over historical controls, whether the chemotherapy is given as adjuvant therapy to the radiotherapy or concurrently with it. The new drugs that have recently been found to be active against NSCLC are now being tested as single agents, in combination regimes and in multimodality strategies for locally advanced disease.[17]

The taxanes, paclitaxel and docetaxel, are giving promising results when used in adjuvant strategies for NSCLC.[9,69] They induce tubulin polymerization, one effect of which is to allow cells to accumulate in the G_2/M phase of the cell cycle, the most radiosensitive phase. Paclitaxel (Taxol) has produced encouraging results in advanced unresectable NSCLC when used concomitantly with radiotherapy.[70] Four ongoing studies have involved the administration of induction chemotherapy, including paclitaxel, followed by the same chemotherapy given concomitantly with radiotherapy.[63,71–73] Niell et al[71] administered two three-week cycles of paclitaxel and cisplatin followed by lower doses of the same chemotherapy weekly during the six weeks of radiotherapy (60 Gy in 30 fractions). They achieved a response rate of 70% to the induction chemotherapy and 89% to the combined treatments. Langer et al[72] used two three-week cycles of paclitaxel, carboplatin and granulocyte colony-stimulating factor (G-CSF) followed by two further three-week cycles of lower doses of the same chemotherapy, given at the same time as radiotherapy. The response rates to the induction therapy and the combined treatment were 81% and 89% respectively. Hainsworth et al[73] initially used two three-week cycles of paclitaxel, cisplatin and etoposide, followed by two three-week cycles of lower doses of the same chemotherapy, given concomitantly with radiotherapy. The induction and combined treatment response rates were 42% and 72% respectively, but the treatment produced a high incidence of severe oesophagitis. They then omitted etoposide from the chemo-radiotherapy, which gave response rates of 46% and 67% and a much reduced incidence of grade 4 oesophagitis. These response rates are very encouraging. Isokangas et al[63] administered three cycles of paclitaxel with carboplatin to patients with locally advanced unresectable NSCLC. The neoadjuvant chemotherapy was followed by radiotherapy and two further concurrent cycles of paclitaxel and cisplatin. This team has reported a preliminary response rate of 87%. In another three studies, chemotherapy involving paclitaxel given concomitantly with radiotherapy is achieving response rates as high as 86%.[74–76] Choy et al[74] administered weekly paclitaxel with radiotherapy, and achieved a response rate of 86%, including two complete responses. However, 37% of the patients experienced grade 3–4 oesophagitis. Adelstein et al[75] administered one 24-hour infusion of paclitaxel and a four-day continuous infusion of cisplatin at the beginning of a course of accelerated hyperfractionated radiotherapy. This strategy achieved a response rate of 63% and allowed some patients to become eligible for surgery. Interestingly, one recent study compared standard thoracic irradiation with or without concomitant cisplatin for locally advanced inoperable NSCLC. No improvement in survival or response rates was detected when cisplatin was added to the radiotherapy, even though cisplatin has long been the mainstay of chemotherapy for NSCLC.[77]

BIOLOGICAL ADJUVANT THERAPIES

Many researchers over the years have tried to harness biological agents as adjuvants to surgery, radiotherapy or chemotherapy in the treatment of cancer.[4]

Adjuvant immunotherapy

Potentiation of the body's natural defence mechanisms is classified as immunotherapy. Takita[78] and Ruckdeschel et al[79] reported that lung cancer patients who developed postoperative empyema survived longer than those who did not. Since then, a number of immunostimulatory agents have been investigated as adjuvant therapy for lung cancer.[80] *Bacillus Calmette–Guérin* (BCG) was shown to improve disease-free survival, but no improvement was found in overall survival.[81–83] *Corynebacterium parvum*, another agent assessed for adjuvant immunotherapy in lung cancer, specifically augments cell-mediated immunity, but the only large-scale trial of this agent as an adjuvant to surgery demonstrated that its use actually decreased survival compared with that for patients who only underwent surgery.[84] Levamisole is an anti-helminthic drug that aug-

ments T-lymphocyte numbers and function, and the chemotactic and phagocytic activity of neutrophils and macrophages. It has been tested in a number of trials as postoperative adjuvant immunotherapy in lung cancer, but few of the trials have demonstrated any improvement in overall survival.[85]

The cytokines are a family of naturally occurring proteins with wide-ranging effects; they include interferons (IFN-α, IFN-β and IFN-γ) and interleukins (e.g. IL-2 and IL-6). In 1990 Bowman et al[86] demonstrated a small increase in survival for patients with advanced NSCLC who were given cisplatin and recombinant IFN-α. In one randomized trial, 179 patients suffering from metastatic NSCLC were given CAP chemotherapy alone or with IFN-α, but the result was statistically inconclusive.[87] Overall response rates were 11% for the CAP group and 22% for the CAP + IFN-α group ($p = 0.14$). Vokes et al[88] conducted a phase I trial of cisplatin, IFN-α and radiotherapy on patients with previously treated refractory disease. They observed encouraging local activity, but with considerable toxicity, and the systemic activity was no more than that seen with cisplatin alone.

In one complete trial of IL-2 as a postoperative adjuvant therapy agent in NSCLC, patients were randomly assigned to receive chemotherapy alone, chemotherapy plus IL-2 plus lymphokine-activated killer (LAK) cells, or a placebo.[89] Improved survival was reported for patients who received immunotherapy, but since the study arms were changed halfway through the trial to immunotherapy with IL-2 and LAK cells, or chemotherapy and radiotherapy, the results are difficult to interpret.

The development of recombinant DNA techniques has allowed a new class of biological agents to be manufactured. $DAB_{309}IL$-2 is fusion of diphtheria toxin and human IL-2.[90] This agent binds to the IL-2 receptors on leukocytes, lymphocytes and some NSCLC cells; it is internalized and causes cell death. Trials of $DAB_{309}IL$-2 are still at the preclinical and phase I stage.

Monoclonal antibodies

Monoclonal antibodies to lung cancer antigens have been developed using recombinant technology. These may become the successors to expensive tumour vaccines against NSCLC, which started to be developed in the 1970s and 1980s, but for which results were not sufficiently encouraging to merit further development.

Antibodies directed against tumour cells can inhibit growth through several mechanisms: recruitment of natural kill (NK) cells; activation of cytotoxic T lymphocytes, neutrophils and macrophages; enhancement of phagocytosis; and binding to cell-specific receptors for growth factors.[91] Sixty or more monoclonal antibodies have been produced against lung cancer antigens, although none of them is specific to lung cancer.

There is obvious potential in using antibodies to carry chemotherapeutic agents to tumour cells. BR96 conjugated to doxorubicin (BR96–DOX) is very active against murine lung cancer xenografts, but has revealed unexpected gastrointestinal toxicity in phase I trials.[92] Finally, a number of growth factors are associated with both NSCLC and SCLC, and antibodies to these growth factors can be produced. Antibodies to growth factors such as transferrin, epidermal growth factor (EGF) and the angiogenesis promoter vascular endothelial growth factor (VEGF) are not yet sufficiently developed for use in adjuvant therapies.

Gene therapy

More than 100 oncogenes and tumour suppressor genes have been identified. It is not yet clear whether it will prove possible to manipulate malignant and premalignant cells at gene level, but great potential exists. Genetically modified tumour cell preparations, expressing cytokines such as IL-2, IL-6, IFN-α and G-CSF have induced tumour regression and even disappearance in murine lung cancer models.[93] Immunizing mice with Ras protein promotes cell-mediated immunity, which may have particular importance in adenocarcinoma, where the presence of *ras* mutations indicates a particularly poor prognosis, as mentioned earlier.

Anti-angiogenic factors

Over 50% of lung cancer patients are estimated to have micrometastases at diagnosis, and their further development depends on the regulation of angiogenesis, the ability to develop vasculature. Anti-angiogenic factors are not directly cytotoxic, and therefore their potential appears to lie in adjuvant therapy.[94] At least 10 endothelial cell inhibitors are being investigated in clinical trials against breast cancer, melanoma and Kaposi's sarcoma. In particular, metalloproteinase inhibitors are being investigated in patients suffering from small cell lung cancer (SCLC) who have already responded to systemic chemotherapy.[4] Metalloproteinases are enzymes that control the turnover and remodelling of the extracellular matrix proteins, and they can facilitate invasion by tumour cells and angiogenesis when overexpressed.[95] Macchiarini et al[96] studied angiogenesis and tumour cell invasion in T1N0M0 NSCLC with respect to the development of metastatic disease. Increases in the numbers of microvessels and of tumour cells in tumour blood vessels were directly related to the development of metastatic disease and therefore survival ($p < 0.001$).

Chemoprevention

Chemoprevention is defined as the use of natural or synthetic chemical agents to reverse, suppress or prevent carcinogenic progression to invasive cancer.[97,98] Chemopreventive agents may be used as either primary or secondary preventative measures; if secondary to other treatment, they may be considered adjuvant therapy. Agents that have been tested for preventative use against lung cancer include the retinoids (vitamin A derivatives), β-carotene and α-tocopherol (vitamin E). Although no benefit has been demonstrated in the ongoing primary prevention trials, a survival advantage has been demonstrated when retinoic acid is used as adjuvant therapy for patients with smoking-related cancers.[99] A trial of retinyl palmitate in patients with resected stage I NSCLC produced a similar result,[100] and the US National Cancer Institute is therefore coordinating a large multi-institutional trial of adjuvant 13-*cis*-retinoic acid (isotretinoin) for patients who have completely resected stage I NSCLC. Another adjuvant strategy that is being employed for SCLC patients who have responded to high-dose conventional chemotherapy is maintenance treatment with IFN-α and 13-*cis*-retinoic acid. IFN-α augments the activity of retinoic acid,[101] and this adjuvant treatment is well tolerated by patients.

CONCLUSIONS

NSCLC is as much an economic challenge as a medical one. The overall prognosis that only 10% of patients will survive five years from diagnosis is dismal. New, more accurate methods of patient selection, new drugs, and new strategies for combined modality therapy are improving prognosis in selected categories of patients.[11]

Meta-analysis has revealed that chemotherapy does improve survival for patients with NSCLC. The side-effects of chemotherapy are manageable, so that patients receiving chemotherapy experience improved quality of life. The full potential of chemotherapy in the treatment of lung cancer has yet to be realized.

Active clinical research must now be encouraged to identify the most effective adjuvant strategies, drugs and methods to combine these with local and biological treatments.

Treatment guidelines now recommend adjuvant or neoadjuvant chemotherapy for stage IA NSCLC within the clinical trial setting, and for stage IB disease, although there are no proven benefits as yet. Adjuvant or neoadjuvant chemotherapy is similarly recommended for patients with stage IIA or B disease who have adequate performance status. Enrolment in clinical trials is encouraged. Some combination of chemotherapy, surgery and radiotherapy is strongly recommended for patients with stage IIIA disease. For all stages, the new drugs with their lower toxicity profiles are recommended.

Treatment guidelines recommend chemotherapy and radiotherapy for stage IIIB disease – either neoadjuvant chemotherapy or chemoradiotherapy, for which there are a number of possible schedules. Surgery can even follow these interventions if there is some chance of complete resection of remaining tumour tissue.

It is now well established that in the great majority of cases NSCLC has disseminated by the time of diagnosis. Neoadjuvant or adjuvant chemotherapy is therefore indicated for most patients. The new generation of active drugs are not only more effective, but also more easily tolerated, so that patients' quality of life is enhanced compared with the older chemotherapy regimes. An improved understanding of prognostic factors for NSCLC and more precise staging methods will ensure that patients are better selected for the most appropriate treatments, whether primary or adjuvant.

REFERENCES

1. Kaiser LR, Friedberg JS, The role of surgery in the multi-modality management of non-small cell lung cancer. *Semin Thorac Cardiovasc Surg* 1997; **9**: 60–79.
2. Feld R, Rubinstein V, Weisenberger TH et al, Sites of recurrence in resected stage I non-small cell lung cancer: a guide for further studies. *J Clin Oncol* 1984; **2**: 1352–8.
3. Non-Small Cell Lung Cancer Collaborative Group, Chemotherapy in non-small cell lung cancer: a meta-analysis using updated data on individual patients from 52 randomised trials. *Br Med J* 1995; **311**: 899–909.
4. Shepherd FA, Alternatives to chemotherapy and radiotherapy as adjuvant therapy for completely resected non-small cell lung cancer. *Lung Cancer* 1997; **17**(Suppl 1): S121–36.
5. Dautzenberg B, Chastang C, Arriagada R et al,

Adjuvant radiotherapy versus combined sequential chemotherapy followed by radiotherapy in the treatment of resected non-small cell lung cancer. *Cancer* 1995; **76**: 779–86.

6. Wada H, Hitomi S, Teramatsu T et al, Adjuvant chemotherapy after complete resection in non-small cell lung cancer. *J Clin Oncol* 1996; **14**: 1048–54.

7. Roth JA, Fossella F, Komaki R et al, A randomised trial comparing peri-operative chemotherapy and surgery with surgery alone in resectable stage IIIA non-small cell lung cancer. *J Natl Cancer Inst* 1994; **86**: 673–80.

8. Rosell R, Gomez-Codina J, Camps C et al, A randomised trial comparing pre-operative chemotherapy plus surgery with surgery alone in patients with non-small cell lung cancer. *N Engl J Med* 1994; **330**: 153–8.

9. Mattson K, Ten Velde G, Krofta K et al, Taxotere® as neoadjuvant therapy for radically-treatable stage III NSCLC. *Proc Am Soc Clin Oncol* 1998; **17**: 494a.

10. Dillman RO, Seagren SL, Propert KL et al, A randomised trial of induction chemotherapy plus high-dose radiation versus radiation alone in stage III non-small cell lung cancer. *N Engl J Med* 1990; **323**: 940–5.

11. Schaake-Koning C, van den Bogaert W, Dalesio O et al, Effects of concomitant cisplatin and radiotherapy on inoperable non-small cell lung cancer. *N Engl J Med* 1992; **326**: 524–30.

12. Roth JA, Atkinson EN, Fossella F et al, Long-term follow-up of patients enrolled in a randomized trial comparing peri-operative chemotherapy and surgery with surgery alone in resectable stage IIIA non-small cell lung cancer. *Lung Cancer* 1998; **21**: 1–6.

13. Bunn PA Jr, Kelly K, New chemotherapeutic agents prolong survival and improve quality of life in non-small cell lung cancer: a review of the literature and future directions. *Clin Cancer Res* 1998; **3**: 1087–100.

14. Lynch TJ Jr, Treatment of stage III non-small cell lung cancer. In: *American Society of Clinical Oncology Educational Book* (Perry MC, ed). American Society of Clinical Oncology: Alexandria, VA, 1998: 265–75.

15. Strauss GM, Langer MP, Elias AD et al, Multimodality treatment of stage IIIa non-small cell lung cancer: a critical review of the literature and strategies for future research. *J Clin Oncol* 1992 **10**: 829–38.

16. Ginsberg RJ, The role of surgery in the treatment of lung cancer. In: *Lung Cancer: Prevention Diagnosis and Treatment* (Hirsch FR, ed). Bristol-Myers Squibb, 1996: 81–96.

17. Giaccone G, New drugs in non-small cell lung cancer, an overview. *Lung Cancer* 1995; **12**(Suppl 1): S155–62.

18. Wozniak AJ, Crowley JJ, Balzerzak SP et al, Randomized phase III trial of cisplatin (CDDP) vs. CDDP plus navelbine (NVB) in treatment of advanced non-small cell lung cancer (NSCLC). An update of a southwest oncology group study (SWOG-9308). *Proc Am Soc Clin Oncol* 1998; **17**: 453a.

19. Gatzemeier U, von Pawel J, Gottfried J et al, Phase III comparative study of high-dose cisplatin (HD-CIS) in patients with advanced non-small cell lung cancer (NSCLC). *Proc Am Soc Clin Oncol* 1998; **17**: 454a.

20. Sandler A, Nemunaitis J, Dehham C et al, Phase III study of cisplatin (C) with or without gemcitabine (G) in patients with advanced non-small cell lung cancer (NSCLC). *Proc Am Soc Clin Oncol* 1998; **17**: 454a.

21. Pawel von J, Roemeling von R, for the International CATAPULT-I Study Group, Survival benefit from Tirazone® (tirapazamine) and cisplatin in advanced non-small cell lung cancer (NSCLC) patients: final results from the international phase III CATAPULT-I trial. *Proc Am Soc Clin Oncol* 1998; **17**: 454a.

22. Belani CP, Natale RB, Lee JS et al, Randomized phase III trial comparing cisplatin/etoposide versus carboplatin/paclitaxel) in advanced and metastatic non-small cell lung cancer (NSCLC). *Proc Am Soc Clin Oncol* 1998; **17**: 455a.

23. Giaccone G, Splinter TAW, Debruyne C et al, Randomised study of paclitaxel–cisplatin versus cisplatin–teniposide in patients with advanced non-small cell lung cancer. *J Clin Oncol* 1998; **16**: 2133–41.

24. Mountain CF, Revisions in the International System for Staging Lung Cancer. *Chest* 1997; **111**: 1710–17.

25. Green MR, Litenibaum RC, Stage IIIA category of non-small cell lung cancer: a new proposal. *J Natl Cancer Inst* 1994; **86**: 586–8.

26. Bonome L, Ciccotosto C, Guidotti A et al, Lung cancer staging: the role of computed tomography and magnetic resonance imaging. *Eur J Radiol* 1996; **23**: 35–45.

27. American Thoracic Society/European Respiratory Society, Pre-treatment evaluation of non-

small cell lung cancer. *Am J Respir Crit Care Med* 1997; **156:** 320–32.

28. Vansteenkiste JF, Stroobants SG, De Leyn PR et al, Potential use of FDG-PET scan after induction chemotherapy in surgically staged IIIa-N$_2$ non-small cell lung cancer: a prospective pilot study. *Ann Oncol* 1998; **9:** 1193–8.

29. Scagliotti GV, Ferrari G, Novello S, Neo-adjuvant chemotherapy prior to surgery in stage III non-small cell lung cancer. *Monaldi Arch Chest Dis* 1997; **6:** 531–4.

30. Pastorino U, Benefits of neo-adjuvant chemotherapy in NSCLC. *Chest* 1996; **109:** 96S–101S.

31. Pisters KMW, Ginsberg RJ, on behalf of BLOT, Phase II trial of induction paclitaxel and carboplatin (PC) in early stage (T2N0, T1-2N1, and selected T3N0-1) non-small cell lung cancer (NSCLC). *Proc Am Soc Clin Oncol* 1998; **17:** 451a.

32. Buccheri G, Ferringo D, Prognostic factors in lung cancer: tables and comments. *Eur Respir J* 1994; **7:** 1350–64.

33. Smit EF, Groen HIM, Splinter TAW et al, New prognostic factors in resectable non-small cell lung cancer. *Thorax* 1996; **51:** 638–46.

34. Volm M, Hahn EW, Mattern J et al, Five-year follow-up study of independent clinical and flow cytometric prognostic factors for the survival of patients with non-small cell lung carcinoma. *Cancer Res* 1988; **48:** 2923–8.

35. Miyamoto H, Harada M, Isobe H et al, Prognostic value of nuclear DNA content and expression of the ras oncogene product in lung cancer. *Cancer Res* 1991; **51:** 6346–50.

36. Filderman AE, Silvestri GA, Gatyonis C et al, Prognostic significance of tumour proliferative fraction and DNA content in stage I non-small cell lung cancer. *Am Rev Respir Dis* 1992; **146:** 707–10.

37. Horin Y, Takahashi T, Kuroishi T et al, Prognostic significance of p53 mutations and 3p deletions in primary resected non-small cell lung cancer. *Cancer Res* 1993; **53:** 1–4.

38. Ebina M, Steinberg S, Mulshine JL et al, Relationship of p53 over-expression and up-regulation of proliferating cell nuclear antigen with the clinical course of non-small cell lung cancer. *Cancer Res* 1994; **54:** 2496–503.

39. Harpole DH, Herndon JE, Wolfe WG et al, A prognostic model of recurrence and death in stage I non-cell cell lung cancer utilizing presentation, histopathology and oncoprotein expression. *Cancer Res* 1995; **55:** 51–6.

40. Van Zandwijk N, Van't Veer LJ, The role of prognostic factors and oncogenes in the detection and management of non-small cell lung cancer. *Oncology* 1998; **12**(1 Suppl 2): 55–9.

41. Xu JH, Quinlan DC, Davidson AG et al, Altered retinoblastoma protein expression and prognosis in early-stage non-small cell lung carcinoma. *J Natl Cancer Inst* 1994; **86:** 695–9.

42. Slebos RJC, Kibbelaar RE, Dalesio O et al, K-ras oncogene activation as a prognostic marker in adenocarcinoma of the lung. *N Engl J Med* 1990; **323:** 561–5.

43. Rosell R, Li S, Skacel Z et al, Prognostic impact of mutated K-ras gene in surgically resected non-small cell lung cancer patients. *Oncogene* 1993; **8:** 2407–12.

44. Stewart LA, Burdett S, Souhami RL, on behalf of the PORT Meta-analysis Trialists Group, Post-operative radiotherapy in non-small cell lung cancer: systematic review and meta-analysis of individual patient data from nine randomised controlled trials. *Lancet* 1998; **352:** 257–63.

45. The Lung Cancer Study Group, prepared by Lad T, Rubinstein L, Sadeghi A, The benefit of adjuvant treatment for resected locally advanced non-small cell lung cancer. *J Clin Oncol* 1988; **6:** 9–17.

46. Niiranen A, Niitamo-Korhonen S, Kouri M et al, Adjuvant chemotherapy after radical surgery for non-small cell lung cancer: a randomised study. *J Clin Oncol* 1992; **10:** 1927–32.

47. Holmes EC, Surgical adjuvant therapy for stage II and stage III adenocarcinoma and large cell undifferentiated carcinoma. *Chest* 1994; **106:** 293S–6S.

48. Dautzenberg B, Arriagada R, Chammard AB et al, A controlled study of postoperative radiotherapy for patients with completely resected nonsmall cell lung carcinoma. *Cancer* 1999; **86:** 265–73.

49. Cameron R, Ginsberg RJ, Induction (pre-operative) therapy and surgery for locally advanced stage IIIa (N2) non-small cell lung cancer. In: *Lung Cancer* (Carney D, ed). Arnold: London, 1995: 78–95.

50. Naruke T, Goya T, Tsuchiya R et al, The importance of surgery to non-small cell lung carcinoma of lung with mediastinal lymph node metastasis. *Ann Thorac Surg* 1988; **46:** 603–10.

51. Martini N, Kris MG, Flehinger BJ et al, Pre-operative chemotherapy for stage IIIa (N2) lung cancer: the Sloan–Kettering experience with 136 patients. *Ann Thorac Surg* 1993; **55:** 1365–74.

52. Burkes RL, Ginsberg RJ, Shepherd FA et al, Induction chemotherapy with mitomycin, vindesine and cisplatin for stage III unresectable non-small cell lung cancer: results of the Toronto phase II trial. *J Clin Oncol* 1992; **10:** 580–6.
53. Rosell R, Font A, Pifarre A et al, The role of induction (neo-adjuvant) chemotherapy in stage IIIA NSCLC. *Chest* 1996; **109:** 102S–6S.
54. Takita H, Regal AM, Antkowiak JG et al, Chemotherapy followed by lung resection in inoperable non-small cell lung carcinomas due to locally far-advanced disease. *Cancer* 1986; **57:** 630–5.
55. Vokes EE, Bitran ID, Hoffman PC et al, Neo-adjuvant vindesine, etoposide, and cisplatin for locally advanced non-small cell lung cancer: final report of a phase 2 study. *Chest* 1989; **96:** 110–13.
56. Sridhar KS, Thurer RJ, Markoe AM et al, Multidisciplinary approach to the treatment of locally and regionally advanced non-small cell lung cancer: University of Miami experience. *Semin Surg Oncol* 1993; **9:** 114–19.
57. Fleck J, Camargo K, Godoy D et al, Chemoradiation therapy versus chemotherapy alone as a neo-adjuvant treatment for stage III non-small cell lung cancer. Preliminary report of a phase III prospective randomised trial. *Proc Am Soc Clin Oncol* 1993; **12:** 333.
58. Weiden PL, Piantadosi S, Pre-operative chemotherapy (cisplatin and fluorouracil) and radiation therapy in stage III non-small cell lung cancer: a phase II study of the Lung Cancer Study Group. *J Natl Cancer Inst* 1991; **83:** 266–73.
59. Strauss GM, Herndon JE, Sherman DD et al, Neo-adjuvant chemotherapy and radiotherapy followed by surgery in stage IIIa non-small cell carcinoma of the lung: report of a Cancer and Leukemia Group B phase II study. *J Clin Oncol* 1992; **10:** 1237–44.
60. Skarin A, Jochelson M, Sheldon T et al, Neo-adjuvant chemotherapy in marginally resectable stage III M0 non-small cell lung cancer: long-term follow-up in 41 patients. *J Surg Oncol* 1989; **40:** 266–74.
61. Reddy S, Lee MS, Bonomi P et al, Combined modality for locally advanced nonsmall cell lung carcinoma: results of treatment and patterns of failure. *Int J Radiat Oncol Biol Phys* 1992; **24:** 17–23.
62. Rusch VW, Albain KS, Crowley JJ et al, Surgical resection of stage IIIA and IIIB non-small cell lung cancer after concurrent induction chemoradiotherapy: a Southwest Oncology Group trial. *J Thorac Cardiovasc Surg* 1993; **105:** 97–106.
63. Isokangas O-P, Joensuu H, Halme M et al, Paclitaxel (Taxol®) and carboplatin followed by concomitant paclitaxel, cisplatin and radiotherapy in inoperable stage III non-small cell lung cancer. *Lung Cancer* 1998; **20:** 127–33.
64. Aamdal S, Wilbe E, Hallen MN et al, Phase I study of concomitant docetaxel (Taxotere®) and radiation in locally advanced non-small cell lung cancer. *Proc Am Soc Clin Oncol* 1997; **16:** 460a.
65. Vokes EE, Combined modality therapy with radiation in NSCLC. *Lung Cancer* 1997; **18**(Suppl 1): 131–2.
66. Splinter TAW, Kirkpatrick A, van Meerbeeck J et al, Randomised trial of surgery versus radiotherapy in patients with stage IIIA non-small cell lung cancer after a response to induction chemotherapy. *Proc Am Soc Clin Oncol* 1998; **17:** 453a.
67. Pritchard RS, Anthony SP, Chemotherapy plus radiotherapy compared with radiotherapy alone in the treatment of locally advanced, unresectable non-small cell lung cancer. *Ann Intern Med* 1996; **125:** 723–9.
68. Sause WT, Scott C, Taylor S et al, Radiation Therapy Oncology Group (RTOG) 88–08 and Eastern Cooperative Oncology Group (ECOG) 4588: preliminary results of a phase III trial in regionally advanced unresectable non-small cell lung cancer. *J Natl Cancer Inst* 1995; **87:** 198–205.
69. Choy H, DeVore R, Paclitaxel, carboplatin and radiation therapy for non-small cell lung cancer. *Oncology* 1998; **12**(1 Suppl 2): 80–6.
70. Akerley W, Choy H, Concurrent paclitaxel and thoracic radiation for advanced non-small cell lung cancer. *Lung Cancer* 1995; **12**(Suppl 2): S107–15.
71. Niell HB, Miller AA, Kumar P et al, Phase I/II trial of paclitaxel (Tax), cisplatin (DDP) and radiation therapy for stage III non-small cell lung cancer (NSCLC). *Proc Am Soc Clin Oncol* 1996; **15:** 389.
72. Langer C, Rosvold I, Kaplan R et al, Induction therapy with paclitaxel (Taxol) and carboplatin (CBDCA) followed by concurrent chemoradiotherapy in unresectable, locally advanced, non-small cell lung carcinoma (NSCLC): preliminary report of FCCC 94–001. *Proc Am Soc Clin Oncol* 1996; **15:** 376.

73. Hainsworth JD, Stroup SL, Gray JR et al, Paclitaxel (1-hour infusion), cisplatin, etoposide and radiation therapy in locally advanced unresectable non-small cell lung cancer (NSCLC). *Proc Am Soc Clin Oncol* 1996; **15:** 379.

74. Choy H, Akerley W, Safran H et al, Phase II trial of weekly paclitaxel and concurrent radiation therapy for locally advanced non-small cell lung cancer. *Proc Am Soc Clin Oncol* 1996; **15:** 371.

75. Adelstein DJ, Rice TW, Becker M et al, Accelerated fractionation radiation, concurrent cisplatin/paclitaxel chemotherapy and surgery for stage III non-small cell lung cancer: preliminary toxicity. *Proc Am Soc Clin Oncol* 1996; **15:** 391.

76. Siddiqui S, Bonomi P, Faber LP et al, Phase I–II trial of escalating doses of paclitaxel, carboplatin, etoposide and simultaneous thoracic radiation + pulmonary resection in stage III non-small cell lung cancer. *Proc Am Soc Clin Oncol* 1996; **15:** 405.

77. Blanke C, Ansari R, Mantravadi R et al, Phase III trial of thoracic irradiation with or without cisplatin for locally advanced unresectable non-small cell lung cancer: a Hoosie, Oncology Group Protocol. *J Clin Oncol* 1995; **13:** 1425–9.

78. Takita H, Effect of post-operative emphysema on survival of patients with bronchogenic carcinoma. *J Thorac Cardiovasc Surg* 1970; **59:** 642–4.

79. Ruckdeschel J, Codish S, Stranaham A et al, Post-operative empyema improves survival in lung cancer. *N Engl J Med* 1972; **287:** 1013–17.

80. Pass H, Pass H, Lung cancer biotherapy: specific and non-specific mechanisms. In: *Lung Cancer: principles and practice* (Pass HI, Mitchell JB, Johnson DH, Turrisi AT, eds). Lippincott-Raven: Philadelphia, 1996: 917–30.

81. Miller AB, Taylor HE, Baker MA et al, Oral administration of BCG as an adjuvant to surgical treatment of carcinoma of the bronchus. *Can Med Assn J* 1979; **121:** 45–54.

82. Mountain CF, Gail MH, Surgical adjuvant intrapleural BCG treatment for stage I non-small cell lung cancer. *J Thorac Cardiovasc Surg* 1981; **82:** 649–57.

83. Ludwig Lung Cancer Study Group, Immunostimulation with intrapleural BCG as adjuvant therapy in resected non-small cell lung cancer. *Cancer* 1986; **58:** 2411–16.

84. Ludwig Lung Cancer Study Group, Adverse effect of intrapleural *Corynebacterium parvum* as adjuvant therapy in resected stage I and II non-

85. small cell carcinoma of the lung. *J Thorac Cardiovasc Surg* 1985; **89:** 842–7.

85. Anthony HM, Mearns AT, Mason MK et al, Levamisole and surgery in bronchial carcinoma patients: increase in deaths from cardiorespiratory failure. *Thorax* 1979; **34:** 4–12.

86. Bowman A, Ferguson RJ, Allan SG et al, Potentiation of cisplatin by alpha-interferon in advanced non-small cell lung cancer (NSCLC): a phase II study. *Ann Oncol* 1990; **1:** 351–3.

87. Rosso R, Ardizoni A, Salvati F et al, Combination chemotherapy and recombinant alfa interferon for metastatic non-small cell lung cancer: a randomised FONICAP trial. *Proc Am Soc Clin Oncol* 1990; **9:** 227.

88. Vokes EE, Haraf DJ, Hoffman PC, Escalating doses of interferon alpha-2A with cisplatin and concomitant radiotherapy: a phase I study. *Cancer Chemother Pharmacol* 1993; **33:** 203–9.

89. Kimura H, Yamaguchi Y, Randomised controlled study with interleukin 2 and lymphokine activated killer cells against post-operative primary lung cancer patients. *Lung Cancer* 1994; **11:** 187 (abst).

90. Nicols J, Waters C, Shaw J, Bacha P, DAB$_{389}$IL-2 mechanism and kinetics of action: in vitro and in vivo preclinical studies. In: *Proceedings of Lilly Oncology Global Medicine Conference, 1995*.

91. Epenetos A (ed), *Monoclonal Antibodies 2: Applications in Clinical Oncology*. Chapman & Hall: London, 1992.

92. Stein R, Goldenberg DM, Prospects for the management of non-small cell carcinoma of the lung with monoclonal antibodies. *Chest* 1991; **99:** 1466–76.

93. Arca MJ, Mule JJ, Change AE, Genetic approaches to adoptive cellular therapy of malignancy. *Semin Oncol* 1996; **23:** 108–17.

94. Folkman J, Clinical applications of research on angiogenesis. *N Engl J Med* 1995; **333:** 1757–63.

95. Brown PD, Giavazzi R, Matrix metalloproteinase inhibitors: a novel class of anti-cancer agents. *Adv Enzyme Regul* 1995; **35:** 293–301.

96. Macchiarini P, Fontanini G, Hardin MJ et al, Blood vessel invasion by tumour cells predicts recurrence in completely resected T1N0M0 non-small cell lung cancer. *J Thorac Cardiovasc Surg* 1993; **106:** 80–9.

97. Lippman SM, Benner SE, Hong WK, Cancer chemo-prevention. *J Clin Oncol* 1994; **12:** 851–73.

98. Hong WK, Lippman SM, Itri LM et al, Prevention of second primary tumours with isotretinoin in squamous cell carcinoma of

the head and neck. *N Engl J Med* 1990; **323:** 795–801.

99. Pastorino U, Infante M, Maioli M et al, Adjuvant treatment of stage I lung cancer with high-dose vitamin A. *J Clin Oncol* 1993; **11:** 1216–22.

100. Bollag W, Holdener E, Retinoids in cancer prevention and therapy. *Ann Oncol* 1992; **3:** 513–26.

101. Mattson K, Ruotsalainen T, Tamminen K et al, Interferon alpha and retinoic acid maintenance therapy for small cell lung cancer. *Chest* 1996; **110:** 1045.

102. Bunn PA Jr, Detterbeck RC, Swisher SG, Waterhouse D, Resectable non-small cell lung cancer: Is surgery enough? Bristol-Myers Squibb Oncology: Princeton, NJ, 1998.

10

Breast cancer: Biologic therapy

Margaret von Mehren, Louis M Weiner

CONTENTS • Introduction • Targets on breast cancer cells • Monoclonal antibodies • Antibody-based therapy • Radioimmunotherapy • Antibody–drug conjugates • Antibody-drug enzyme prodrug therapy (ADEPT) • Bispecific antibody therapy • Immunotoxins • New structures for antibody-based tumor targeting • Vaccine therapy • Conclusions

INTRODUCTION

The most common malignancy in women is breast cancer, with an estimated lifetime risk of 8.4–9.4%.[1] Owing to the increased awareness of the value of screening for this disease, a greater number of women are having early lesions detected and treated. Selected adjuvant chemotherapeutic and hormonal strategies have increased disease-free and overall survival in women at risk for the development of metastatic disease.[2] In spite of these improvements in the diagnosis and treatment of breast cancer, significant numbers of patients die of breast cancer annually. New approaches such as antibody-based therapies and vaccine strategies have shown promise in the metastatic setting, but these treatments have the best chance to be effective in the adjuvant and minimal disease settings. Breast cancer cells contain surface antigens and mutated proteins that can serve as therapeutic targets and immunogens. The rationale for these approaches and preclinical and clinical data will be reviewed in this chapter. Examples of strategies in other tumor types with potential relevance to the treatment of breast cancer will be described.

TARGETS ON BREAST CANCER CELLS

c-erbB-2 (HER2/neu)

The c-erbB-2 protooncogene encodes for a receptor tyrosine kinase that is a member of the heregulin family, which comprises the epidermal growth factor receptor (EGFR), c-ErbB-2 (HER2), c-ErbB-3 and cErbB-4.[3] The neu protooncogene was originally discovered by detecting a murine humoral response to a 185 kDa protein following inoculation of mice with rat tumors, stimulated by in utero nitrosoethylurea injections.[4] Its human homologue c-erbB-2 was discovered through the similarity of its protein product c-ErbB-2 to EGFR.[5–7] The protein receptor, when transfected into fibroblasts, transformed the phenotype of these cells.[8,9] The endogenous ligand is unknown. However, c-ErbB-2 has been shown to mediate intracellular signals when dimerized with c-ErbB-3 (HER3) and c-ErbB-4 (HER4), or when bound with heregulin.[10,11] Unlike the normal cellular homologue, which is not oncogenic, HER2 contains a point mutation in the transmembrane portion of the molecule.[12,13] Inserting truncated forms of c-ErbB-2 or overexpressing the protein results in a transformed phenotype.[8,14] In human tissues, c-ErbB-2 is detected in secretory epithelial tissues and the basal layer of skin.[15,16] c-ErbB-2 is also overexpressed in approximately 30% of adenocarcinomas,[17–21] as well as comedo, large cell and ductal carcinoma in situ.[22] HER2 has become a target for antibody-based therapies because of its role in oncogenesis and its overexpression in particular tumor types compared with normal host tissues.

Epidermal growth factor receptor (EGFR)

EGFR is a 170 kDa transmembrane glycoprotein that is overexpressed in 40% if breast cancers. This receptor has a number of ligands, including epidermal growth factor (EGF) and the transforming growth factor alpha (TGF-α). Overexpression of EGFR and its ligands has been found in breast carcinoma cell lines and human carcinomas, providing evidence for the existence of an autocrine growth loop.[23–25] For example, murine and human epithelial cells transformed with the c-Ha-*ras* protooncogene are found to have elevated levels of TGF-α. When a TGF-α-neutralizing antibody is added to the in vitro system, 50–80% of the anchorage-independent growth is inhibited.[26]

Carcinoembryonic antigen (CEA)

CEA is an 18 kDa glycoprotein present on endodermally derived neoplasms and in the digestive organs of the human fetus.[27,28] Adenocarcinomas expressing this antigen do not stimulate an immune response, because CEA is present in fetal development. CEA is a member of the immunoglobulin superfamily located on chromosome 19, and is believed to be involved with intercellular interactions.[29] CEA is felt to be an adhesion molecule, and may allow tumor cells to attach to normal cells in the metastatic process.[30] Targeting CEA may therefore be important in the prevention of metastases. CEA has been reported to be expressed in 68–88% of breast adenocarcinomas.[31]

Carbohydrate targets

Carbohydrate and mucin molecules are also found on cell surfaces. Lewis-Y (Le^y) is a carbohydrate antigen found on the surface of many carcinomas, including those derived from breast, lung, colon, rectum and prostate. Mucin molecules are found on most carcinoma cells, and differ from those found on normal cell surfaces as a result of incomplete glycosylation.[32] The carcinoma-associated mucins have shorter carbohydrate side-chains, thus exposing the core peptide and glycopeptide determinants.[33] A series of epitopes have been described, including Tf (β-D-Gal-(1–3)-α-GalNAc), Tn (N-acetyl-D-galactosamine-α-O-Ser/Thr), sialyl-Tn (dAcNeu α2-6αGalNAc-O-Ser/Thr), and MUC1.

EGP-2/GA733-2

A series of murine antibodies, identified by immunizing mice with cell lines from gastrointestinal cancers, have been found to recognize closely related tumor-associated epitopes. These antibodies detect a 38 kDa surface glycoprotein variously referred to as EGP-2, GA733-2 or Ep-CAM. The normal distribution of EGP-2 is on the baso-lateral surface of nonsquamous epithelium of the lower respiratory tract, lower gastrointestinal tract, tubules of the kidney, surface epithelium of the ovary, exocrine and endocrine pancreas, hair follicles, secretory tubules of sweat glands, bile ducts, and thymic epithelium. EGP-2 expression is also associated with various cancers, such as those derived from the colon, rectum, pancreas, lung and breast. Although the antigen is abundantly expressed, it is not shed in the circulation.[34] Various groups have cloned genes that transcribe proteins recognized by these antibodies.[35,36] EGP-2 has been shown to have homology to proteins involved with cell–cell, as well as cell–matrix interactions. Cells transfected with this gene demonstrate enhanced in vitro intercellular adhesion.[37]

Transferrin receptor

The transferrin receptor is comprised of two identical transmembrane subunits linked by disulfide bonds. Its expression is controlled both by post-transcriptional iron response elements on mRNA and at the transcription level. When the receptor complexes with a ligand, it is rapidly internalized via endocytosis. The ligand is altered in the acidic pH of the endosome, and becomes unbound in the endosome cytosol. The endosome is then recycled within minutes.[38] The rapid internalization and regeneration on the cell surface makes this receptor ideal for targeting drugs, toxins or radioisotopes conjugated to antibodies. Transferrin receptors are expressed on breast carcinoma cells.[39]

Mutated *ras*

The *ras* protooncogenes encode a conserved family of 21 kDa proteins,[40] which function in signaling pathways involved with cell growth and differentiation.[41] Ras binds to the inner aspect of the outer cellular membrane, associates with guanosine nucleotides and has GTPase activity. There are three known *ras* genes, H-*ras*, K-*ras*, and N-*ras* located on different chromosomes,[42] with the majority of mutations found at codon 12.[43] Specific activating mutations or overexpression of these oncogenes transform cells.[44] Reports on the presence of *ras* mutations in normal mammary tissue and breast cancers are conflicting. Some describe one of the *ras* mutations in most breast cancers, with K-*ras* being more common than the other mutated forms,[45] while others described it as a rare occurrence.[43]

In summary, these proteins and glycoproteins provide targets for antibody- and vaccine-based therapies. Some of these proteins are found on normal cells, but are overexpressed on tumor cells, such as EGFR and HER2. They have been shown to transform cells in vitro. The transferrin receptor has been targeted because of its ability to rapidly internalize ligands bound to it, providing a means to get radioactive or chemotherapeutic agents specifically within a cell. Lastly, mutated protooncogenes associated with malignant cell transformation are unique tumor targets.

MONOCLONAL ANTIBODIES

The primary impetus behind the development of therapeutic and diagnostic strategies using monoclonal antibodies (MAbs) has been the specific targeting properties of these molecules. By specifically binding to tumor-associated antigens, antibodies can induce one of several biologic responses with limited toxicity to normal tissues. Antibodies may direct antitumor effects by inducing apoptosis,[46] interfering with ligand–receptor interactions[47] or preventing the expression of proteins that are critical to the neoplastic phenotype. Alternatively, they may induce an anti-idiotype network,[48] complement-mediated cytotoxicity[49] or antibody-directed cellular cytotoxicity.[50]

Initial clinical trials with MAbs led to some striking examples of antitumor effects,[51] but the majority have served to illustrate the obstacles to successful therapy (Table 10.1). Most of the Mabs employed in clinical trials have been derived from mice, and patients exposed to them have developed human anti-mouse antibody (HAMA) responses, thus limiting the number of treatments that patients can receive.[52] There has also been extensive description of the barriers that impede antibody distribution within tumors, such as (1) disordered vasculature, (2) increased hydrostatic pressure within tumors and (3) heterogeneity of antigen distribution within tumors.[53] If antibodies do reach their targets, there is little evidence that they efficiently mediate in vivo antibody-dependent cytotoxicity. For this to occur, sufficient numbers of effector cells, such as macrophages, natural killer (NK) cells or cytotoxic T cells, must be activated in the tumor.[54] Finally, many tumors are known to secrete compounds that downregulate the immune response.[55,56] Preclinical and clinical data with improved molecules that address these impediments continue to demonstrate an emerging

Table 10.1 Obstacles to antibody therapy

- Immune response against foreign antibody
- Abnormal tumor vasculature
- Increased hydrostatic pressure within tumors
  Heterogeneic antigen expression
- Lack of effector cells within tumor

ecules are better able to reach tumor targets, but also are cleared more rapidly via renal excretion.[59] Antibody molecules can be made to be less immunogenic by 'humanizing' their backbone structures.[60] The advent of phage display library techniques has also allowed for rapid screening and production of useful antibodies.[61] These molecules have also been engineered to attach toxins, cytokines, radiolabeled elements or genes, thus broadening the utility of these molecules to serve as delivery vehicles for cancer therapeutics.

Another advance has been the development of bispecific antibodies (BsAbs) that consist of two antibodies with specificity for distinct antigens.[62] These constructs have been synthesized by covalently linking two monoclonal antibodies[63] or monoclonal antibody fragments,[64] by the production of hybrid hybridomas,[65] or by engineering recombinant bispecifics.[66] This allows targeting of two distinct tumor antigens found on tumor cells or the simultaneous engagement of a tumor-associated antigen and a cytotoxic trigger molecule on effector cells. The rationale for the first approach is the hypothesis that if

role for antibody-based therapy as a component of the oncologic armamentarium.

A variety of molecules apart from the conventional immunoglobulin molecule are available for clinical development (Figure 10.1). Smaller fragments that contain intact immunoglobulin-binding sites, such as F(ab')$_2$ and Fab, do not contain the Fc binding domain of the molecule.[57,58] scFv molecules contain the heavy and light chains of the binding site(s) joined by a short linker. These smaller mol-

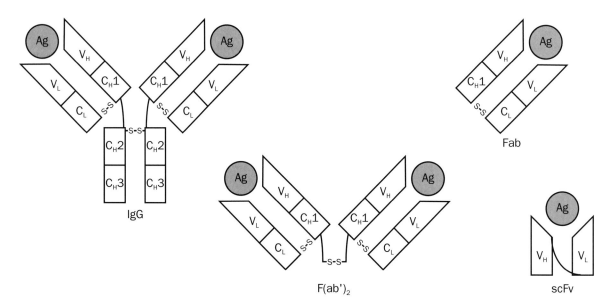

Figure 10.1 Structures of the immunoglobulin G molecule and smaller antibody fragments: F(ab')$_2$, Fab and ScFv. F(ab')$_2$, and Fab can be produced by enzymatic digestion, while other constructs are produced primarily by recombinant engineering. Ag, antigen.

two different antigens on tumor cells are bound then the antibody is more likely to interrupt normal cellular metabolism by interfering with the function of the ligand.[67] The second approach allows for targeting of an immune effector cell directly to a tumor cell, enhancing the immune response against the tumor. The majority of BsAbs are of the latter type. Many of these molecules are still undergoing preclinical testing, while others have reached clinical trials. The following will review the recent advances in the development of antibody-based strategies in breast cancer or model systems for breast cancer therapy.

ANTIBODY-BASED THERAPY

Preclinical and clinical trials have examined a multitude of antibodies with specificity for breast cancer-associated antigens (Table 10.2). Not all of these antibodies have reached clinical testing, but results of those studies that have reached clinical testing will be reviewed, along with the preclinical data on promising antibodies.

FC-2.15 is a murine antibody developed with specificity for human breast carcinomas and their proliferating cells.[68] It recognizes three proteins, with molecular weights of 160, 130

Table 10.2 Preclinical and clinical Mabs for breast cancer-associated antigens		
Antigen	**Antibody**	**Ref**
Unknown	FC-2.15	68
Carcinoembryonic antigen (CEA)	MN-14	74
c-ErbB-2 (HER2)	4D5	84
	rhuMAb HER2	75
	FRP5	225
	ICR62	85
	520C9	67
EGP-2	17-1A	68
Breast mucin	Mc1	226
	Mc3	226
	Mc5	226
	BrE-1	226
	BrE-2	226
	BrE-3	115
	B1	226
	B3	227
Lewis^y (Le^y)	BR64	171
	BR96	171
Tag-72	CC49	117
Pancarcinoma	RS7	107
Anti-adenocarcinoma	L6	108

and 115 kDa in cell lysates of human breast cancer cells as well as in colon, squamous and thyroid tumors. It also recognizes three proteins from lysates generated from neutrophils, with molecular weights of 250, 185 and 115 kDa. Eleven patients (five breast cancer patients) with tumors positive by immunohistochemistry with FC-2.15 were treated with antibody infusions every other day for a total of four infusions. Initially infusions were administered over four hours. However, hypotension, tachycardia and tachypnea were observed at doses administered at 3 mg/h. Subsequently infusion rates were decreased to 0.05 mg/h to allow for dose escalation. Patients were noted to develop neutropenia beginning within one hour after commencing the infusion and resolving one hour after discontinuation of antibody infusion. One patient receiving 0.05 mg/kg/h developed fever at hour 27 and was found to be neutropenic and bacteremic owing to *Pseudomonas aeruginosa*. Based on this patient, infusions were subsequently delivered over 20 h every other day, to allow for recovery of neutrophil counts between infusions. Patients otherwise tolerated therapy with fever, shortness of breath (especially in patients with pulmonary infiltrative disease) and asymptomatic thrombocytopenia. All patients developed HAMA responses. One patient with metastatic breast cancer to lung, liver and bone, refractory to chemotherapy, had significant improvement in her pain and shortness of breath as well as a decrease in the size of hepatic nodules and stabilization of pulmonary nodules following one cycle of therapy. Three months later, the patient was found to have progressive disease. A second course of therapy was well tolerated without evidence of an allergic response following prophylaxis with diphenhydramine. The patient did not have a second clinical response.

17-1A, an antibody that recognizes EGP-2, has undergone extensive clinical testing, primarily in patients with malignancies of the gastrointestinal tract. Phase I studies demonstrated that the antibody therapy was well tolerated and objective responses were observed.[69–71] A prospective multicenter randomized study in patients with stage III colorectal carcinoma has been completed.[72] Patients were randomized to receive observation or 17-1A therapy after curative surgery. Treatment consisted of 500 mg 17-1A intravenously (i.v.) postoperatively, followed by four doses of 100 mg i.v. every four weeks. At five years, 36% of patients treated had died from all causes, compared with 51% in the non-treated group. The recurrence rate was 48.7% in the treated group, compared with 66.5% in the non-treated group. The results of this study suggest that multi-institutional studies with antibody-based therapies are feasible. They also demonstrate an effect of antibody therapy in an adjuvant setting where there is minimal residual disease. Intergroup trials are ongoing to confirm these results.

A means to circumvent an immune response to a mouse antibody is to humanize the antibody.[60] The first step in this process is to determine the amino acids within the variable region of the antibody that are important for binding to the antigen. These amino acids or amino acid sequences are known as the complementarity-determining regions (CDR) of the Ab. Once these regions are known, a recombinant immunoglobulin is made by engineering the appropriate DNA sequences into the framework of a human immunoglobulin gene. This construct is then placed into a cellular system that can transcribe the recombinant DNA construct, glycosylate the translated protein, and secrete it into the culture supernatant for purification.

This approach has been evaluated with antibodies against breast mucins,[73] hu-BrE-3 and hu-Mc3. In preclinical studies hu-BrE-3 and hu-Mc3 were found to have similar reactivity and affinity for their antigens, as well as unaltered biodistribution in murine models. A humanized version of the murine anti-carcinoembryonic-antigen (CEA) antibody MN-14 has been produced and ^{131}I-conjugated.[74] The iodinated form of the antibody has been utilized in imaging studies in patients with CEA-expressing tumors. The humanized antibody has similar biodistribution, tumor targeting, pharmacokinetic and dosimetry properties as the murine parent antibody. A patient with an elevated titer of human anti-mouse antibody has received three injections of hMN-14 without complications. Three patients who initially received two injections of MN-14, followed by hMN-14, developed a humoral response to hMN-14; this was not seen in patients receiving hMN-14 alone, demonstrating that the humanized antibody is less antigenic.

rhuMAb HER2,[75] also known as Herceptin, is a humanized antibody derived from 4D5, a murine monoclonal antibody that recognizes c-ErbB-2. Basegla et al[75] have reported the results of a phase II trial in women with metastatic breast cancer, and have demonstrated an objective response rate of 11.6%, with responses seen in the liver, mediastinum, lymph nodes and chest wall lesions. Patients received 10 or more treatments with the antibody, and none developed an antibody response against rhuMAb HER2. Cobleigh et al[76] treated 222 women with metastatic breast, finding an objective response rate of 16%. The median response duration was 9.1 months, with a median overall survival of 13 months, which is superior to those reported for second-line chemotherapy in metastatic breast cancer. In both of these trials, there were a significant number of women who had stable disease: 32.6% and 30% respectively.

A phase III trial comparing cytotoxic chemotherapy with Herceptin has been completed.[77] Patients receiving initial therapy for metastatic breast cancer were treated with doxorubicin or epirubicin and cyclophosphamide, or with paclitaxel if they had received an anthracycline in the adjuvant setting. Patients were then randomized to receive chemotherapy alone or in combination with weekly antibody therapy. There was an improvement in the response rates for combination therapy from 42.1% to 64.9% for the anthracycline-based regimens and from 25.0% to 57.3% for the taxane regimen. Myocardial dysfunction such as is seen with anthracycline therapy was observed with increased frequency in patients receiving antibody with doxorubicin or epirubicin. Preclinical data have demonstrated that Herceptin does not have synergistic or additive effects with all chemotherapies; in particular, there is evidence of inhibition when

it is combined with 5-fluorouracil.[78] Based on these clinical trials, Herceptin has been approved by the US Food and Drug Administration for the treatment of women with metastatic breast cancer who overexpress HER2/Neu alone or in combination with paclitaxel. Herceptin is only the second antibody to receive FDA approval for use in cancer therapy. Phase III adjuvant studies are now beginning to evaluate the impact of Herceptin in patients whose breast cancers overexpress HER2/Neu.

The rationale for using antibody-based therapies, apart from their selective targeting of tumor cells, comes from preclinical observations in which antibody therapy alone in the absence of effector cells has resulted in a change in phenotype of malignant cells. Studies utilizing Mab 7.16.4, which recognizes rat Neu, were found to decrease cell surface expression of c-ErbB-2 but not to decrease intracellular production of the protein.[79] This decrease persisted with continued exposure to the antibody, but was not seen when monovalent F(ab) fragments were used, since there was no crosslinking of receptors. Also, cultures of transformed cells grown in soft agar in the presence of antibody were no longer capable of developing large colonies, and grew in a similar fashion to the wild-type cells, which were not producing c-ErbB-2. Therefore the antibody treatment led to loss of the transformed phenotype. It did not, however, have a cytotoxic effect, since colonies were able to grow if the antibody was removed from the culture medium.

N28, an anti-c-ErbB-2 antibody, has stimulatory effects on c-ErbB-2-expressing tumors in vivo, in contrast to N29, which also recognizes c-ErbB-2.[80] Evaluation in vitro demonstrated that these antibodies bind to different epitopes on c-ErbB-2 and lead to different intracellular events.[81] Treatment of c-ErbB-2-expressing cells in vitro by N29, but not N28, led to loss of transformed phenotype in 60–90% of cells, and was associated with translocation of the receptor from the cell membrane to cytoplasmic and perinuclear sites. There was also lipid and casein production, as is seen in normal glandular tissue of the breast in cells treated with N29, but not N28. Cells treated with N28 were shown to have marked increased phosphorylation of c-ErbB-2 compared with minimal phosphorylation of c-ErbB-2 in cells exposed to N29.

By using 4D5, a murine antibody against c-ErbB-2 subsequently humanized as rhuMAb HER2, the intracellular signaling pathways elicited by antibody binding c-ErbB-2 were evaluated.[82] In breast cancer cell lines overexpressing c-ErbB-2, in vitro growth was inhibited by 60–80% after seven days of continuous exposure to 4D5 compared with non-overexpressing cell lines. After a 15 min exposure to 4D5, there was increased phosphorylation of c-ErbB-2 itself, as well as 56 kDa protein, thought to be a downstream substrate. There was also an increase in c-*fos* mRNA, a second messenger for some kinases, known to regulate factors controlling cell cycle progression. In contrast, when 4D5 was added for 15 h, there was reduced c-ErbB-2 phosphorylation beyond what would be seen due to internalization of the receptor alone. This inhibition was seen even in the presence of growth factors such as EGF or TGF-α.[83] It has also been demonstrated in vitro that treatment with 4D5 leads to enhanced sensitivity to the cytotoxic effects of tumor necrosis factor α (TNF-α), which is lost in breast cancer cell lines overexpressing c-ErbB-2.[84]

Targets for antibody therapy in the past have focused on tumor-associated antigens that could be recognized by a MAb and target the immune system to destroy tumor cells. With growing knowledge of signaling pathways, antibodies are being developed to target receptors important for growth or the compounds that bind these receptors. Preclinical studies by Tosi et al[85] have demonstrated the ability of anti-EGFR antibodies to block tyrosine kinase activation of the EGFR. They have also demonstrated, in cells that overexpress EGFR, the ability of these antibodies to disrupt a known autocrine loop involving TGF-α. Another example of an EGFR MAb is ICR62, which has been extensively characterized by Modjtahedi and colleagues and recently tested in a phase I trial of squamous cell cancers of the head and neck, and lung.[86] Modjtahedi et al

have shown that this antibody can effectively block the binding of the EGFR ligands to this receptor, and that it inhibits the in vitro growth of tumor cell lines overexpressing EGFR. This growth inhibition is due to terminal differentiation of the EGFR-overexpressing cell lines. In the phase I study, patients were treated with one dose of ICR62, with minimal side-effects. The administered antibody localized to tumor, as assessed by biopsy. Further studies with multiple doses are planned, with the goal of duplicating the in vitro observations of terminal differentiation.

Other antibodies against EGFR have been shown to have affinities for the receptor similar to its natural ligands, EGF and TGF-α. When the human–mouse chimeric MAb C255 binds to EGFR, it inhibits the normal tyrosine kinase function of this receptor, affecting cells' ability for signal transduction.[87] Another pathway that can be targeted in eukaryotic cells involves the cyclic adenosine monophosphate (c-AMP)-dependent protein kinase. There are two isoforms of this kinase, PKAI and PKAII, which differ in their regulatory subunits.[88] PKAII predominates in resting cells, whereas PKAI is found in rapidly dividing cells and malignant cells. PKAI has also been shown to be induced by transforming factors such as TGF-α, Ras and c-ErbB-2.[89,90] In an in vivo model utilizing a human colon cancer cell line, mice treated with MAb C225 in combination with 8-chloro-c-AMP, a selective inhibitor of PKAI, there was a statistically significant improvement in survival in animals treated with the combination in comparison to either agent alone. Furthermore, when tumors were analyzed immunohistochemically following treatment, there was a marked reduction in EGF-related growth factors such as TGF-α, basic fibroblast growth factor (bFGF), vascular endothelial growth factor (VEGF) and amphiregulin. PCNA index was decreased from control values of 60% to 3%.[91]

Resistance to chemotherapy has been linked to the overexpression of c-ErbB-2 and EGFR.[92–94] The role of antibodies that block these receptors in decreasing drug resistance has been evaluated. Antibodies directed against EGFR have been shown to increase the toxicity of doxorubicin and cisplatin;[95,96] there are conflicting studies revealing enhanced cytotoxicity of chemotherapeutic agents and radiation therapy[97–99] with EGF. Of interest in the former studies was the lack of evidence demonstrating increased drug uptake or cell cycle arrest to explain the enhanced cytotoxicity observed. Studies utilizing antibody against c-ErbB-2 have demonstrated enhancement of cisplatin cytotoxicity.[100,101] Arteaga et al[102] attempted to elucidate the mechanism underlying this phenomenon. In vitro studies demonstrated increased DNA adduct formation when cells were treated with anti-c-ErbB-2 antibody with cisplatin, compared with cisplatin alone. This was not due to the intracellular accumulation of cisplatin, but rather appeared to be mediated via intracellular signaling caused by the antibody binding to the c-ErbB-2 receptor, leading to phosphorylation of the receptor and the downstream signal, phospholipase C-γ1.

Recent data have also suggested that antibody therapy may enhance the efficacy of radiation therapy.[103,104] There is evidence of decreased DNA repair in breast cancer cell lines overexpressing HER2/Neu treated with recombinant humanized monoclonal antibodies against HER2 and radiation therapy; this effect is not seen in lines that do not overexpress HER2/Neu. Phase I studies with recurrent squamous cell cancer with C225 have demonstrated safety; further studies will be needed to assess whether the combination of antibody and radiation therapy is superior to radiation alone.

RADIOIMMUNOTHERAPY

Antibodies can also be used to deliver radioactive compounds to the cell.[105,106] RS7, a pancarcinoma IgG1 murine antibody radioconjugated to iodine-131 (^{131}I) has been studied in a murine model.[107] Animals with established 100 mm^3 tumors were treated with 250 µCi of labeled RS7. There was a 60% resolution of tumors within two weeks, followed by complete remissions (CRs). Seventy percent of animals treated with 270 µCi with 200–300 mm^3 tumors

achieved CRs. No significant systemic toxicity was observed.

DeNardo and colleagues have developed a humanized anti-adenocarcinoma antibody, chimeric L6 (ChL6).[108] It has been chelated with various radioisotopes, including ^{131}I, and tested in the clinical setting.[109,110] Initial phase I studies in patients with chemotherapy-refractory metastatic breast cancer demonstrated a 50% response rate; however, because of myelosuppression, particularly thrombocytopenia, doses of radiation could not be escalated above 60–70 mCi/m^2. More recent studies have escalated doses to 150 mCi/m^2, followed by autologous stem cell transplantation. The clinical course of three patients has been reported. Patients were given 200 mg of unconjugated antibody prior to ^{131}I-ChL6 treatment to block binding by normal vascular endothelium. Patients also received Lugol's solution beginning three days prior to and continuing for 14 days to block the uptake of radioactive iodine by the thyroid. One patient received only one course of therapy, because of progressive disease. Another patient received two cycles, but subsequently developed HAMA, without objective response. A third patient was able to receive three cycles of therapy with the addition of cyclosporine to inhibit the formation of HAMA. Cumulative radiation doses were calculated to be 3100 and 11 200 cGy to lungs and tumor respectively. This patient had an improvement in her performance status, a decline in her tumor markers, and relief of bone pain for nine months.

In a subsequent study, patients received up to four doses at monthly intervals of ^{131}I-ChL6 at doses of 20–70 mCi/m^2. Four of six patients treated at 60 mCi/m^2 were able to receive more than one cycle of therapy without experiencing grade 4 hematologic toxicity. Granulocyte colony-stimulating factor (G-CSF) at 5 µg/kg was added on days 7–17 in two other patients treated at this dose level. In these two heavily pretreated patients, the addition of G-CSF did not ameliorate the hematologic toxicity. Only one patient was treated at 70 mCi/m^2, with significant grade 4 hematologic toxicity developing during the fourth treatment cycle. There were four of ten patients who had a partial response lasting three weeks to five months, with an overall survival of 2.3–9.0 months.[111]

Utilizing a new conjugation method, this group is evaluating ^{90}Y-ChL6.[112] Yttrium-90 (^{90}Y) has more energetic β-emissions, and the conjugation method (DOTA) binds metallic radionuclides with quite exceptional stability. Therapy with this antibody and paclitaxel in a murine model utilizing human breast cancer xenografts has demonstrated synergistic activity.[113] This activity is schedule-dependent, with increased cures and complete responses when paclitaxel is delivered 6–24 h following antibody therapy, rather than when given prior to the antibody infusion.

Mucin may be an attractive target for radioimmunotherapy. For radioimmunotherapy to be effective, it is likely to require multiple doses. Therefore the antigen of interest should not be downmodulated, or cells selected out that are antigen-negative. Mc5, a murine antibody recognizing a tandem repeat of MUC-1, was radiolabeled with ^{131}I and tested in a human breast cancer xenograft model. Mice were treated when the grafts reached 100 mm^3 with a single dose of 1.5 mCi labeled antibody. Tumor growth was inhibited by 96% compared with controls at 26 days following treatment. Three of 18 animals treated every 22–25 days for four doses were cured of their tumors. On assessing for expression of MUC-1, there was no significant loss of expression.[114]

BrE-3, a MAb directed against human epithelial mucin, has also been investigated in the clinical setting.[115] Preclinical studies in immunodeficient murine models using human xenografts of tumors expressing intermediate to low levels of milk fat globule treated with ^{90}Y-labeled antibody, resulted in eradication of established tumors.[116] A phase I study was conducted employing escalating doses of ^{90}Y-BrE-3 in heavily pretreated metastatic breast cancer patients, whose tumors were reactive with BrE-3 antibody. In vivo the ^{90}Y dissociates from the antibody and becomes incorporated into bone, resulting in a higher radiation dose to the bone marrow tissue than to other tissues. To minimize hematologic toxicity, 15 days following treatment with 1.5 mg/m^2 BrE-3 labeled with 15 mCi/m^2 or 20 mCi/m^2 ^{90}Y, patients were reinfused with autologous stem cells or bone marrow and treated with G-CSF. Patients tolerated therapy well, without significant acute toxicities. The only severe delayed toxicities were hematologic. Patients at both dose levels developed grade 4 thrombocytopenia, while grade 4 neutropenia was only seen at the higher dose level. Patients simultaneously received ^{111}In-labeled antibody to determine localization of the antibody. Known areas of tumor were imaged in eight of the nine treated patients, including brain metastases in two of the patients. Four patients had partial responses; responding sites included lymph nodes, skin and bone marrow. Another patient had palliation of bone disease transiently, but no objective response. Further dose escalations are planned with this compound, and a humanized construct of this antibody is being developed.

Cytokine therapy has been combined with antibodies as a means of increasing the expression of tumor antigen. Interferon-α (IFN-α), for example, has been combined with the radiolabeled TAG-72 antibody CC49.[117] Patients were randomized to receive 3×10^6 U IFN-α subcutaneously daily for 14 days, or no interferon, followed by ^{131}I-labeled CC49. Patients receiving the interferon were found to have significant increases in their TAG-72 antigen expression by tumors, as well as improved localization of CC49 MAb. The efficacy of this therapy is undergoing study.

ANTIBODY–DRUG CONJUGATES

Systemic toxicity of cytotoxic chemotherapy may be reduced if the drug is targeted to the tumor directly via an antibody. This approach has been evaluated with daunorubicin (daunomycin),[118,119] doxorubicin,[120] methotrexate,[121,122] vinca alkaloids[123] and chlorambucil.[124] BR64 and BR96 are antibodies with specificity for Le^y antigen. They have been linked to doxorubicin via an acid-labile conjugation, to give BR64–DOX and BR96–DOX respectively. These conjugates release free doxorubicin when in the acidic environment of lysosomes or endosomes. This is an attractive approach for patients with breast cancer, since doxorubicin is considered the most active agent in breast cancer. The targeted delivery of doxorubicin to tumor cells expressing the Le^y antigen limits systemic toxicity, including cardiotoxicity, which often limits the amount of doxorubicin that can be used to treat patients. Preclinical models of BR64–DOX with human MCF7 breast carcinomas have demonstrated superior efficacy of the antibody conjugate compared with the antibody alone in both prolonged delay in tumor growth and in an increase in tumor regression and cures.[125]

The doxorubicin derivative maleimido-caproyl doxorubicin hydrazone has been conjugated to the human chimeric form of the BR96 MAb. This construct is stable in plasma, but when it is internalized into an acidic cellular compartment, doxorubicin is then liberated. Preclinical studies demonstrated complete and partial responses in mice bearing pre-existing MCF-7 carcinomas, with repeated doses being superior to single-dose therapy.[126] Human clinical trials with this agent have been performed.[127] Patients with advanced carcinomas expressing Le^y were treated weekly for three weeks with BR96–DOX. Doses were escalated to deliver 500 mg/m^2/week of antibody and 15 mg/m^2/week of doxorubicin. Dose-limiting toxicity was vomiting with hematemesis, caused by superficial hemorrhagic gastritis. The vomiting was dose-related, and unrelieved by antiemetic therapy, but was less severe with repetitive dosing. Minimal hematologic toxicity was observed, and no cardiovascular side-effects were seen. Owing to expression of Le^y on pancreatic tissues, patients were evaluated for evidence of pancreatitis; mild elevations of amylase and lipase were observed.

ANTIBODY-DIRECTED ENZYME PRODRUG THERAPY (ADEPT)

Another means to harness antibody therapy is the tumor delivery of enzymes that can activate prodrugs.[128] Antibody-directed enzyme prodrug therapy (ADEPT) allows for the antibody-mediated tumor localization of an enzyme, followed by the systemic delivery of a relatively non-toxic prodrug, which is enzymatically cleaved to its active form at the tumor site. This not only allows for the killing of the cells bound by the antibody, but also of adjacent tumor cells. The activated prodrug can also diffuse into the tumor mass more readily than the large antibody–enzyme conjugate, and allows for deeper penetration of the drug. The antibody may also be used to transport 'suicide enzymes', such as ribonucleases, deoxyribonucleases, or proteins with similar activities such as α-sarcin, mitogillin and colicins; these enzymes destroy RNA and DNA, resulting in the death of the cell.

An example of this strategy utilizes antibodies covalently linked to alkaline phosphatase (Aϕ) which can convert the prodrugs of etoposide, doxorubicin and mitomycin. L6, an antibody specific for a carbohydrate antigen on adenocarcinomas, and 1F5, which recognizes CD20 on B lymphocytes, have been conjugated to Aϕ and tested for their antitumor effects in vitro and in vivo.[129] Etoposide was 100-fold more toxic than etoposide phosphate when treating H3347 human colon cancer cells. In the presence of L6–Aϕ conjugated antibody, the cytotoxicity of etoposide phosphate was enhanced. Improved cytotoxicity was not observed using 1F5–Aϕ conjugate. The specific interaction of the relevant conjugate with H3347 cells is required for prodrug-enhanced cytotoxicity. In vivo studies demonstrated greater antitumor effects using L6–Aϕ with etoposide phosphate rather than etoposide alone, partially owing to the limited doses of etoposide that could be given because of host toxicity.

The prodrug 5-fluorocytosine (5-FC) is converted to 5-fluorouracil (5-FU) by cytosine deaminase, a microbial enzyme. This system has been evaluated in vivo with human adenocarcinomas treated with an antibody–enzyme conjugate (L6–CD) followed by 5-FC.[130] The maximum tolerated dose (MTD) of 5-FC was 2.4 g/kg when given without L6–CD, with no demonstrable serum levels of 5-FU. The MTD of 5-FC decreased to 120 mg/kg when animals were treated with L6–CD. The toxicity of 5-FC with antibody conjugate was decreased by clearing unbound L6–CD with an anti-idiotype antibody prior to administration of 5-FC, thus limiting conversion of 5-FC to 5-FU within the vascular compartment. Levels of 5-FU within tumor samples were 17 times higher in the conjugate-treated animals than in those treated with systemic 5-FU.

BISPECIFIC ANTIBODY THERAPY

Bispecific antibodies (BsAbs) have been developed by combining two antibodies with specificity for two tumor-associated antigens; alternatively, they have combined an antibody with specificity for a tumor antigen with one specific for a trigger molecule on an immune effector cell. Ring and colleagues screened BsAbs with specificity to mucin, three different glycoproteins, transferrin receptor and c-ErbB-2. In vitro assays employing the breast cancer cell line SKBR3 revealed greater than 30% growth inhibition using a BsAb with speci-

ficities for anti-c-ErbB-2 and anti-transferrin receptor.[67] When combined with the iron chelator deferoxamine, there was enhanced growth inhibition achieved with lower doses of antibody and deferoxamine than observed when either one is used alone.[131]

More extensive work has been done in the construction, evaluation and in vivo testing of bispecifics which target tumor-associated antigens and effector cells. These antibodies have targeted either T-cell receptors or Fcγ receptors found on antigen presenting cells (Table 10.3). These antibodies target effector cells to tumor cells, natural killer (NK) cells or macrophages (Mφ). When T-cell receptors are bound, the T-cell is activated, leading to the production of IFN-γ and TNF-α, which may be responsible for part of the bystander effect seen in animal models, where cytotoxicity is not restricted to cells bound by antibody. Binding of T-cell receptors by these antibodies triggers cytotoxicity regardless of the antigen specificity of the T cell.[132,133] Also, the T cells do not require binding of the major histocompatibility complex (MHC)

Table 10.3 Cytotoxic trigger molecules

Receptor	Location[a]	Cytotoxic trigger
FcγRI	Monocytes, PMN	Yes
FcγRII	PMN, monocytes, Mφ, B, T cells, dendritic cells, platelets	Yes
FcγRIIIA	NK cells, Mφ	Yes
FcγRIIIB	PMN	No
TCR/CD3	T cells	Yes
CD2	T cells	Yes
CD44	T cells	Yes
CD59	T cells	Yes
CD69	T cells	Yes

[a] PMN, polymorphonuclear neutrophils; Mφ, macrophages; NK, natural killer.

for activation; MHC expression is often down-regulated on tumor cells, resulting in inefficient presentation to the immune system.[134] In vitro, utilizing a bispecific antibody against EGP-2 and various T-cell receptors, CD3, CD5 or CD28, there was T-cell activation. When interleukin-2 (IL-2) was added, there was further activation of T cells. However, combinations of antibodies targeting all three receptors resulted in complete activation of T cells, which could not be further enhanced by IL-2. This observation may allow for optimal T-cell activation in vivo without the added toxicities of IL-2 therapy.[135]

Two BsAbs with specificity for FcγR and c-ErbB-2 have been characterized and are undergoing clinical trials. MDX–H2A is the fusion of two murine MAbs: MAb22, which recognizes FcγRI, and 520C9, which is specific for c-ErbB-2.[136] The binding site of MAb22 to FcγRI is distinct from that for the human Fc portion of Ig molecules. This allows for binding of the Fc receptor in vivo even if the receptor is occupied by an Ig molecule, while retaining FcγRI-dependent functions such as antibody-dependent cell-mediated cytotoxicity (ADCC), phagocytosis, superoxide generation and enzyme release. In vivo assays of polymorphonuclear neutrophils (PMN) and monocytes from patients with G-CSF showed an upregulation of FcγRI compared with control samples from patients not treated with G-CSF. Based on the observation of an increased effector cell population with G-CSF therapy, clinical trials using HER2/Neu × FcγRI bispecific antibodies[137] have been conducted. MDX–H210, a half-humanized bispecific antibody targeting FcγRI and HER2/Neu, was given weekly for four treatments. Therapy was tolerated without any dose-limiting toxicity up to 20 mg/m². Seven of ten patients had stable disease.[138]

In a phase Ia/Ib trial, patients with advanced breast and ovarian cancer overexpressing c-ErbB-2 were given one dose of antibody. Most patients developed fever and mild hypotension. One-third of patients were noted to have a one- to twofold increase in transaminases 48–72 h following therapy, which resolved spontaneously by days 4–7. Rapid, transient decreases

in monocytes were also observed. With increasing doses from 0.35 to 10 mg/m², an increasing percentage of monocytes bound BsAb. TNF-α levels increased, but not in a dose-dependent manner, during hours 1–3. Subsequently, IL-6 and G-CSF increased from 3 to 6 h post infusion; their secretion required a threshold dose of antibody, but levels did not rise at higher antibody doses. Biopsies demonstrated mononuclear cell infiltrates and antibody localization 48 h following infusion. Ten patients were evaluable for clinical responses. One patient with breast cancer noted a tumor flare and erythema following injection, and subsequently had a decrease in the size of subcutaneous metastases and axillary adenopathy. A lymphangitic lung infiltrate in this patient remained unchanged. Another patient with ovarian cancer had a 50% reduction in cervical lymph nodes, but progression of intraabdominal disease was demonstrated by the development of intestinal obstruction.

Preclinical data have demonstrated the ability of bispecific antibodies that bind tumor and FcγRIII to redirect lysis by large granular lymphocytes in the presence of competing human Ig.[139,140] We have evaluated 2B1, which recognizes c-ErbB-2 and FcγRIII.[141] In a phase I study, patients with c-ErbB-2-overexpressing tumors were treated with six infusions of antibody over eight days, within minimal toxicities.[142] Immune activation was demonstrated by increases in circulating TNF-α, IL-6 IL-8, and to a lesser extent granulocyte–monocyte colony-stimulating factor (GM-CSF) and IFN-α. A unique observation made in this group of patients was the development of an antibody response against the intracellular domain of c-ErbB-2.[143] These results suggest that BsAb-promoted cytolysis led to processing of c-ErbB-2 via FcγRIII, leading to antigen presentation. This would suggest that 2B1 therapy can immunize patients in vivo against c-ErbB-2.

Various groups are developing smaller bispecific antibody constructs to optimize penetration into tumor tissues. One such construct is the CD3/17-1A bispecific molecules constructed by linking the variable heavy- and light-chain domains of antibodies with specificity for CD3, the T-cell receptor, and for the EGP-2 antigen found on many carcinomas of epithelial origin.[144]

IMMUNOTOXINS

An immunotoxin (IT) is an engineered drug that consists of a targeting monoclonal antibody linked to a protein toxin.[145] ITs were originally constructed using chemical crosslinking agents to couple the toxin to the antibody, resulting in a large protein structure with a molecular mass of 175 000 kDa or more. More recently, ITs have been cloned and expressed in bacterial expression systems as single-chain IT fusion proteins linking the variable region of the antibody to the toxin.[146] The antibody component binds to the target on the malignant cell and is internalized, and the toxin or drug incapacitates the cell. Many compounds have been developed targeting various antigens linked to several different toxins as outlined in Table 10.4.

The toxins used most commonly have been ricin, diphtheria toxin (DT) and *Pseudomonas* exotoxin (PE). Ricin and DT contain two chains: A and B. In ricin, the A chain is responsible for the toxic effects via N-glycosidase activity, which inactivates the 60S ribosomal subunit.[147] The A chain of DT and domain 3 of PE have adenosine diphosphate ribosylation activity, which inactivates ribosomal elongation factor 2, and inhibits protein translation.[148,149] The B chains and domains 1 and 2 of PE are required for toxin binding to the cell surface and translocation to the correct cytoplasmic compartment.

Initial constructs with ricin and DT isolated the A chain by reduction of the disulfide bonds between the two chains.[150] PE was treated with

Table 10.4 Immunotoxins

Target	Antibody	Toxin[a]	Ref
Breast mucins	B3 (Fv)	PE38	228
	B3 (Fab)	PE38[M]	229
Lewis[y]	BR96sFv	PE40	174
EGFR	DAB$_{389}$EGF	DT	230
c-ErbB-2	scFv (FRP5)	ETA	231
	e23	PE	232
	W900H1	SAP	233
	W800E0	PE	233
Transferrin receptor	HB21	PE	234
	TFR (Fv)	PE40/DT	235
	E6	PE/DT/EDN	236, 237
	454A12	Ricin A chain	232
	5E9	Gelonin	238
55 kDa protein on breast cancer cells	260F9	Ricin A chain	168, 239
42 kDa protein on breast cancer cells	317G5	Ricin A chain	240

[a] PE, *Pseudomonas* exotoxin; DT, diphtheria toxin; ETA, exotoxin A; SAP, sapronin; EDN, eosinophil-derived neurotoxin.

2-iminothiolane, which reduced its binding to the PE receptor cell surfaces, but also allowed conjugation to antibody structures.[151] With the development of cloning techniques, genetically engineered constructs include sequences for binding and translocation, but delete portions irrelevant to the toxic event. For example, mutant forms of DT are more effective than those with the A chain alone, because they contain the translocation sequences.[152,153] This strategy has not always been successful, because of poor internalization or inappropriate intracellular translocation. Recombinant ITs, engineered with specific intracellular translocation sequences, can target the appropriate intracellular compartment where the toxin is active.[154,155] Other 'toxins' employed include chemotherapeutic agents and cytokines.[156]

Preclinical data in vitro and in vivo and human clinical trials have identified challenges to the successful clinical use of ITs. Selecting an epitope on the antigen of interest closer to the cell surface appears to aid in improved internalization.[157–159] Immunotoxins have also been found to have limited in vivo stability owing to rapid clearance by the liver. Strategies have been developed to limit the recognition of the glycosylated proteins by the reticuloendotheial system,[160–162] reduction of the proteins by glutathione,[163] and complex formation with α_2-macroglobulin.[164] The large size of the initial constructs composed of whole MAbs and intact toxin proteins limited their ability to penetrate tumors; molecules are now being generated with sFv linked to the active moiety of the toxin. Treatment with ITs has been associated with unanticipated toxicities.[165–168] The development of humoral responses has limited the ability to give repeated doses of the drugs. Other common toxicities have included fever, anorexia, malaise, arthralgias and myalgias. A vascular leak syndrome characterized by weight gain, edema, dyspnea and hypoalbuminemia was seen in several studies utilizing different antibodies. The syndrome has been hypothesized to be due to endothelial damage secondary to high concentrations of toxin,[169] and others have demonstrated binding of the immunotoxin to Fc receptors on monocytes,

which may induce the release of vasoactive compounds.[168] Neurologic toxicities, including sensorimotor neuropathies associated with axonal loss and demyelination, have also been observed. Cases of rhabdomyolysis and acrocyanosis, manifested as reversible distal digital skin necrosis, have also been reported.[170]

One IT that has been successfully developed is based on BR96,[171] a murine IgG3 MAb that recognizes the Le^y antigen. This antibody was found to be tumor-selective; initial screens of the antibody revealed that it bound to a myriad of neoplasms, but to a limited number of normal tissues; including the esophagus, stomach and intestines, as well as acinar cells of the pancreas. It is rapidly internalized into lysosomes and endosomes by tumor cells, and is able to mediate both antibody and complement-dependent cytotoxicity, growth inhibition, and cell death.

BR96 sFv has been conjugated to PE40[172] (BR96 sFv–PE40) and also to doxorubicin[127] (BR96–DOX: see the earlier discussion on antibody–drug conjugates). When this IT binds to cells bearing Le^y, protein synthesis is inhibited in a manner dependent upon the number of surface receptors.[173] BR96 sFv-PE40 has also been evaluated in murine and rat xenograft models using the human breast carcinoma cell line H3396[172] and MCF-7.[174] The IT is capable of eliminating tumors in a dose- and schedule-dependent manner. Large tumors were cured when treated with 0.625 mg/kg intravenously every four days for a total of five doses. Preclinical toxicology studies revealed hepatotoxicity and vascular leak syndrome, which could be abrogated by premedicating with dexamethasone.[175] Other constructs targeting c-ErbB-2 are under development.[176]

Another approach to targeted therapy links the therapeutic agent to the natural ligand for a receptor found on cancer cells. For example, heregulin binds HER3[177] and HER4.[178] The fusion protein HAR–TX β2 joins a chimeric heregulin β2 ligand with PE40.[179] The fusion protein binds to, and is cytotoxic to, breast cancer cells that express the heregulin ligands on their surface. This binding requires the presence of HER4 for the cytotoxic effect, although the fusion protein can bind to cells that express only HER3.[180] Another construct, HRGβ2/PE40, was found to be cytotoxic in cell lines with c-ErbB-3 alone or in conjunction with c-ErbB-2 or c-ErbB-4, as well as cells expressing c-ErbB-4 alone.[181]

The intracellular target of the toxin can also be targeted. Early ITs with PE were found to be inactive when the ligand was placed at the carboxy terminus of PE. Analysis revealed that the amino acids at the end of the molecule, REDLK, are critical for the cytotoxicity of the molecule. These critical amino acids were changed to a similar sequence, KDEL, known to retain proteins in the lumen of the endoplasmic reticulum, where protein synthesis occurs. Constructs combining an sFv directed against the IL-2 receptor and PE, PE–KDEL or PE–(KDEL)$_3$ were compared. There was two or three times greater cytotoxicity in vitro and in vivo with the PE–KDEL molecules than with PE alone.[182]

NEW STRUCTURES FOR ANTIBODY-BASED TUMOR TARGETING

The tumor-targeting vehicle has been evaluated as a means to increase delivery of antibody to tumor. Recent advances in the formulation of liposomes have resulted in their decreased uptake by the reticuloendothelial system, thus increasing their circulation time.[183] A humanized anti-c-ErbB-2 Fab' fragment, derived from the antiproliferative antibody rhuMAb HER2, has been formulated in liposomes with or without doxorubicin.[184] In vitro, these conjugates demonstrate specific binding to and internalization by c-ErbB-2-overexpressing tumors. Liposomes have also been formulated to contain both the antibody fragment and doxorubicin. In a murine model, doxorubicin was shown to be specifically targeted to a human breast cancer xenograft.

The newest approach to altering tumor growth using antibodies is the use of intrabodies, which are intracellular antibodies synthesized by the cell and targeted to inactivate specific proteins within specific compartments of the cell.[185] The first example of this techno-

logy in cancer therapy derives from Deshane and colleagues, who have developed a plasmid encoding as scFv that binds c-ErbB-2 within the endoplasmic reticulum. The plasmid was introduced into tumor cells using a modified adenovirus vector. The downregulation of cell surface receptor resulted in loss of the transformed phenotype. Using this strategy, a human ovarian cancer cell line lost its ability to form colonies in soft agar, and subcutaneous xenografts of this tumor line were eradicated.[186]

More recently, ribonucleases (RNases) have been evaluated as candidate toxins.[187,188] RNases from eosinophils[189,190] and pancreatic tissue[191] have been found to be cytotoxic to mammalian cells and to prolong survival in animal tumor models. Rybak and colleagues have initially evaluated bovine pancreatic ribonuclease A, and more recently angiogenin, a human protein with homology to pancreatic RNase. Angiogenin has been linked to an anti-transferrin antibody (CH2.5–Ang). CH2.5–Ang supernatants selectively inhibit protein synthesis of cells from the leukemia cell line K562 by 50% following a 24 h incubation. This toxicity could be blocked by adding excess parental antibody to the supernatant. These observations suggest that CH2.5–Ang is effective only when it is internalized into cells. Angiogenin is an attractive toxin to employ, since it is of human origin and should not be as immunogenic as catalytic toxins derived from prokaryotes.

Another approach has been to modify T cells to specifically recognize the antigen of interest. The T-cell receptor contains α/β heterodimers that provide the specificity for the binding of the T cell. These chains are complexed with invariant CD3γ, δ, ε and ζ chains. Studies have demonstrated that crosslinking of the ζ chain leads to signaling of the T-cell receptor. In an attempt to make a T cell with particular specificity, the ζ-chain gene linked to a sFv that recognizes c-ErbB-2 was transfected into cytotoxic T lymphocytes (CTL).[192] In vitro, the transfected T cells are stimulated specifically by c-ErbB-2 and are capable of lysing tumor cells expressing c-ErbB-2 irrespective of the presence of MHC molecules. The transfected T cells have been shown to be active in a nude mouse model. Tumors decreased in size, but were not completely eradicated when transfected CTL were given to tumor-bearing mice – this may be due to an insufficient number of transfected T cells within the tumor.

VACCINE THERAPY

Since the discovery of immunization techniques, vaccines to prevent cancer recurrence have been sought. Unlike infections, cancers arise from cells that the immune system recognizes as self, and therefore does not usually find immunogenic. Attempts at vaccination utilizing irradiated autologous tumor cells or cell lysates mixed with adjuvants have for the most part been unsuccessful in the tumor systems in which they have been tried. A small number of antigens have been identified that appear to be tumor-specific and have been recognized by humoral immune responses in cancer patients. These include glycolipids (T, Tn, sialyl-Tn),[193] glycoproteins (MUC1),[194] and cell cycle or signal transduction proteins (HER2/Neu, p53).[195,196] Other antigens that have been evaluated are proteins expressed on tumor cells, which had been expressed at an embryonic stage, such as CEA. A new approach employs vaccination with heat-shock proteins.[197] Cells, when stressed by heat or glucose deprivation, express a series of proteins that are capable of eliciting T-cell responses. Alternatively, vaccincation utilizing DNA of an antigen of interest has also been evaluated.

Vaccines are utilized to present an antigen to the immune system so that a humoral and/or cellular response develops. The antigen must be incorporated, processed and presented by an antigen-presenting cell (APC) such as a dendritic cell, macrophage or monocyte. APCs present antigens to T cells to stimulate a cellular response, and to B cells to induce a humoral response. Processing of the antigen involves uptake of the antigen followed by proteolytic cleavage of the protein. Peptide fragments are then presented on the cell surface in a groove of the MHC receptor. There are ongoing investigations in many laboratories determining the antigenic epitopes associated with different MHC receptors.

There has recently been interest in targeting cellular responses, since many preclinical in vivo studies suggest that T cells are more effective in causing tumor regressions than is antibody production by B-cell-mediated humoral responses. When an antigen is presented to a naive CD4[+] T cell, two signals are required for the T cell to be stimulated to divide and differentiate to produce an adaptive immune response.[198] An APC presents the protein antigen as peptide fragments in the groove of an MHC molecule to the T-cell receptor. CD8[+] T cells recognize 8- to 10-amino-acid peptides within the groove of MHC class I molecules. These peptides are derived from proteins degraded intracellularly by the APC.[199] CD4[+] T cells recognize peptides 13–18 amino acids in length from the extracellular environment that are presented via MHC class II molecules.

The role of tumor cell vaccines in an adjuvant setting has been evaluated in breast cancer.[200] Patients with stage II breast cancer were randomized to receive cyclophosphamide, methotrexate and 5-FU (CMF), CMF with Bacille Calmette–Guérin (BCG), or CMF with BCG and allogeneic tumor cell vaccines. The tumor cell vaccines were derived from the breast cancer cell lines MDA-MB-157, MDA-MB-231 and 631. Patients received CMF every four weeks. BCG was given as four intradermal injections weekly from week 3 to week 13, and then every other week for two years. Those receiving BCG and tumor vaccine received the injection on week 3 as 20 intradermal injections in the axilla and lower abdomen. The first vaccination consisted of 10^8 irradiated cells. On week 5, the patients received the same number of cells, which were unirradiated. Starting with week 7, the dose was decreased to 10^7 cells, given weekly until week 15, at which time it was decreased to every other week for a year. Toxicities included increased fatigue with BCG. Patients receiving tumor cell vaccine developed ulceration at at least one site of injection, and many had multiple draining sites. The vaccine arm was suspended when 14 of 41 patients contracted hepatitis B, thought to be due to contaminated human A-gamma serum used in the processing of the vaccine. Patients were followed for five years. There were no statistically significant differences in the recurrence rate and overall survival at that time in the tumor vaccine group.

One epitope that has been investigated in tumor vaccines is derived from cell surface mucin molecules. Utilizing a breast cancer murine model, Longenecker and his colleagues have demonstrated specific humoral and cellular responses to mucin epitopes when animals were immunized with sialyl-Tn.[201] Prior to vaccination, animals were pretreated with low doses of cyclophosphamide to eliminate T-suppresser lymphocytes. A phase I clinical trial has been conducted in patients with metastatic breast cancer.[202] Patients were treated with 300 mg/m^2 of cyclophosphamide three days prior to vaccination. Sialyl-Tn conjugated to keyhole limpet hemocyanin at doses of 25, 100 or 500 µg was mixed with DETOX adjuvant and injected in two divided doses. Four patients received 25 µg and six patients 100 µg given at two-weekly intervals; one patient received a dose of 500 µg, which had to be reduced to 25 µg on subsequent immunizations because of an extensive delayed-type hypersensitivity (DTH) reaction. Patients received between two and eight immunizations. Titers of both IgM (1:640 to 1:10 240) and IgG (1:160 to 1:20 480) against sialyl-Tn documented the development of a humoral response. Ten of the twelve patients' sera following immunization showed enhanced in vitro complement-mediated cytotoxicity. Therapy was well tolerated, apart from DTH reactions, which usually occurred 24–48 h following the initial injection. Half of the patients had recall reactions at injection sites following subsequent immunizations. Five of the patients developed fluctuant granulomas at their injection sites 2–10 weeks following injection, which subsequently ulcerated. Patients had minimal nausea and vomiting with the cyclophosphamide. Three patients with extensive disease had progression while on therapy, although one of these patients had a mixed response, with disappearance of cutaneous chest wall disease but progression of pleuropulmonary disease. Another patient with lymph node metastases also had a mixed response, with resolution of supraclavicular adenopathy, stable disease in other neck lymph nodes, but progression of axillary lymph nodes. Two patients had stable pulmonary metastases 13 and 15 months following therapy, although one of these patients was found to have brain metastases 3.5 months following therapy. Two patients had partial responses of lung nodules and cervical adenopathy.

Several approaches to vaccination against CEA have been studied. Based on the network hypothesis of Lindenmann and Jerne,[203,204] exposure to a foreign antigen results in the production of an antibody response, Ab1, with specificity for the antigen. A subsequent Ab2 response may occur against the antigen-specific portions of Ab1, which now resembles portions of the original antigen. This Ab2 has been termed an anti-idiotypic antibody; immunizing patients with Ab2 provides the specific immunologic epitope to be presented. This approach has the potential advantages of allowing for immunization of antigens that are not readily available in sufficient quantity or purity, or when the antigen is not protein.[205]

Foon et al[206] have utilized 3H1, a murine monoclonal anti-idiotypic antibody against CEA in patients with CEA-positive advanced colorectal carcinomas. Patients were treated every other week with intracutaneous injections of 1, 2 or 4 mg of precipitated antibody for a total of four doses. Following immunization, the sera from 9 of 12 patients contained antibodies against 3H1. These newly generated antibodies were able to bind to autologous and allogeneic tumor samples positive for CEA. Seven of twelve patients demonstrated specific CD4$^+$ T-cell proliferation responses to 3H1 following immunization that had been absent prior to therapy. However, these immunologic responses were not accompanied by demonstrable clinical responses. Therapy was complicated by mild local reactions at the injection site, fever and chills.

Antibody-based therapies have also induced the development of an anti-idiotypic antibody response[207] that has been demonstrated to correlate with clinical outcome.[208,209] One mechanism that has been proposed for this benefit is the induction of a T-cell response with specificity for the induced Ab2. Twenty-four patients with metastatic colorectal cancer were treated with murine monoclonal antibody 17-1A and evaluated prospectively for T-cell responses.[210] At baseline, three patients had T-cell responses with specificity for Ab2. Following therapy, two of the three demonstrated augmented responses, whereas the third patient lost the T-cell response. Four patients, initially without a T-cell response, developed a response. The five patients who demonstrated a clinical benefit from therapy – four with a new response and one with an augmented response – all had T-cell induction or augmentation from baseline.

Polynucleotide vaccine therapy involves intramuscular injections with plasmid DNA in non-replicating vectors. Preclinical mouse studies have examined the dose schedule of CEA cDNA in a cytomegaloviral plasmid with the early promoter/enhancer.[211,212] A threshold dose of 50 µg of DNA given one to three times weekly was required to produce consistent humoral and cellular responses. Immunized animals were able to withstand challenges by inoculation with CEA-expressing tumors. Several hypotheses have been generated to explain the mechanism whereby these polynucleotide vaccines may work. First, the myocytes may function as APCs with intracellular synthesis of CEA with subsequent MHC class I peptide display; this would elicit T-cell activation and cell surface expression of the antigen, resulting in a B-cell response as well. Alternatively, the myocytes may serve as a source of CEA for draining lymph nodes. CEA would be recognized by B cells and processed by APCs for presentation to T cells. Both mechanisms may play a role, with an initial response within the lymph node to intact CEA and a booster effect by the myocytes expressing CEA. As this vector is non-replicating, yet is able to elicit humoral and cellular responses without the use of adjuvants, it has potential advantages over other vector-based vaccine strategies. Further preclinical studies are ongoing in animals with preexisting colon and breast tumors, as well as phase I clinical trials in patients with colorectal carcinoma.

CEA can also be expressed by viral vectors containing the cDNA for CEA. One such construct has utilized a vaccinia virus vector (rV–CEA).[213] In animal studies, mice were both protected from tumor challenge and showed tumor regression following vaccination with rV–CEA.[214] This vaccine has also elicited specific T-cell responses in mice, non-human primates and patients with advanced colorectal carcinoma.[215] To enhance response to vaccination with this construct, preclinical studies are focusing on the coadministration of agents that can enhance the efficacy of vaccination. When mice with palpable tumors are vaccinated with one dose of 10^7 plaque-forming units (pfu) rV–CEA, there is complete regression of tumors in 20% of animals. When mice received five days of intraperitoneal (i.p.) injections of 1 µg of IL-2 starting three days after vaccination, there was a 60% rate of complete tumor regression. Doses of 0.1 µg and 5 µg were not as effective, with 10% and 30% complete regression respectively.[216]

B7 is a costimulatory molecule that binds to CD28 on T cells, resulting in the production of IL-2 and IFN-γ by a T-helper 1 (Th1) cellular response. IL-2 from this interaction is important for the induction of an antigen-specific cytotoxic T-cell response. Tumor cells that have been transfected with B7 can induce a specific T-cell response in the absence of Th1 lymphocytes. Hodge et al[217] vaccinated tumor-bearing mice with varying ratios of vaccinia vectors containing CEA (rV–CEA) and B7 (rV–B7). They examined T-cell responses, and found a dose-dependent response when the mice were vaccinated with rV–CEA and control vector, but no response when they were vaccinated with rV–B7 and control vector. However, animals receiving rV–CEA and rV–B7 had increased T-cell lymphoproliferative responses especially at a 3:1 ratio of rV–CEA to rV–B7. There were also similar trends with in vitro cytotoxicity assays using CEA-bearing tumor cells. Clinical trials utilizing this approach are now being completed.

Mutant Ras epitopes have been analyzed in vitro for their ability to induce cytolytic T cells. Peptides have been shown to induce a T-cell response when presented via class I or class II MHC molecules and cytolytic T cells.[218,219] MHC class I restricted T cells with specificity for a Ras peptide have been shown to protect mice from challenge with a *ras*-expressing tumor.[220]

The use of heat-shock proteins (HSPs) in vaccinations may have advantages over other approaches. Although HSPs are not antigenic themselves, they complex with a wide variety of tumor-related proteins. HSPs are non-polymeric, and bind to the antigenic proteins irrespective of MHC haplotype; this allows vaccines derived in this manner to be used in the entire population. It is unnecessary to determine the specific antigen(s) in formulating the vaccine, since homogeneous HSP-peptide complexes can be purified easily. HSP-peptide vaccines are also multivalent, presenting more than one epitope for immunologic recognition. This approach also allows for the development of individualized vaccines by extracting HSP from individual tumor samples. Preclinical models have evaluated immunizations with HSPs.[221,222] There was a dose-dependent protection against tumor challenge on immunizing against HSP derived from tumor cells, which was not seen when HSP derived from normal tissues was used to immunize animals. This protection is derived from the induction of MHC I restricted CTLs.

A new trend in vaccine strategies has come from observations in animal studies in which tumors have been transfected with genes for various cytokines, including growth factors and interleukins. The immunization of tumor-bearing animals with such gene-modified tumors has led to the eradication of many tumors and demonstration of antitumor immune responses. Attempts to employ these strategies in the clinical setting are ongoing, utilizing retroviral vectors as vehicles for the delivery of the cytokines.

Another approach to vaccination involves the immunization of patients with APCs that present the immunogen against which an immune response is desired. Using peptide-pulsed dendritic cells, T-cell-dependent responses can be stimulated. Following the demonstration that CD34$^+$ cells can differentiate into dendritic cells in the presence of TNF-α

and GM-CSF, this strategy has become much more feasible. In vitro, it has been shown to be effective in presenting peptide sequences derived from c-ErbB-2, and is currently being evaluated in patients with stage III and IV breast cancer.[223]

The development of vaccine strategies may add to the armementarium of therapeutic options for breast cancer patients, particularly as part of adjuvant therapy. As many of the epitopes being chosen as targets are not unique to cancer cells, there is the potential for the development of an autoimmune response. Initial trials to date have not demonstrated such a response. However, in an in vivo murine model system, immunizing with a cDNA vaccine expressing rat HER2/*neu*, there was an increase in the fetal loss in pregnant females that had been successfully vaccinated, in contrast to unvaccinated controls. There was no evidence of autoimuune responses within epithelial tissues, where low levels of HER2/*neu* are found in intestines and in the kidney.[224]

CONCLUSIONS

The past decade has seen an increased understanding of immune recognition and processing of antigens. This new knowledge, combined with advances in recombinant technology, has led to the production of a wide array of new agents. Antibody-based agents have improved targeting capabilities and have been combined with new therapeutic moieties. We have moved into a new therapeutic era with the documented efficacy of Herceptin as a single agent and in combination with chemotherapy. Vaccine strategies have a wealth of new immunogenic agents to be evaluated. Most encouraging is the evidence from recent clinical trials that these immunologic agents are effective in breast cancer patients. These results lead to renewed enthusiasm that new immunologic agents and strategies will find a role in the therapy of breast cancer patients.

REFERENCES

1. Schouten LJM, Straatman H, Kiemeney LALM, Verbeck ALM, Cancer incidence: life table risk versus cumulative risk. *J Epidemiol Comm Health* 1994; **48:** 596–600.

2. Early Breast Cancer Trialists' Collaborative Group, Systemic treatment of early breast cancer by hormonal, cytotoxic or immunotherapy: 133 randomized trials involving 31,000 recurrences and 24,000 deaths among 75,000 women. *Lancet* 1992; **339:** 1–15, 71–85.

3. Lupu R, Cardillo M, Harris L et al, Interaction between erbB-receptors and heregulin in breast cancer tumor progression and drug resistance. *Semin Cancer Biol* 1995; **6:** 135–45.

4. Schubert D, Heinemann S, Carlisle W et al, Clonal cell lines from the rat central nervous system. *Nature* 1974; **249:** 224–7.

5. King CR, Kraus MH, Aaronson SA, Amplification of a novel c-*erb*B-related gene in a human mammary carcinoma. *Science* 1985; **229:** 974–6.

6. Coussens L, Yang-Feng TL, Liao YC et al, Tyrosine kinase receptor with extensive homology to EGF receptor shares chromosomal location with *neu* oncogene. *Science* 1985; **230:** 1132–9.

7. Yamamoto T, Ikawa S, Akiyama T et al, Similarity of protein encoded by the human c-*erb*B-2 gene to epidermal growth factor receptor. *Nature* 1986; **319:** 230–7.

8. DiFore PP, Pierce JH, Kraus MH et al, *erb*B-2 is a potent oncogene when over-expressed in NIH/3T3 cells. *Science* 1989; **237:** 178–82.

9. Hudziak RM, Schlessinger J, Ullrich A, Increased expression of the putative growth factor receptor p185 HER2 causes transformation and tumorigenesis of NIH/3T3 cells. *Proc Natl Acad Sci USA* 1987; **84:** 7159–63.

10. Wallasch C, Weiß FU, Niederfellner G et al, Heregulin-dependent regulation of HER2/*neu* oncogene is signaling by heterodimerization with HER3. *EMBO J* 1995; **14:** 4267–75.

11. Plowman GD, Green JM, Culouscou JM et al, Heregulin induces tyrosine phosphorylation of HER2/P180erbB4. *Nature* 1993; **366:** 473–5.

12. Schechter AL, Stern DF, Vaidyanathan L et al, The *neu*-oncogene: an *erb*B related gene encoding a 185,000 Mr tumor antigen. *Nature* 1984; **312:** 513–16.

13. Bargmann CI, Hung M-C, Weinberg RA, Multiple independent activations of the *neu* oncogene by a point mutation altering the transmembrane domain of p185. *Cell* 1986; **45:** 649–57.

14. Scott GK, Robles R, Park JW et al, A truncated intracellular HER2/*neu* receptor produced by alternative RNA processing affects growth of human carcinoma cells. *Mol Cell Biol* 1993; **13:** 2247–57.

15. Press MF, Cordon-Cardo C, Slamon DJ, Expression of the HER-2/*neu* proto-oncogene in normal human and fetal tissues. *Oncogene* 1990; **5:** 953–62.

16. Cohen JA, Weiner DB, More KF et al, Expression pattern of the *neu* (NGL) gene-encoded growth factor receptor protein (p185^{neu}) in normal and transformed epithelial tissues. *Oncogene* 1989; **4:** 81–8.

17. McGuire HC Jr, Greene MI, The *neu* (c-erbB-2) oncogene. *Semin Oncol* 1989; **16:** 148–55.

18. Tahara E, Growth factors and oncogenes in human gastrointestinal carcinomas. *J Cancer Res Clin Oncol* 1990; **116:** 121–31.

19. Schneider PM, Hung MC, Chiocca SM, Differential expression of the c-erbB-2 gene in human small cell and non-small cell lung cancer. *Cancer Res* 1989; **49:** 4968–71.

20. Haldane JS, Hird V, Hughes CM, c-erbB-2 oncogene in ovarian cancer. *J Pathol* 1990; **162:** 231–7.

21. Frankel AE, Ring DB, Tringale F, Tissue distribution of breast cancer-associated antigens defined by monoclonal antibodies. *J Biol Resp Modif* 1985; **4:** 273–86.

22. Klijn JGM, Berns PMJJ, Schmitz PIM, Foekens JA, The clinical significance of epidermal growth factor receptor (EGFR) in human breast cancer: a review of 5232 patients. *Endocrine Rev* 1992; **13:** 3–17.

23. Salmon DS, Kim N, Saeki T, Ciardiello F, Transforming growth factor-α: an oncodevelopmental growth factor. *Cancer Cells* 1990; **2:** 389–97.

24. Barrett-Lee PJ, Travers MT, Lugmani Y, Coombs RC, Transcripts for transforming growth factors in human breast cancer: clinical correlates. *Br J Cancer* 1990; **61:** 612–17.

25. Lundy J, Scuss A, Stanick D et al, Expression of *neu* protein, EGF and TGFα in breast cancer. *Am J Pathol* 1991; **138:** 1527–34.

26. Ciardiello F, McGeady ML, Kim N et al, Transforming growth factor-α expression is enhanced by an activated c-Ha-*ras* protooncogene but not by c-*neu* protooncogene, and overexpression of the transforming growth factor-α

complementary DNA leads to transformation. *Cell Growth Diff* 1990; **1:** 407–20.

27. Gold O, Freedman SO, Demonstration of tumor specific antigens in human colonic carcinomata by immunological tolerance and absorption techniques. *J Exp Med* 1965; **121:** 439–62.

28. Zimmerman W, Weber B, Ortlieb B et al, Chromosomal localization of the carcinoembryonic antigen gene family and differential expression in various tissues. *Cancer Res* 1988; **48:** 2550–4.

29. Thompson J, Zimmerman W, The carcinoembryonic antigen gene family: structure, expression, and evolution. *Tumour Biol* 1988; **9:** 63–83.

30. Benchinol S, Fuks A, Jothy S et al, Carcinoembryonic antigen, a human tumor marker functions as an intercellular adhesion molecule. *Cell* 1989; **57:** 327–34.

31. Kuhajda FP, Offutt LE, Mendelsohn G, The distribution of carcinoembryonic antigen in breast carcinoma. Diagnostic and prognostic implications. *Cancer* 1983; **52:** 1257–64.

32. Hanisch FF, Uhlenbruek G, Egge H, Peter-Katalinic J, A B72.3 second-generation monoclonal antibody (CC49) defines the mucin-carried carbohydrate epitope Galβ(1→3) [NeuAcα(2→6)]. *Biol Chem* 1989; **370:** 21–6.

33. Springer GF, T and Tn, general carcinoma autoantigens. *Science* 1984; **224:** 1198–206.

34. Moldenhauer G, Momburg F, Moller P et al, Epithelium-specific surface glycoprotein of M_r 34,000 is a widely distributed human carcinoma marker. *Br J Cancer* 1987; **56:** 714–21.

35. Perz MS, Walker LE, Isolation and characterization of a cDNA encoding the KS1/4 epithelial carcinoma marker. *J Immunol* 1989; **142:** 3662–7.

36. Simon B, Podolsky DK, Moldenhauer G et al, Epithelial glycoprotein is a member of a family of epithelial-cell surface antigens homologous to nidogen, a matrix adhesion protein. *Proc Natl Acad Sci USA* 1990; **87:** 2755–9.

37. Litvinov SV, Velders MP, Bakker HAM et al, Ep-CAM: a human epithelial antigen is a homophilic cell–cell adhesion molecule. *J Cell Biol* 1994; **125:** 437–46.

38. Cook JD, Skikne BS, Baynes RD, Serum transferrin receptor. *Annu Rev Med* 1993; **44:** 63–74.

39. Elliott RL, Elliott MC, Wang F, Head JF, Breast carcinoma and the role of iron metabolism. A cytochemical, tissue culture, and ultrastructural study. *Ann NY Acad Sci* 1993; **698:** 159–66.

40. Bos JL, *Ras* oncogenes in human cancer. A review. *Cancer Res* 1989; **49:** 4682–9.

41. Bourne HR, Sanders DA, McCormick F, The GTPase superfamily: a conserved switch for diverse cell functions. *Nature* 1990; **348:** 125–32.

42. Stavnezer E, Fogh I, Wigler MH, Three human transforming genes are related to the viral *ras* oncogenes. *Proc Natl Acad Sci USA* 1983; **80:** 2112–16.

43. Abrams SI, Hand PH, Tsang KY, Schlom J, Mutant *ras* epitopes as targets for cancer vaccines. *Semin Oncol* 1996; **23:** 118–34.

44. Chang EH, Furth ME, Scolnick EM, Lowy DR, Tumorigenic transformation of mammalian cells induced by a normal human gene homologous to the oncogene of Harvey sarcoma virus. *Nature* 1982; **297:** 479–83.

45. Gulbis B, Galand P, Immunodetection of the p21-*ras* products in human normal and preneoplastic tissues and solid tumors: a review. *Human Pathol* 1993; **24:** 1271–85.

46. Trauth BC, Klas C, Peters AM et al, Monoclonal antibody-mediated tumor regression by induction of apoptosis. *Science* 1989; **245:** 301–10.

47. Waldman TA, Monoclonal antibodies in diagnosis and therapy. *Science* 1991; **252:** 387–94.

48. O'Connell MJ, Chen ZJ, Yang H et al, Active specific immunotherapy with antiidiotypic antibodies in patients with solid tumors. *Semin Surg Oncol* 1989; **5:** 441–7.

49. Houghton AN, Mintzer D, Cordon-Cardo C et al, Mouse monoclonal IgG3 antibody detecting GD3 ganglioside: a phase I trial in patients with malignant melanoma. *Proc Natl Acad Sci USA* 1985; **82:** 1242–6.

50. Steplewski Z, Lubeck MD, Koprowski H, Human macrophages armed with murine immunoglobulin G2a antibodies to tumors destroy human cancer cells. *Science* 1983; **221:** 865–7.

51. Miller RA, Maloney DG, Warnke R, Levy R, Treatment of B-cell lymphoma with monoclonal anti-idiotype antibody. *N Engl J Med* 1982; **306:** 517–22.

52. Khazaeli MB, Conry RM, LoBuglio AF, Human immune response to monoclonal antibodies. *J Immunother* 1994; **15:** 42–52.

53. Jain RK, Baxter LT. Mechanisms of heterogeneous distribution of monoclonal antibodies and other macromolecules in tumors: significance of elevated interstitial pressure. *Cancer Res* 1988; **48:** 7022–32.

54. Badger CC, Anasetti C, Davis J, Bernstein ID, Treatment of malignancy with unmodified antibody. *Pathol Immunopathol Res* 1987; **6:** 419–34.

55. Holland G, Zlotnik A, Interleukin-10 and cancer. *Cancer Invest* 1993; **11**: 751–8.

56. Nørgaard P, Hougaard S, Poulsen HS, Thomsen M, Transforming growth factor β and cancer. *Cancer Treat Rev* 1995; **21**: 367–403.

57. Porter RR, Separation of fractions of rabbit gamma-globulin containing the antibody and antigenic combining sites. *Nature* 1958; **182**: 670–1.

58. Nisonoff A, Wissler FC, Lipman LN, Properties of the major component of a peptic digest of rabbit antibody. *Science* 1960; **132**: 1770–1.

59. Adams GP, McCartney JE, Tai MS et al, Highly specific in vivo tumor targeting by monovalent and divalent forms of 741F8 anti-c-erbB-2 single chain Fv. *Cancer Res* 1993; **53**: 4026–34.

60. Winter G, Harris WJ, Humanized antibodies. *Trends Pharmacol Sci* 1993; **15**: 139–43.

61. Marks C, Marks JD, Phage libraries – a new route to clinically useful antibodies. *N Engl J Med* 1996; **335**: 730–3.

62. de Palazzo IG, Gercel-Taylor C, Kitson J, Weiner LM, Potentiation of tumor lysis by a bispecific antibody that binds to CA19-9 antigen and the Fcγ receptor expressed by human large granular lymphocytes. *Cancer Res* 1990; **50**: 7123–8.

63. Segal DM, Wunderlich JM, Targeting of cytotoxic cells with heterocrosslinked antibodies. *Cancer Invest* 1988; **6**: 83–92.

64. DeSilva BS, Wilson GS, Solid phase synthesis of bifunctional antibodies. *J Immunol Meth* 1995; **188**: 9–19.

65. Staertz UD, Bevan MJ, Hybrid hybridoma producing a bispecific monoclonal antibody that can focus effector T-cell activity. *Proc Natl Acad Sci USA* 1986; **83**: 1453–7.

66. Carter P, Ridgway J, Zhu Z, Toward the production of bispecific antibody fragments for clinical applications. *J Hematother* 1995; **4**(5): 43–70.

67. Ring DB, Hsieh-Ma ST, Shi T, Reeder J, Antigen forks: bispecific reagents that inhibit cell growth by binding selected pairs of tumor antigens. *Cancer Immunol Immunother* 1994; **39**: 41–8.

68. Mordoh J, Silva C, Albarellos M et al, Phase I clinical trial in cancer patients of a new monoclonal antibody FC-2.15 reacting with tumor proliferating cells. *J Immunother* 1995; **3**: 151–60.

69. Douillard JY, Lehur PM, Vignoud J et al, Monoclonal antibodies specific immunotherapy of gastrointestinal tumors. *Hybridoma* 1986; **5**(Suppl 1): S139–49.

70. Sears HF, Atkinson B, Herlyn D et al, The use of monoclonal antibody in a phase I clinical trial of human gastrointestinal tumors. *Lancet* 1982; **i**: 762–5.

71. Sears HF, Steplewski Z, Herlyn D, Koprowski H, Effects of monoclonal antibody immunotherapy on patients with gastrointestinal adenocarcinoma. *J Biol Resp Modif* 1983; **3**: 138–50.

72. Riethmuller G, Schneider-Gaclicke E, Schlimok G et al, Randomized trial of monoclonal antibody for adjuvant therapy of resected Dukes' C colorectal carcinoma. *Lancet* 1994; **343**: 1177–83.

73. Ceriani RL, Blank EW, Corito JR, Peterson JA, Biologic activity of two humanized antibodies against two different breast cancer antigens and comparison to their original murine forms. *Cancer Res* 1995; **55**(Suppl): 5852s–6s.

74. Sharkey RM, Juweid M, Shevitz J et al, Evaluation of a complementarity-determining region-grafted (humanized) anti-carcinoembryonic antigen monoclonal antibody in preclinical and clinical studies. *Cancer Res* 1995; **55**(Suppl): 5935–45.

75. Basegla J, Tripathy D, Mendelsohn J et al, Phase II study of weekly intravenous recombinant humanized anti-p185[HER2] monoclonal antibody in patients with HER2/*neu*-overexpressing metastatic breast cancer. *J Clin Oncol* 1996; **14**: 737–44.

76. Cobleigh MA, Vogel CL, Tripathy D et al, Efficacy and safety of Herceptin™ (humanized anti-HER2 antibody) as a single agent in 222 women with HER2 overexpression who relapsed following chemotherapy for metastatic breast cancer. *Proc Am Soc Clin Oncol* 1998; **17**: A376.

77. Slamon D, Shak S, Paton V et al, Addition of Herceptin™ (humanized anti-HER2 antibody) to first line chemotherapy for HER2 overexpressing metastatic breast cancer (HER2+/MBC) markedly increases anticancer activity: a randomized multinational controlled phase III trial. *Proc Am Soc Clin Oncol* 1998; **17**: A377.

78. Pegram M, Hsu S, Lewis G et al, Inhibitory effects of combinations of HER-2/neu antibody and chemotherapeutic agents used for treatment of human breast cancers. *Oncogene* 1999; **18**: 2241–51.

79. Drebin JA, Link VC, Stern DF et al, Down modulation of an oncogene protein product and reversion of the transformed phenotype by monoclonal antibodies. *Cell* 1985; **41**: 695–706.

80. Stanovski I, Hurwitz E, Leitner D et al, Mechanistic aspects of the opposing effects of monoclonal antibodies to the *erb*B-2 receptor on tumor growth. *Proc Natl Acad Sci USA* 1991; **88:** 8691–5.

81. Bacus SS, Stancovski I, Huberman E et al, Tumor-inhibitory monoclonal antibodies to the HER2/neu receptor induce differentiation of human breast cancer cells. *Cancer Res* 1992; **52:** 2580–9.

82. Scott GK, Dodson JM, Montgomery PA et al, p185^HER2 signal transduction in breast cancer cells. *J Biol Chem* 1991; **266:** 14300–5.

83. Kumar R, Shepard HM, Mendelsohn J, Regulation of the c-*erb*B-2 gene product by a monoclonal antibody and serum growth factor(s) in human mammary carcinoma cells. *Mol Cell Biol* 1991; **11:** 979–86.

84. Hudziak RM, Lewis GD, Winget M et al, p185^HER2 monoclonal antibody has antiprolifera-tive effects in vitro and sensitizes human breast tumor cells to tumor necrosis factor. *Mol Cell Biol* 1989; **9:** 1165–72.

85. Tosi E, Valota O, Negri DRM et al, Anti-tumor efficacy of an anti-epidermal-growth-factor-receptor monoclonal antibody and its F(ab')₂ fragment against high- and low-EGFR-express-ing carcinomas in nude mice. *Int J Cancer* 1995; **62:** 643–50.

86. Modjtahedi H, Hickish T, Nicolson M et al, Phase I trial and tumour localization of the anti-EGFR monoclonal antibody ICR62 in head neck or lung cancer. *Br J Cancer* 1996; **73:** 228–35.

87. Gill GN, Kawanmoto T, Cochet C et al, Monoclonal anti-epidermal growth factor receptor antibodies which are inhibitors of epi-dermal growth factor binding and antagonists of epidermal growth factor-stimulated tyrosine protein kinase activity. *J Biol Chem* 1984; **259:** 7755–60.

88. Taylor SS, Buechler JA, Yonemoto W, cAMP-dependent protein kinase: framework for a diverse family of regulatory enzymes. *Annu Rev Biochem* 1990; **50:** 7093–100.

89. Tortora G, Ciardiello F, Ally S et al, Site-selective 8-chloro-adenosine 3',5'-monophos-phate inhibits transforming growth factor alpha transformation of mammary epithelial cells by restoration of the normal mRNA patterns for cAMP-dependent protein kinase regula-tory subunit isoforms which show disruption upon transformation. *J Biol Chem* 1990; **265:**1016–20.

90. Ciardiello R, Pepe S, Bianco C et al, Down-regulation of RI alpha subunit of the cAMP-dependent protein kinase induces growth inhibition of human mammary epithe-lial cells transformed by c-HA-ras and c-erbB-2 proto-oncogenes. *Int J Cancer* 1993; **53:** 438–43.

91. Ciardiello F, Damiano R, Bianco C et al, Antitumour activity of combined blockade of epidermal growth factor receptor and protein kinase A. *J Natl Cancer Inst* 1996; **88:** 1770–6.

92. Benz CC, Scott GK, Sarup JC et al, Estrogen-dependent, tamoxifen-resistant tumorigenic growth of MCF-7 cells transfected with HER2/neu. *Breast Cancer Res Treat* 1992; **24:** 85–95.

93. Alfred DC, Clark GM, Tandon AK et al, Her-2/neu in node-negative breast cancer: prognostic significance of overexpression influ-enced by the presence of in situ carcinoma. *J Clin Oncol* 1992; **10:** 599–602.

94. Meyres MB, Merluzzi VJ, Spengler BA, Biedler JL, Epidermal growth factor receptor is increased in multidrug-resistant chinese ham-ster and mouse tumor cells. *Proc Natl Acad Sci USA* 1986; **83:** 5521–5.

95. Aboud-Pirak E, Hurwitz E, Pirak ME et al, Efficacy of antibodies to epidermal growth fac-tor receptor against KB carcinoma cells in vitro and in nude mice. *J Natl Cancer Inst* 1988; **80:** 1605–11.

96. Baselga J, Norton L, Masui H et al, Antitumour effects of doxorubicin in combination with anti-epidermal growth factor receptor monoclonal antibodies. *J Natl Cancer Inst* 1993; **85:** 1327–33.

97. Amagase H, Kakimoto M, Hashimoto K et al, Epidermal growth factor receptor-mediated selective cytotoxicity of antitumor agents towards human xenografts and murine syn-geneic solid tumors. *Jpn J Cancer Res* 1989; **80:** 670–8.

98. Kwok TT, Sutherland RM, Epidermal growth factor reduces resistance to doxorubicin. *Int J Cancer* 1991; **49:** 73–6.

99. Kwok TT, Sutherland RM, Enhancement of sen-sitivity of human squamous carcinoma cells to radiation by epidermal growth factor. *J Natl Cancer Inst* 1989; **81:** 1020–4.

100. Hancock MC, Langton BC, Chan T et al, A monoclonal antibody against the c-erbB-2 protein enhances the cytotoxicity of *cis*-diamminedichlortoplatinum against human breast and ovarian tumor cell lines. *Cancer Res* 1991; **51:** 4575–80.

101. Pietras RJ, Fendly VR, Chazin VR et al, Antibody to HER-2/*neu* receptor blocks DNA repair after cisplatin in human breast and ovarian cancer cells. *Oncogene* 1994; **9:** 1829–38.

102. Artega CL, Winnier AR, Poirier MC et al, p195$^{c-erbB-2}$ signaling enhances cisplatin-induced cytotoxicity in human breast carcinoma cells: association between an oncogenic receptor tyrosine kinase and drug-induced DNA repair. *Cancer Res* 1994; **54:** 3758–65.

103. Pietras RJ, Poen JC, Gallardo D et al, Monoclonal antibody in HER-2/neu receptor modulates repair of radiation-induced DNA damage and enhances radiosensitivity of human breast cancer cells overexpressing this oncogene. *Cancer Res* 1999; **59:** 1347–55.

104. Wheeler RH, Spencer S, Bucksbaum D, Robert F, Monoclonal antibodies as potentiators of radiotherapy anbd chemotherapy in the management of head and neck cancer. *Curr Opin Oncol* 1999; **11:** 187–98.

105. Smellie WB, Dean CJ, Sacks NPM et al, Radioimmunotherapy of breast cancer xenografts with monoclonal antibody ICR12 against c-erbB-2 p185: comparison of iodogen and *N*-succinimidyl 1-methyl-3-(tri-*n*-butylstannyl)benzoate radioiodination methods. *Cancer Res* 1995; **55**(Suppl): 5842s–6s.

106. Juweid M, Sharkey RM, Behr T et al, Targeting and initial radioimmunotherapy of medullary thyroid carcinoma with ^{131}I-labeled monoclonal antibodies to carcinoembryonic antigen. *Cancer Res* 1995; **55**(Suppl): 5946s–51s.

107. Shih LB, Yuan H, Aninipot R et al, In vitro and in vivo reactivity of an internalizing Ab, RS7, with human breast cancer. *Cancer Res* 1995; **55**(Suppl): 5857s–63s.

108. Adams GP, DeNardo GP, Amin A et al, Comparison of the pharmacokinetics in mice and the biologic activity of murine L-6 and human-mouse chimeric Ch L-6 antibody. *Antibody Immunoconj Radiopharm* 1992; **5:** 81–95.

109. DeNardo SJ, Mirick GR, Kroger LA et al, The biologic window for ChL6 radioimmunotherapy. *Cancer* 1994; **73**(Suppl): 1023–32.

110. Richman CR, DeNardo SJ, O'Grady LF, DeNardo GL, Radioimmunotherapy for breast cancer using escalating fractionated doses of ^{131}I-labeled chimeric L6 antibody with peripheral blood progenitor cell transfusions. *Cancer Res* 1995; **55**(Suppl): 5916s–20s.

111. Denardo SJ, O'Grady LF, Richman CR et al, Radioimmunotherapy for advanced breast cancer using I-131-ChL6 antibody. *Anticancer Res* 1997; **17:** 1745–52.

112. Denardo SJ, Richman CM, Goldstein DS et al, Yttrium-90/indium-111-DOTA-peptide-chimeric-L6: pharmacokinetics, dosimetry and initial results in patients with incurable breast cancer. *Anticancer Res* 1997; **17:** 1735–44.

113. Denardo SJ, Kukis DL, Kroger LA et al, Synergy of Taxol and radioimmunotherapy with yttrium-90-labeled chimeric L6 antibody: efficacy and toxicity in breast cancer xenografts. *Proc Natl Acad Sci USA* 1997; **94:** 4000–4.

114. Peterson JA, Blank EW, Cerrani RL, Effects of multiple repeated dose of immunotherapy on target antigen expression (breast MUC-1 mucin) in breast carcinomas. *Cancer Res* 1987; **57:** 1103–8.

115. Schrier DM, Stemmer SM, Johnson T et al, High dose ^{90}Y mx-diethylenetriaminepentaacetic acid (DPTA)–BrE-3 and autologous hematopoetic stem cell support (AHSCS) for the treatment of advanced breast cancer: a phase I trial. *Cancer Res* 1995; **55**(Suppl): 5921–4.

116. Blank EW, Pant KD, Chan CM et al, A novel anti-breast epithelial mucin MoAb (BrE-3). *Cancer* 1992; **5:** 38–44.

117. Murray JL, Macey DJ, Grant EJ et al, Enhanced TAG-72 expression and tumor uptake of radiolabeled monoclonal antibody CC49 in metastatic breast cancer patients following α-interferon treatment. *Cancer Res* 1995; **55**(Suppl): 5925s–8s.

118. Arnon R, Sela M, In vitro and in vivo efficacy of conjugates of daunomycin with anti-tumor antibodies. *Immunol Rev* 1982; **62:** 5–27.

119. Dillman RO, Johnson DE, Shawler DL, Koziol JA, Superiority of an acid-labile daunorubicin–monoclonal antibody immunoconjugate compared to free drug. *Cancer Res* 1988; **48:** 6097–102.

120. Yang MH, Reisfeld RA, Doxorubicin conjugated with a monoclonal antibody directed to a human melanoma-associated proteoglycan suppresses the growth of established tumor xenografts in nude mice. *Proc Natl Acad Sci USA* 1988; **85:** 1189–93.

121. Kukarni PN, Blair AH, Ghose TI, Covalent binding of methotrexate to immunoglobulins and the effect of antibody-linked drug on tumor growth in vivo. *Cancer Res* 1981; **41:** 2700–6.

122. Shih LB, Sharkey RM, Primus FJ, Goldenberg DM, Site-specific linkage of methotrexate to monoclonal antibodies using an intermediate carrier. *Int J Cancer* 1988; **41:** 832–9.

123. Starling JJ, Maciak RS, Law KL et al, In vivo activity of a monoclonal antibody–*Vinca* alkaloid immunoconjugate directed against a solid tumor membrane antigen characterized by heterogeneous expression and noninternalization of antibody–antigen complexes. *Cancer Res* 1991; **51**: 2965–72.

124. Smyth MJ, Pietersz GA, Classon BJ, McKenzie IFC, Specific targeting of chlorambucil to tumors with the use of monoclonal antibodies. *J Natl Cancer Inst* 1986; **76**: 503–10.

125. Meyer DL, Law KL, Payne JK et al, Site-specific prodrug activation by antibody–beta-lactamase conjugates: preclinical investigation of the efficacy and toxicity of doxorubicin delivered by antibody-directed catalysis. *Bioconj Chem* 1995; **6**: 440–6.

126. Trail PA, Willner D, Lasch SJ et al, Cure of xenografted human carcinomas by BR96–doxorubicin immunoconjugates. *Science* 1993; **261**: 212–15.

127. Giantonio BJ, Gilewski TA, Bookman MA et al, A phase I study of weekly BR96–DOX in patients with advanced carcinoma expressing the Lewis[y] antigen. *Proc Am Soc Clin Oncol* 1996; **15**: 443.

128. Deonarain MP, Spooner RA, Epenetos AA, Genetic delivery of enzymes for cancer therapy. *Gene Ther* 1995; **2**: 235–44.

129. Senter PD, Sauliner MG, Schreiber GJ et al, Anti-tumor effects of antibody–alkaline phosphatase conjugates in combination with etoposide phosphate. *Proc Natl Acad Sci USA* 1988; **85**: 4842–6.

130. Wallace PM, MacMaster JF, Smith VF et al, Intratumoral generation of 5-fluorouracil mediated by an antibody–cytosine deaminase conjugate in combination with 5-fluorocytosine. *Cancer Res* 1994; **54**: 2719–23.

131. Hsieh-Ma ST, Shi T, Reeder J, Ring DB, In vitro tumor growth inhibition by bispecific antibodies to human transferrin receptor and tumor-associated antigens is augmented by the iron chelator deferoxamine. *Clin Immunol Immunopathol* 1996; **80**: 185–93.

132. Staertz UD, Kanagawa O, Bevan MJ, Hybrid antibodies can target sites for attack by T-cells. *Nature* 1985; **314**: 628–31.

133. Perez P, Hoffman RW, Shaw S et al, Specific targeting of cytotoxic T-cells by anti-T$_3$ linked to anti-target cell antibody. *Nature* 1985; **316**: 354–6.

134. Pantel K, Schlimok G, Kutter D et al, Frequent down-regulation of major histocompatability class I antigen expression on individual micrometastatic carcinoma cells. *Cancer Res* 1991; **51**: 4712–15.

135. Kroesen B-J, Bakker A, Van Lier RAW et al, Bispecific antibody-mediated target cell-specific costimulation of resting T cells via CD5 and CD28. *Cancer Res* 1995; **55**: 4409–15.

136. Valone FH, Kaufman PA, Guyre PM et al, Phase Ia/Ib trial of bispecific antibody MDX-210 in patients with advanced breast or ovarian cancer that overexpresses the proto-oncogene HER-2/*neu*. *J Clin Oncol* 1995; **13**: 2281–92.

137. Stockmeyer B, Valerius T, Repp R et al, Preclinical studies with FCγR bispecific antibodies and granulocyte colony-stimulating factor primed neutrophils as effector cells against HER-2/*neu* overexpressing breast cancer. *Cancer Res* 1997; **57**: 696–701.

138. Posey JA, Raspet R, Verma H et al, A pilot trial of GM-CSF and MDX-H210 in patients with erbB-2-positive advanced malignancies. *J Immunother* 1999; **22**: 371–9.

139. de Palazzo IG, Gercel-Taylor C, Kitson J, Weiner LM, Potentiation of tumor lysis by a bispecific antibody that binds to CA19-9 antigen and the Fcγ receptor expressed by human by large granular lymphocytes. *Cancer Res* 1990; **50**: 7123–8.

140. Ferrini S, Prigione I, Miotti S et al, Bispecific monoclonal antibodies directed to CD16 and to a tumor-associated antigen induce target cell lysis by resting NK cells and a subset of NK clones. *Int J Cancer* 1990; **48**: 227–33.

141. Weiner LM, Holmes M, Richeson A et al, Binding and cytotoxicity characteristics of the bispecific murine monoclonal antibody 2B1. *J Immunol* 1993; **151**: 2877–86.

142. Weiner LM, Clark JI, Davey M et al, Phase I trial of 2B1, a bispecific monoclonal antibody targeting c-erbB-2 and FcγRIII. *Cancer Res* 1995; **55**: 4586–93.

143. Gralow J, Weiner L, Ring D et al, HER-2/*neu* specific immunity can be induced by therapy with 2B1, a bispecific monoclonal antibody binding to HER-2/*neu* and CD16. *Proc Am Soc Clin Oncol* 1995; **14**: A1807.

144. Mack M, Reithmuller G, Kuffer P, A small bispecific antibody construct expressed as functional single-chain molecule with high tumor cell cytotoxicity. *Proc Natl Acad Sci USA* 1995; **92**: 7021–5.

145. Wawryzynczak EJ, Systemic immunotoxin therapy of cancer: advances and approaches. *Br J Cancer* 1991; **64:** 624–30.

146. Siegall CB, Single-chain fusion toxins for the treatment of breast cancer: antitumor activity of BR96 sFv–PE40 and heregulin–PE40. *Rec Res Cancer Res* 1995; **140:** 51–60.

147. Endo Y, Mitsui K, Motizuki M et al, The mechanism of action of ricin and related toxic lectins on eukaryotic ribosomes. *J Biol Chem* 1987; **262:** 5908–12.

148. Murphy JR, van der Spek JC, Targeting diphtheria toxin to growth factor receptors. *Semin Cancer Biol* 1995; **6:** 259–65.

149. Hwang J, Fitzgerald DJ, Adhya S, Pastan I, Functional domains of *Pseudomonas* exotoxin identifies by deletion analysis of the gene expressed in *E. coli. Cell* 1987; **48:** 129–36.

150. Cumber AJ, Forrester JA, Foxwell BM et al, Preparation of antibody–toxin conjugates. *Meth Enzymol* 1987; **151:** 139–45.

151. Fitzgerald DJ, Construction of immunotoxins using *Pseudomonas* exotoxin A. *Meth Enzymol* 1985; **112:** 207–25.

152. Colombatti M, Greenfield L, Youle RJ, Cloned fragment of diphtheria toxin linked to T cell-specific antibody identifies regions of B chain active in cell entry. *J Biol Chem* 1986; **261:** 3030–5.

153. Johnson VG, Wilson D, Greenfield L et al, The role of the diphtheria toxin receptor in cytosol translocation. *J Biol Chem* 1988; **263:** 1295–300.

154. Kihara A, Pastan I, Cytotoxic activity of chimeric toxins containing the epidermal growth factor-like domain of heregulins fused to PE38 KDEL, a truncated recombinant form of *Pseudomonas* exotoxin. *Cancer Res* 1995; **55:** 71–7.

155. Kreitman RJ, Puri RK, Pastan I, Increased antitumor activity of circularly permuted interleukin 4-toxin in mice with interleukin 4 receptor-bearing human carcinoma. *Cancer Res* 1995; **55:** 3357–63.

156. Ozello L, De Rosa CM, Blank EW et al, The use of natural interferon alpha conjugated to a monoclonal antibody anti-mammary epithelial mucin (Mc5) for the treatment of human breast cancer xenografts. *Breast Cancer Res Treat* 1993; **25:** 265–76.

157. May RD, Finkelman FD, Wheeler HT et al, Evaluation of ricin A chain-containing immunotoxins directed against different epitopes on the δ-chain of cell surface associated IgD on murine B cells. *J Immunol* 1990; **144:** 3637–42.

158. Press OW, Martin PJ, Thorpe PE, Vitetta ES, Ricin A chain-containing immunotoxins directed against different epitopes on the CD2 molecule differ in their ability to kill normal and malignant T cells. *J Immunol* 1988; **141:** 4410–17.

159. Till M, May RD, Uhr JW et al, An assay that predicts the ability of monoclonal antibodies to form potent ricin A chain-containing immunotoxins. *Cancer Res* 1988; **48:** 1119–23.

160. Thorpe PE, Wallace PM, Knowles PP et al, Improved antitumor effects of immunotoxins prepared with deglycosilated ricin A-chain and hindered disulfide linkages. *Cancer Res* 1988; **48:** 6396–403.

161. Wawrzynczak EJ, Davies AJS, Strategies in antibody therapy of cancer. *Clin Exp Immunol* 1990; **82:** 189–93.

162. Wawrzynczak EJ, Cumbe AJ, Henry RV, Parnell GD, Comparative biochemical cytotoxicity and pharmacokinetic properties of immunotoxins made with native ricin A chain, ricin A_1 chain and recombinant A chain. *Int J Cancer* 1991; **47:** 130–5.

163. Cumbers AJ, Westwood JH, Henry RV et al, Structural features of the antibody–A chain linkage that influence the activity and stability of ricin A chain immunotoxins. *Bioconj Chem* 1992; **3:** 397–401.

164. Ghetie M-A, Uhr JW, Vitetta ES, Covalent binding of human $α_2$-macroglobulin to deglycosylated ricin A chain and its immunotoxins. *Cancer Res* 1991; **51:** 1482–7.

165. Chaudhery VK, Jinno Y, Gallo MG et al, Mutagenesis of *Pseudomonas* exotoxin in identification of sequences responsible for animal toxicity. *J Biol Chem* 1990; **265:** 16306–10.

166. Bookman MA, Godfrey C, Padavic H et al, Antitransferrin receptor immunotoxin therapy: phase I intraperitoneal trial. *Proc Am Soc Clin Oncol* 1990; **9:** 187.

167. Gould BJ, Borowitz MJ, Graves ES et al, Phase I study of an anti-breast cancer immunotoxin by continuous infusion: report of a targeted toxic effect not predicted by animal studies. *J Natl Cancer Inst* 1989; **81:** 775–81.

168. Weiner LM, O'Dwyer J, Kitson J et al, Phase I evaluation of an anti-breast carcinoma monoclonal antibody 260F9-recombinant ricin A chain immunoconjugate. *Cancer Res* 1989; **49:** 4062–7.

169. Frankel AE, Tagge EP, Willingham MC, Clinical trials of targeted toxins. *Semin Cancer Biol* 1995; **6:** 307–17.

170. Stone MJ, Sarscille EA, Fay JW et al, A phase I study of bolus versus continuous infusion of the anti-CD19 immunotoxin IgG–HD36–dgA, in patients with B-cell lymphoma. *Blood* 1996; **88:** 1188–97.

171. Hellström I, Garrigues HJ, Garrigues U, Hellström KE, Highly tumor-reactive internalizing, mouse monoclonal antibodies to Le^y-related cell surface antigens. *Cancer Res* 1990; **50:** 2183–90.

172. Siegall CB, Chace D, Mixan B et al, In vitro and in vivo characterization of BR96 sFv-PE40. *J Immunol* 1994; **152:** 2377–84.

173. Friedman PN, McAndrew SJM, Gawlak SL et al, BR96 sFv–PE40, a potent single-chain immunotoxin that selectively kills carcinoma cells. *Cancer Res* 1993; **53:** 334–9.

174. Friedman PN, Chace DF, Trail PA, Siegall CB, Antitumor activity of the single-chain immunotoxin BR96 sFv–PE40 against established breast and lung tumor xenografts. *J Immunol* 1993; **150:** 3054–61.

175. Siegall CB, Ligitt D, Chace D et al, Prevention of immunotoxin-mediated vascular leak syndrome in rats with retention of antitumor activity. *Proc Natl Acad Sci USA* 1994; **91:** 9514–18.

176. King CR, Kaspryk PG, Fischer PH et al, Preclinical testing of an anti-*erb*B-2 recombinant toxin. *Breast Cancer Res Treat* 1996; **38:** 19–25.

177. Carraway KL III, Sliwkowski MX, Akita RW et al, The erbB3 gene product is a receptor for heregulin. *J Biol Chem* 1994; **269:** 14303–6.

178. Plowman GD, Green JM, Culouscou JM et al, Heregulin induces tyrosine phosphorylation of HER4/p180^{erbB4}. *Nature* 1993; **366:** 473–5.

179. Seigall CB, Single-chain fusion toxins for the treatment of breast cancer: antitumor activity of BR96 sFv–PE40 and heregulin–PE40. *Rec Res Cancer Res* 1996; **140:** 51–60.

180. Seigall CB, Bacus SS, Cohen BD et al, HER4 expression correlates with cytotoxicity directed by a heregulin–toxin fusion protein. *J Biol Chem* 1995; **270:** 7625–30.

181. Fiddes RJ, Janes PW, Sanderson GM et al, Heregulin (HRG)-induced mitogenic signaling and cytotoxicity of a HRG/PE40 ligand toxin in human breast cancer cells. *Cell Growth Diff* 1995; **6:** 1567–77.

182. Seetharam S, Chaudharry VK, Pastan I, Increased cytotoxic activity of *Pseudomonas* exotoxin and two chimeric toxins ending in KDEL. *J Biol Chem* 1991; **266:** 17376–81.

183. Huang SK, Mayhew EM, Gilani S et al, Pharmacokinetics and therapeutics of sterically stabilized liposomes in mice bearing C-26 colon carcinoma. *Cancer Res* 1992; **52:** 6774–81.

184. Park JW, Hong K, Carter P et al, Development of anti-p185^{HER2} immunoliposomes for cancer therapy. *Proc Natl Acad Sci USA* 1995; **92:** 1327–31.

185. Deonarain MP, Epenetos AA, Targeting enzymes for cancer therapy: old enzymes in new roles. *Br J Cancer* 1994; **70:** 786–94.

186. Deshane J, Cabrera G, Grim JE et al, Targeted eradication of ovarian cancer mediated by intracellular expression of anti-erbB-2 single chain antibody. *Gynecol Oncol* 1994; **59:** 8–14.

187. Rybak SM, Saxena SK, Ackerman EJ, Youle RJ, Cytotoxic potential of ribonuclease and ribonuclease hybrid proteins. *J Biol Chem* 1991; **266:** 21202–7.

188. Rybak SM, Hoogenboom HR, Meady MH et al, Humanization of immunotoxins. *Proc Natl Acad Sci USA* 1992; **89:** 3165–9.

189. Slifman NR, Loegering DA, McKean DJ, Gleich GJ, Ribonuclease activity associated with human eosinophil-derived neurotoxin and eosinophilic cationic protein. *J Immunol* 1986; **137:** 2913–17.

190. Gullberg U, Widegren B, Arnason U et al, The cytotoxic eosinophil cationic protein (ECP) has ribonuclease activity. *Biochem Biophys Res Commun* 1986; **139:** 1239–42.

191. Roth J, Ribonuclease activity and cancer: a review. *Cancer Res* 1963; **23:** 657–66.

192. Wels W, Groner B, Hynes NE, Intervention in receptor tyrosine kinase-mediated pathways: recombinant antibody fusion proteins targeted to ErbB2. *Curr Top Microbiol Immunol* 1996; **213:** 113–28.

193. Cote RJ, Morrissey DM, Houghton AN et al, Specificity analysis of human monoclonal antibodies reactive with cell surface and intracellular antigens. *Proc Natl Acad Sci, USA* 1986; **83:** 2959–63.

194. Barnd DL, Gupta RK, Metzgar RS, Finn OJ, Specific, MHC-unrestricted recognition of tumor-associated mucins by human cytotoxic T cells. *Proc Natl Acad Sci USA* 1989; **86:** 7159–65.

195. Disis ML, Calenoff E, McLaughin G et al, Existent T cell and antibody immunity to HER-2/neu protein in patients with breast cancer. *Cancer Res* 1994; **54:** 16–22.

196. Crawford LV, Pim DC, Bulbrook RD, Detection of antibodies against the cellular protein p53 in sera from patients with breast cancer. *Int J Cancer* 1982; **30:** 403–8.

197. Blachere NK, Srivastava PK, Heat shock protein-based vaccines and related thoughts on immunogenicity of human tumors. *Semin Cancer Biol* 1995; **6**: 349–55.

198. Janeway CA, Bottomly K, Signals and signs for lymphocyte responses. *Cell* 1994; **76**: 275–85.

199. Rothbard JB, Gefter ML, Interactions between immunogenic peptides and MHC proteins. *Annu Rev Immunol* 1991; **9**: 527–65.

200. Giuliano AE, Sparks FC, Patterson K, Adjuvant chemo-immunotherapy in stage II carcinoma of the breast. *J Surg Oncol* 1986; **31**: 255–9.

201. Fung PY, Madej SM, Koganty R, Longenecker BM, Active specific immunotherapy of a murine mammary adenocarcinoma using a synthetic tumor-associated glycoconjugate. *Cancer Res* 1990; **50**: 4308–14.

202. MacLean GD, Reddish M, Koganty RR et al, Immunization of breast cancer patients using a synthetic sialyl-Tn glycoconjugate plus Detox adjuvant. *Cancer Immunol Immunother* 1993; **36**: 215–22.

203. Lindenmann J, Speculations on Ids and homobodies. *Ann Immunol* 1973; **124**: 171–84.

204. Jerne NK, Towards a network theory of the immune system. *Ann Immunol* 1974; **125C**: 373–89.

205. Chapman PB, Anti-idiotypic monoclonal antibody cancer vaccines. *Semin Cancer Biol* 1995; **6**: 367–74.

206. Foon KA, Chakraborty M, John WJ et al, Immune response to the carcinoembryonic antigen in patients treated with an anti-idiotype antibody vaccine. *J Clin Invest* 1995; **96**: 334–42.

207. Clarke JI, Alpaugh RK, von Mehren M et al, Induction of multiple anti-c-erbB-2 specificities accompanies a classical idiotypic cascade following 2B1 bispecific monoclonal antibody treatment. *Cancer Immunol Immunother* 1997; **44**: 265–72.

208. Frödin J-E, Faxas ME, Haström B et al, Induction of anti-anti idiotypic antibodies in patients treated with the mouse monoclonal antibody 17-1A (ab₁). Relation to the clinical outcome: an important antitumoral effector function? *Hybridoma* 1991; **10**: 421–32.

209. Cheung NK, Cheung IY, Canet A et al, Antibody response to murine anti-GD₂ monoclonal antibodies: correlation with patient survival. *Cancer Res* 1996; **54**: 2228–33.

210. Fagerberg J, Hjelm A-L, Ragnhammar P et al, Tumor regression in monoclonal antibody-treated patients correlates with the presence of

anti-idiotypic-reactive T lymphocytes. *Cancer Res* 1995; **55**: 1824–7.

211. Conry RM, LoBuglio AF, Kantor J et al, Immune response to a carcinoembryonic antigen polynucleotide vaccine. *Cancer Res* 1994; **54**: 1164–8.

212. Conry RM, LoBuglio AF, Loechel F, A carcinoembryonic antigen polynucleotide vaccine has in vivo antitumor activity. *Gene Ther* 1995; **2**: 59–65.

213. Tsang KY, Zremba S, Nieroda CA et al, Generation of human cytotoxic T-cells specific for human carcinoembryonic antigen (CEA) epitopes from patients immunized with recombinant vaccinia–CEA (rV–CEA) vaccine. *J Natl Cancer Inst* 1995; **87**: 982–90.

214. Kaufman H, Schlom J, Kantor J, A recombinant vaccinia virus expressing human carcinoembryonic antigen (CEA). *Int J Cancer* 1991; **48**: 900–7.

215. Conry RM, Saleh MN, Schlom J, LoBuglio AF, Breaking tolerance to carcinoembryonic antigen with a recombinant vaccinia virus in man. *Proc Am Assoc Cancer Res* 1995; **36**: A492.

216. McLaughlin JP, Schlom J, Kantor JA, Greiner JW, Improved immunotherapy of a recombinant carcinoembryonic antigen vaccinia vaccine when given in combination with interleukin-2. *Cancer Res* 1996; **56**: 2361–7.

217. Hodge JW, McLaughin JP, Abrams SI et al, Admixture of a recombinant vaccinia virus containing the gene for the costimulatory molecule B7 and a recombinant vaccinia virus containing a tumor-associated antigen gene results in enhanced specific T-cell responses and antitumor immunity. *Cancer Res* 1995; **55**: 3598–603.

218. Abrams SI, Dobrzanski MJ, Wells DT et al, Peptide-specific activation of cytolytic CD4⁺ T lymphocytes against tumor cells bearing mutated epitopes of K-*ras* p21. *Eur J Immunol* 1995; **25**: 2588–97.

219. Skipper J, Stauss HJ, Identification of two cytotoxic T lymphocyte-recognized epitopes in the Ras protein. *J Exp Med* 1993; **177**: 1493–8.

220. Fenton RG, Taub DD, Kwak LW et al, Cytotoxic T-cell response and in vivo protection against tumor cells harboring activated *ras* proto-oncogenes. *J Natl Cancer Inst* 1993; **85**: 1294–302.

221. Udono H, Srivastava PK, Comparison of tumor-specific immunogenicities of stress-induced proteins gp96 hsp 90, and hsp70. *J Immunol* 1994; **152**: 5398–403.

222. Blachere NE, Udono H, Janetzki S et al, Heat

shock protein vaccines against cancer. *J Immunother* 1993; **14:** 352–6.

223. Bernhard H, Disis ML, Hermfell S et al, Generation of immuno-stimulatory dendritic cells from human CD34⁺ hematopoetic progenitor cells of the bone marrow and peripheral blood. *Cancer Res* 1995; **55:** 1099–104.

224. Venazi FM, Petrelli C, Concetti A, Amici A, *neu*/HER-2 cDNA vaccination and pregnancy loss. *Ann NY Acad Sci* 1995; **772:** 274–7.

225. Harwerth IM, Wels W, Schlegel J et al, Monoclonal antibodies directed to the *erb*B-2 receptor inhibit in vivo tumour cell growth. *Br J Cancer* 1993; **68:** 1140–5.

226. Peterson JA, Conto JR, Taylor MR, Ceriani RL, Selection of tumor-specific epitopes on target antigens for radioimmunotherapy of breast cancer. *Cancer Res* 1995; **55:** 5847s–51s.

227. Pastan I, Lovelace ET, Gallo MG et al, Characterization of monoclonal antibodies B1 and B3 that react with mucinous adenocarcinomas. *Cancer Res* 1991; **51:** 3781–7.

228. Benhar I, Pastan I, Identification of residues that stabilize the single-chain Fv of residues that stabilize the single-chain Fv of monoclonal antibodies B3. *J Biol Chem* 1995; **270:** 23373–80.

229. Choe M, Webber KO, Pastan I, B3(Fab)–PE38ᴹ: a recombinant immunotoxin in which a mutant form of *Pseudomonas* exotoxin is fused to the Fab fragment of monoclonal antibody B3. *Cancer Res* 1994; **54:** 3460–7.

230. Murphy JR, vander Spek JC, Targeting diphtheria toxin to growth factor receptors. *Semin Cancer Biol* 1995; **6:** 259–67.

231. Wels W, Harwerth IM, Muller M et al, Selective inhibition of tumor cell growth by a recombinant single-chain antibody–toxin specific for the erbB-2 receptor. *Cancer Res* 1992; **52:** 6310–17.

232. King CR, Kaprzyk PG, Fischer PH et al, Preclinical testing of an anti-erbB-2 recombinant toxin. *Breast Cancer Res Treat* 1996; **38:** 19–25.

233. DiLazzaro C, Digiesi G, Tecce R et al, Immunotoxins to the HER 2 oncogene produce: functional and ultrastructural analysis of their cytotoxic activity. *Cancer Immunol Immunother* 1994; **39:** 318–24.

234. Debinski W, Pastan I, Monovalent immunotoxin containing truncated form of *Pseudomonas* exotoxin as potent antitumor agent. *Cancer Res* 1992; **52:** 5379–85.

235. Batra JK, Fitzgerald DJ, Chaudhary VK, Pastan I, Single chain immunotoxins directed at the human transferrin receptor containing *Pseudomonas* exotoxin A or Diphtheria toxin: anti-TFR(Fv)–PE40 and DT388–anti-TFR(Fv). *Mol Cell Biol* 1991; **11:** 2200–5.

236. Newton DL, Nicholls PJ, Rybak SM, Youle RJ, Expression and characterization of recombinant human eosinophil-derived neurotoxin and eosinophil-derived neurotoxin–anti-transferrin receptor sFv. *J Biol Chem* 1994; **269:** 26739–45.

237. Nicholls PJ, Johnson VG, Andrew SM et al, Characterization of single-chain antibody (sFv)–toxin fusion proteins produced in vitro in rabbit reticulocyte lysate. *J Biol Chem* 1993; **268:** 5302–8.

238. Scott CF, Goldmacher VS, Lambert JM et al, An immunotoxin composed of a monoclonal anti-transferrin receptor antibody linked by a disulfide bond to the ribosome-inactivating protein gelonin: potent in vitro and in vivo effects against human tumors. *J Natl Cancer Inst* 1987; **79:** 1163–72.

239. Gould BJ, Borowitz MJ, Groves ES et al, Phase I study of an anti-breast cancer immunotoxin by continuous infusion: report of a targeted toxic effect not predicted by animal studies. *J Natl Cancer Inst* 1989; **81:** 775–81.

240. Yu YH, Crews JR, Cooper K et al, Use of immunotoxins in combination to inhibit clonogenic growth of human breast carcinoma cells. *Cancer Res* 1990; **50:** 3231–8.

11

Soft tissue sarcoma

Alexander MM Eggermont

INTRODUCTION

Soft tissue sarcomas (STS) are tumours of mesenchymal origin, and account for about 1% of all adult malignant tumours in the USA. Each year, about 6000 new cases of STS are diagnosed, and 3300 patients die of metastatic STS.[1] About 60% of these tumours occur in the extremities. The results of primary surgical treatment are hampered by the often large size of these tumours at presentation. In extremities, local failure rates of 35% and high amputation rates of up to 50% were not unusual in the recent past, while results are even worse for sarcomas in the head and neck region and retroperitoneum.[2–4] Apart from size, it has been clearly shown that tumour grade is the most important prognostic factor: deep-seated grade 3 tumours (high grade) larger than 5 cm have a failure rate greater than 60%.[5] Because tumours are often large at initial presentation, and because of the high local failure rate, high amputation rate and high systemic failure rate, many attempts have been directed at the development of adjuvant treatment strategies focusing on improvement of one or more of these failure patterns. First we shall briefly discuss developments in systemic adjuvant therapy in STS. Since no biologics have been involved in adjuvant trials in STS, this section will be very brief.

Management of extremity sarcomas has focused on how to avoid amputation or functionally mutilating surgery. It is in this field that the application of a biologic agent, namely tumour necrosis factor α (TNF-α) has been successfully developed and has established itself.[6–9] It can play an important role in the management of locally advanced or irresectable STS of the limbs. In this chapter, we shall focus on these new developments, and we shall speculate, on the basis of (pre)clinical observations, about the ways in which the use of TNF-α may be extended in the future in the management of STS.

SYSTEMIC ADJUVANT THERAPY FOR SYSTEMIC MICROMETASTASES IN SOFT TISSUE SARCOMA

The development of effective adjuvant treatment against systemic micrometastases is of prime importance in attempting to improve the overall cure rate of STS patients after resection of the primary tumour. Over the past 20 years, 11 trials have been conducted either with doxorubicin alone[10–14] or with combination chemotherapy.[15–20] In spite of a significant impact on disease-free survival in 5 out of these 11 trials, a significant prolongation of overall survival in the treatment arm was only observed in 2 of the 11. In these 2 trials, only small numbers of patients were randomized, so one can only conclude that at present there is no proof that adjuvant chemotherapy is beneficial to the STS patient and that adjuvant chemotherapy remains investigational. Biologic agents have not been part of the adjuvant chemotherapy strategies in STS, in contrast to the situation in osteosarcoma. In this latter disease, muramyl tripeptide phosphatidylethanolamine (MTP–PE), a potent activator of monocyte activity,[21] has been shown to have activity in its liposomal-encapsulated form.[22] It can be combined with ifosfamide,[23] and at present is being evaluated in an adjuvant phase III trial in osteosarcoma in the USA.

ADJUVANT STRATEGIES FOR LIMB SALVAGE AND LOCAL CONTROL IN EXTREMITY SOFT TISSUE SARCOMAS

Although control and prevention of distant metastases is still a major concern, limb salvage has become all the more important in the light of evidence that amputations do not improve survival rates in patients with large (>5 cm) deep-seated high-grade sarcomas.[24] Local recurrence rates vary according to the initial surgical procedure, and improved local control has been reported to correlate with better survival.[25] However, several studies have shown that marginal excisions with a high risk for local recurrence do not influence survival significantly.[24,26–29] Treatment options for locally advanced extremity STS may consist of an amputation or a limb-sparing extensive surgical procedure followed by radiation therapy. This combination may mutilate and compromise limb function considerably.

Induction intraarterial/intravenous chemotherapy: multimodality induction therapy

Preoperative induction intraarterial regional chemotherapy for extremity sarcomas was developed at UCLA in the 1970s,[30] and Suit et al[31] reported on the use of preoperative radiotherapy in 1981. Eilber and colleagues at UCLA combined preoperative (intraarterial or systemic) chemotherapy and radiotherapy to improve resectability rates – a strategy employed and reported on by many other groups.[32–38] In the course of time, the multidisciplinary programme at UCLA developed highly successful treatment schedules combining preoperative chemotherapy and radiotherapy followed by resectional surgery and often by further adjuvant chemotherapy. The most important conclusions from the UCLA programme, as reviewed by Eilber et al[39] are as follows:

- Local control improves when both preoperative chemotherapy and radiotherapy are applied.
- Preoperative radiotherapy utilizing 35 Gy is associated with excellent local control (9% local recurrences), but causes too many complications (fractures); 17.5 Gy is not effective enough (20% local recurrences), and 28 Gy is adequate (14% local recurrences, no fractures).
- Intraarterial chemotherapy is no more effective than intravenous chemotherapy.
- High-dose ifosfamide followed by doxorubicin and cisplatin in combination with 28 Gy radiotherapy increases complete response (CR) rates from about 8% in all previous protocols to about 40%.

It must be pointed out that these results were often achieved in patients who had undergone incomplete (debulking) resections of their tumours. This high rate of CRs was thus achieved upon relatively small tumours. Much lower CR rates are observed in trials of systemic induction chemotherapy involving 'untouched', often large, tumours such as in the trial reported by Rouësse et al[40] from the

Table 11.1 Isolated limb perfusion (ILP) for irresectable soft tissue sarcomas with cytostatic drugs only

Drugs	Number of ILPs	CR (%)	PR (%)	NC/PD (%)	Limb salvage (%)	Local recurrence (%)	Ref
Melphalan/Act-D/ mechlorethamine	17	0	35	65	ns	ns	46
Melphalan/Act-D/ mechlorethamine, various	51	6	12	82	84	ns	47
1. ILP + surgery (melphalan/Act-D)	30	ns	ns	ns	58	36	48
2. ILP + XRT + surgery (cisplatin)	20	ns	ns	ns	94	32	48
3. ILP + i.a. doxorubicin + surgery (doxorubicin)	17	ns	ns	ns	94	34	48
Cisplatin	17	0	18	82	ns	ns	49
Melphalan/ doxorubicin	13	7	0	93	61	ns	50
Doxorubicin	22	0	74[a]	26	91	28	51

Abbreviations: CR, complete response; PR, partial response; NC/PD, no change/progressive disease; Act-D, actinomycin D (dactinomycin); XRT, X-ray therapy; i.a., intraarterial; ns, not significant.
[a] No clinical response data; PR only based on radiological and/or histopathological estimates of necrosis. No patients with multiple tumors; 28% of patients had systemic metastases.

Institut Bergonié and in the study reported by Pezzi et al[41] from the MD Anderson Cancer Center. According to these reports, various multidrug regimens resulted in an overall response of 60%, with CR rates of 6–11%.

As conventional postoperative radiation therapy may be added in cases with marginal or positive resection margins, other radiation techniques may also be used. Amputation may also be avoided, and local control improved by applying brachytherapy techniques to the tumour bed in the context of marginal resections.[42]

Induction chemotherapy by isolated limb perfusion

Yet another strategy is to perform an isolated limb perfusion (ILP) with cytostatic agents. This technique, first described by Creech et al,[43] exposes tumours to drug concentrations more than 20 times higher than after systemic therapy to maximize tumour reduction.[44] Melphalan, the standard drug for ILP in the treatment of melanoma in-transit metastases,[45] has also been used in the treatment of extremity STS. ILP may render an irresectable tumour resectable and reduce the local recurrence rate. In cases with widespread metastases, it can be used palliatively for alleviation of pain and to avoid ablative surgery.[46,47] The results of ILP with melphalan as well as other drugs in patients with irresectable or locally advanced extremity STS, followed by a delayed resection of the tumour (remnant), are summarized in Table 11.1. In general, only low clinical response rates (CRs invariably below 10%; partial responses (PRs) up to 35%) have been reported.[48–53] Doxorubicin and melphalan were investigated in the ILP setting in the Netherlands, and only one CR (7%) and no PRs were observed, while three amputations had to be performed because of doxorubicin-related toxicity.[50] In a study from Italy, over 50% necrosis in STS tumours after ILP with doxorubicin was observed in 16 of 23 patients (74%), but no clinical response data were provided and, most importantly, no complete remissions were observed.[51]

Most other reports on the use of ILP in STS patients concern adjuvant ILPs in situations where the sarcomas had already been (non-radically) resected, or were resected immediately after the limb perfusion.[52–55] These reports therefore do not give information on response rate or on the role of ILP in limb salvage. Because of the modest results achieved by ILP with cytostatic drugs alone, this procedure has been abandoned in most centres for the management of locally advanced extremity STS.

Biochemotherapy: application of tumour necrosis factor α in ILP

Tumour necrosis factor α

The observation that tumour necrosis factor α (TNF-α) can cause acute haemorrhagic necrosis of tumour nodules in syngeneic (murine) and xenogeneic (human) tumour systems after local or systemic injection,[56–58] at doses 10–50-fold higher than the maximum tolerated dose observed after intravenous (i.v.) administration in cancer patients,[59] indicates that this potent but highly toxic agent may only achieve the necessary levels when administered in patients in an isolated perfusion setting where regional drug levels 20–50 times higher than after i.v. administration have been demonstrated in humans.[44]

TNF-α is a cytokine produced mainly by activated macrophages.[46] In vitro, about one-third of human epithelial cancer cell culture lines are very sensitive to the cytolytic effects of TNF-α, while one-third show cytostasis and one-third are relatively resistant. The inhibitory effects of TNF-α on normal cells require 100–10 000-fold higher concentrations.[60,61] Administration of TNF-α in vivo can cause acute haemorrhagic necrosis of tumour nodules in murine syngeneic and xenogeneic transplantation tumour systems.[56–59] The antitumour effects of TNF-α in vivo probably result from both direct and indirect mechanisms. TNF-α is a pleiotropic agent, and has a profound effect on the function of effector cells of the immune system,[59] on the activation of the coagulation system,[62,63] and on the generation and activation of heamatopoietic cells, and it has been demonstrated to be a primary mediator of endotoxic shock. Pharmacological doses of TNF-α induce the secretion of various other cytokines, such as granulocyte–macrophage colony-stimulating factor (GM-CSF), interleukin (IL)-1 and IL-6, and classical hormones, as well as small-molecule mediators of inflammation. In phase I–II studies, TNF-α has been found to be very toxic when administered systemically.[64–73] The maximum tolerated dose was reported to vary between 200 and 400 $\mu g/m^2$, depending on the number of doses given and whether the TNF-α was given as an i.v. bolus or a continuous infusion. Toxicity consists mainly of fevers with rigours and chills, hypotension, fatigue, nausea, anorexia, leukopenia and thrombocytopenia, and transient hepatic and renal toxicity. The severity of the toxicity associated with the higher systemic doses of TNF-α (>75 $\mu g/m^2$) is

Table 11.2 Isolated limb perfusion (ILP) for soft tissue sarcomas with TNF-α + cytostatic drugs

Drugs	Number of ILPs	CR (%)	PR (%)	NC/PD (%)	Limb salvage (%)	Local recurrence (%)	Ref
TNF-α + IFN-γ + melphalan	20	55[a]	40[a]	5[a]	90	11	7
TNF-α + melphalan	8	100[b]	0	0	63.5	0	80
TNF-α + melphalan	9	67[b]	22[b]	11[b]	89	ns	81
TNF-α + IFN-γ + melphalan	55[c]	18[d] 36[a]	64[d] 51[a]	18[d] 13[a]	84	13[c]	8
TNF-α ± IFN-γ + melphalan	186[e]	18[d] 29[a]	57[d] 53[a]	25[d] 18[a]	82	22[e]	9

Abbreviations: TNF-α, tumour necrosis factor α; IFN-γ, interferon-γ, CR, complete response; PR, partial response; NC/PD, no change/progressive disease; ns, not significant.
[a] Response rate is compilation of clinical response + histopathological response: CR: 100% necrosis; PR: >50–99% necrosis.
[b] Response rate based on % necrosis after resection.
[c] 24% of patients had multiple tumours; 16% had known systemic metastases.
[d] Clinical response rates (according to WHO measurement criteria).
[e] 23% of patients had multiple tumours; 13% had known systemic metastases.

dose-limiting. This is unfortunate, since the antitumour properties of TNF-α appear to require the maximum tolerable doses. Therefore the clinical use of TNF-α may be restricted to locoregional applications such as ILP, since intralesional administration only allows for a modest increase in the dose.[74] In an isolated perfusion system, the combination with chemotherapy and hyperthermia can be expected to further enhance antitumour activity.[75–79]

Successful use of TNF-α in ILP in STS patients
Lejeune and Liénard pioneered the application of TNF-α in the ILP setting. The initial results with high CR rates after treatment of 19 stage IIIA melanoma patients with in-transit metastases

and 4 patients with locally advanced extremity STS were published in 1992.[6] In a multicentre study protocol, standard rules for the perfusion technique, resection of residual tumour, and for pre- and postoperative evaluation were defined. The results of the initial experience with the triple regimen, i.e. TNF-α + interferon-γ (IFN-γ) + melphalan, were reported in 1993 and 1996.[7,8] Two other European groups, one from the UK and one from Italy, reported small studies in 1993 and in 1995.[80,81] The results of 200 perfusions in an eight-centre European cooperative study in patients with locally advanced STS of the extremities treated mainly with TNF-α + melphalan have been reported,[9] and will be discussed here. The results of these reports are summarized in Table 11.2. Here we shall discuss in detail the two large series.[8,9]

The European experience

In eight European cancer centres, from 1991 until the end of 1995, a total of 200 ILPs were performed in 186 patients with locally advanced extremity STS that were considered to be unresectable or only resectable at the cost of significant loss of limb function. The composition of this series of patients is unusual, and demonstrates that most patients were referred because amputation was considered the only option. This is underlined by unusual characteristics such as the facts that large single tumours (median size 16 cm) were present in 143 patients (77%), multifocal primary or multiple recurrent tumours were present in 43 patients (23%) (ranging from 2 to more than 100 tumours), and 25 patients (13%) had known systemic metastases at the time of the ILP. Most (161/186) tumours were high grade (110 grade III, 51 grade II), and there were 25 grade I sarcomas (always very large, recurrent or multiple).

ILP consisted of a 90 minutes long perfusion, 3 mg (arm)–4 mg (leg) TNF-α and 10 mg/l leg volume or 13 mg/l arm volume of melphalan at mild hyperthermia (39–40°C). The first 55 patients also received IFN-γ (0.2 mg) in the perfusate as well as subcutaneously on the two days prior to the operation. Throughout the perfusion period, any potential leakage of the drugs was monitored using a radioactive ^{125}I-albumin tracer. Continuous monitoring was performed with a precordial scintillation probe.

Tumour response and limb salvage

A major tumour response was seen in 82% of the patients, rendering most of these large sarcomas subsequently resectable. The key parameters defining outcome of treatment were clinical and pathological response, final outcome of treatment, and limb salvage. Clinical response rates were 33 CR (18%), 106 PR (57%), 42 no change (NC) (22%) and 5 progressive disease (PD) (3%). Final outcome as defined by clinical plus pathological responses were 54 CR (29%), 99 PR (53%), 29 NC (16%) and 4 PD (2%). At a median follow-up of almost 2 years (22 months) (range 6–58 months), limb salvage was achieved in 82%. In 126 patients with a single tumour, the tumour remnant was resected and

in 14 patients (11%) a local recurrence developed after 3–24 months. In the other 60 patients, no resection was performed (because of multiple tumours, systemic metastases, refusal to be amputated), and local tumour control was obtained in 33 patients (55%) while recurrences occurred in 27 patients (45%). Limb salvage was often still achieved as patients were already dying of systemic disease. Additional radiation therapy was given in only 39/186 patients (21%). The limb had to be amputated in 34 patients (18%): in 6 in spite of an excellent response, and in 28 because of insufficient response to the ILP or because of local tumour recurrence 4–24 months after ILP.

Regional toxicity was comparable to that observed with perfusions using melphalan alone; systemic toxicity was moderate or less, and was easily manageable. Almost all patients developed fever, sometimes with chills, within four hours of the ILP, and were treated effectively with paracetamol or indomethacin. Most patients developed a hyperdynamic state, and went through a phase of slightly lowered blood pressure that was easily managed by administering fluid and did not require the administration of vasopressor drugs.

Conclusions on efficacy

When one compares the response rates obtained using TNF-α-based ILPs (82% in the 186-patient series, 100% (all CRs) in the small UK series and 89% in the Italian report, as compiled in Table 11.2), it is clear that the response rates are far superior to the response rates historically reported after ILP with chemotherapy alone (Table 11.1) or after intraarterial or intravenous induction chemotherapy, as discussed earlier in this chapter. Moreover, in these chemotherapy series, the median tumour size is much lower and patients with multiple tumours are usually not included, whereas almost 25% of the patients in the TNF-α ILP series had multiple tumours. Obviously, only a randomized trial comparing the various approaches would give an answer as to which method is most effective and in which patients one or another procedure is most appropriate, but this will not be an easy trial to carry out.

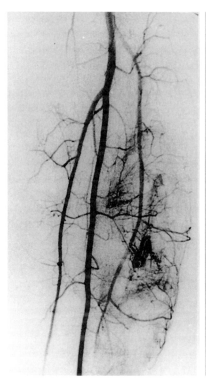
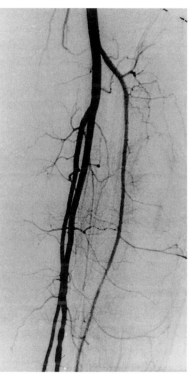

Figure 11.1 Typical angiographic observations before and after isolated limb perfusion (ILP) with TNF-α. The pre-ILP angiogram of a hypervascular grade III MFH in the right lower leg of a 40-year-old man is shown on the left. The tumour was fixed to the vessels and the bone, and had invaded the popliteal nerve causing popliteal nerve palsy (dropping foot). On the post-ILP angiogram (two weeks after ILP), the disappearance of all tumour-associated vessels is striking, whereas no damage seems to have been inflicted upon the normal vessels. The patient had a quick clinical response, with softening of the tumour and over 50% regression, rendering the tumour mobile again. Resection of the tumour remnant, eight weeks after ILP, revealed 100% necrosis.

ILP with TNF-α + melphalan seems of particular palliative value in patients with widespread metastatic disease and with an uncontrollably rapidly growing tumour, threatening the limb. In all but 2 of 25 such patients, a single ILP provided rapid and life-lasting (two or more years) local control. The introduction of TNF-α in ILP for locally advanced extremity STS marks the development of an effective new treatment option in the management of this disease.

Efficacy of TNF-α in ILP for melanoma and various carcinomas

High CR and PR rates have also been reported in various histologies (>20) of STS and in melanoma (complete remission rates in melanoma varying from 64% to 91% have been reported[6,81–83]), predicting that response to ILP with TNF-α may depend upon factors apart from tumour type, and suggesting that TNF-α mediates its antitumour effects via the vascular

bed of the tumours. This seems indeed to be the case, since responses in various carcinomas have also been noted after ILP with TNF-α + melphalan, including squamous cell carcinomas, Merkel cell carcinomas, and soft tissue metastases of renal cell cancer, osteosarcoma and lymphoma (AMM Eggermont, unpublished observations).

Clinical observations and histological studies of the antitumour effects

Antitumour effects after TNF-α-containing ILPs can be extremely rapid. This indicates that the TNF-α-mediated collapse of the tumour vascular bed may play an essential role in the antitumour mechanism. The selective destructive effects of TNF-α ILP on tumour-associated vessels have been illustrated elsewhere by pre- and post-perfusion angiographs. Figure 11.1 shows an example of the typical angiographic appearance in patients with hypervascular large extremity sarcomas with an extended tumour-associated vascular bed, which has completely disappeared on angiography one to two weeks after the ILP. Moreover, in sarcoma patients, magnetic resonance spectrometry studies have clearly shown virtually complete metabolic shutdown of the tumour within 16 hours after the perfusion, confirming the likelihood that TNF-α is mediating its most important effects on the vasculature of the tumour.[84] At the histopathological level, these intravascular effects such as platelet aggregation, erythrostasis, and endothelial and vascular destruction have been described based on observations of sequential biopsies in melanoma and sarcoma patients.[85–87] These observations resemble many of the TNF-α related phenomena reported in experimental tumour systems.[88,89]

Observations on TNF-α-based ILPs in animal tumour models

Synergy with chemotherapy

In Rotterdam, rat extremity tumour models of non-immunogenic soft tissue sarcomas (BN175) and of osteosarcomas (ROS-1) have been developed. In both tumour systems, highly synergistic antitumour effects are observed when an ineffective dose of TNF-α is combined with a dose of melphalan that when used alone in ILP causes only temporary growth arrest. The combination of TNF-α + melphalan always has a highly synergistic antitumour effect, resulting in a complete remission rate of 70–80%.[90,91] Histopathologically, extensive haemorrhagic necrosis is observed after ILP with the combination, but not after ILP with melphalan alone.[92] Early endothelial damage and platelet aggregation in the tumour vessels are observed after ILP with TNF-α + melphalan, and this is believed to lead to ischaemic (coagulative) necrosis, which is in line with observations in human patients.

Our observations confirm that TNF-α exerts its major effect on larger tumours with well-developed vasculature, in contrast to small tumours (diameter < 3 mm) with lack of a developed capillary bed.[93,94] It was shown that sarcomas of 4–5 mm diameter are less susceptible to TNF-α than those of 8–9 mm diameter.[93]

Role of anoxia

In the BN175 sarcoma model in the rat, it has been shown that a non-oxygenated limb perfusion with TNF-α alone has remarkable antitumour effects, in contrast to the lack of impact on tumour growth of an oxygenated ILP. The potentiating effect is so strong, resulting in CRs in most rats, that, in spite of indications that TNF-related toxicity towards the normal tissues is also increased, this phenomenon needs to be explored further.[95]

Role of interferon-γ

Another observation made in the BN175 rat sarcoma model regards interferon (IFN)-γ. Many reports in the literature have shown potentiation of the antitumour activity of TNF-α by IFN-γ both in vitro[96] and in vivo.[97] In our sarcoma models, the antitumour effects of TNF-α + melphalan ILP were not further enhanced by the addition of subcutaneous administration with IFN-γ or by the addition of IFN-γ to the perfusate.[98] This is in line with our experience in patients with sarcoma.[7–9]

Role of neutrophils

Sequential morphological analysis in our tumour models has revealed a more intense polymorphonuclear neutrophil (PMN) infiltration in tumours when melphalan was combined with TNF-α compared with series treated with melphalan alone. We observed that total body irradiation and the related reduction in white blood cell count decreased the response to an ILP with TNF-α + melphalan significantly, and reduced it to the level of effects obtained with melphalan alone. Therefore these data strongly suggest an important role for neutrophils in the immediate effects of TNF-α.[99]

Role of nitric oxide

Nitric oxide (NO) is an important molecule in the maintenance of both vascular tone and the integrity of the vascular wall, and is strongly produced in experimental and human tumours. Its inhibition could lead to hypoxia and an enhancement of TNF-α early vascular effects in the tumour. Moreover NO inhibits platelet aggregation, and inhibition of the synthesis of

NO may facilitate platelet aggregation and thus enhance TNF-α effects. The typical TNF-α tumour response was observed when NO synthase was inhibited by L-NAME during ILP. Inhibition of NO may augment TNF-α vascular effects, through hypoxia in the tumour and abrogation of the protective effects of NO such as inhibition of platelet aggregation.[100]

Conclusion
In conclusion, we can state that our isolated limb perfusion models in the rat permit us to investigate the mechanisms by which TNF-α exerts its antitumour effects in this system and to determine agents and manipulations through which the activity of TNF-α can be enhanced. It is hoped that this will result in clinical applications of TNF-α that may improve the outcome of treatment in cancer patients.

FUTURE PERSPECTIVES

Development of organ perfusion models

The isolated limb perfusion system should be considered as a model system in which to develop new treatment strategies with TNF-α. Since a number of organs can be perfused in a similar fashion, it stands to reason that isolated lung,[101] liver[102,103] and kidney[104] perfusion models have been developed to investigate the applicability and efficacy of TNF-α in these systems. Isolated lung perfusions are of particular interest as a treatment option for sarcoma patients, since the lungs are usually the primary and sometimes the sole site of distant metastases in STS.

Systemic treatment with TNF-α: tumour targeting of TNF-α

It has been demonstrated in the preclinical TNF-α programme in Rotterdam that TNF-α may regain its potential as a targetable agent in systemic treatment regimens. Both TNF-α and melphalan can be encapsulated in Stealth liposomes with good encapsulation efficiency.[70] A

preferential localization of Stealth liposomes in the BN175 STS was observed, reaching almost 10% of the injected dose at 12 hours after injection. Seventy-two hours after injection of the liposomes, up to 15% of the injected dose could still be detected in the circulation, and there was a tumour localization of 4% at that time point. With the combination of Stealth liposome-encapsulated TNF-α and DOX-SL, we observed significant antitumour effects in our model after systemic treatment for the first time.[105] Moreover, much less toxicity was observed after the repeated administration of TNF-α liposomes than after repeated injections of equal doses of free TNF-α. These findings will prompt research into the treatment of other tumours at sites (lung and liver) other than the extremities with a combination of liposomal agents.

CONCLUSIONS

At the present time, biologic agents are not widely used in the systemic treatment of soft tissue sarcomas. The activity of TNF-α in the setting of isolated limb perfusion in combination with melphalan has received much attention lately, and has shown the power of the concept of biochemotherapy that is directed against both the tumour cell component as well as the stromal component of sarcomas – and this can improve the response rates of large, otherwise often refractory tumours spectacularly. Whether this will lead to the development of more effective regional applications such as isolated lung perfusions for STS metastases to the lung remains to be seen. Whether TNF-α will eventually find its way back into systemic treatment, by making use of tumour targeting strategies such as encapsulation in liposomes, is also uncertain but is an attractive concept to work on.

REFERENCES

1. Boring CC, Squires TS, Tong T, Montgomery S, Cancer Statistics, 1994. *CA Cancer J Clin* 1994; **44:** 7–26.
2. Shiu M, Castro E, Hadju S, Surgical treatment of 297 soft tissue sarcomas of the extremity. *Ann Surg* 1975; **182:** 597–602.
3. Wanebo H, Kones R, MacFarlane J, Eilber F, Head and neck sarcoma: report of head and neck sarcoma registry. *Head and Neck* 1992; **Jan–Feb:** 1–7.
4. Binder SC, Katz B, Sheridan B, Retroperitoneal liposarcoma. *Ann Surg* 1978; **187:** 257–61.
5. Costa J, Wesley R, Gladstein E, Rosenberg SA, The grading of soft tissue sarcoma: results of a clinicopathologic correlation in a series of 163 cases. *Cancer* 1984; **53:** 530–41.
6. Liénard D, Ewalenko P, Delmotte JJ et al, High-dose recombinant tumor necrosis factor alpha in combination with interferon gamma and melphalan in isolation perfusion of the limbs for melanoma and sarcoma. *J Clin Oncol* 1992; **10:** 50–62.
7. Eggermont AMM, Liénard D, Schraffordt Koops H et al, Treatment of irresectable soft tissue sarcomas of the limbs by isolation perfusion with high dose TNF-α in combination with gamma-interferon and melphalan. In: *Tumor Necrosis Factor: Molecular and Cellular Biology and Clinical Relevance* (Fiers W, Buurman WA, eds). Karger Verlag: Basel, 1993: 239–43.
8. Eggermont AMM, Schraffordt Koops H, Lienard D et al, Isolated limb perfusion with high dose tumor necrosis factor α in combination with IFNγ and melphalan for irresectable extremity soft tissue sarcomas: a multicenter trial. *J Clin Oncol* 1996; **14:** 2656–65.
9. Eggermont AMM, Schraffordt Koops H, Klausner J et al, Isolated limb perfusion with tumor necrosis factor-α and melphalan in 186 patients with locally advanced extremity sarcomas: the cumulative multicenter European experience. *Ann Surg* 1996; **224:** 756–65.
10. Wilson RE, Wood WC, Lerner HL et al, Doxorubicin chemotherapy in the treatment of soft tissue sarcoma: combined results of two randomized trials. *Arch Surg* 1986; **121:** 1354–9.
11. Antman K, Ryan L, Borden E et al, Pooled results from three randomized adjuvant studies of doxorubicin versus observation in soft tissue sarcoma: 10 year results and review of the literature. In: *Adjuvant Therapy of Cancer VI* (Salmon SE, ed). WB Saunders: Philadelphia, 1990, 529–43.
12. Alvegard TA, Sigurdsson H, Mouridsen H et al, Adjuvant chemotherapy with doxorubicin in high grade soft tissue sarcoma: a randomized trial of the Scandinavian Sarcoma Group. *J Clin Oncol* 1989; **7:** 1504–13.
13. Eilber FR, Giuliano AE, Hurth JF, Morton DL, A randomized prospective trial using postoperative chemotherapy (Adriamycin) in high grade soft tissue sarcoma. *Am J Clin Oncol* 1988; **11:** 39–45.
14. Gherlinzoni F, Pignatti G, Fontana M, Giunti A, Soft tissue sarcomas: the experience of at the Istituto Ortopedico Rizzoli. *Chir Organi Mov* 1990; **75:** 150–4.
15. Benjamin RS, Terjanian TO, Genoglio CJ et al, The importance of combination chemotherapy for adjuvant treatment of high risk patients with soft tissue sarcomas of the extremities. In: *Adjuvant Therapy of Cancer V* (Salmon SE, ed). Grune & Stratton: New York, 1987: 735–44.
16. Edmonson JH, Fleming TR, Ivans JC et al, A randomized study of systemic chemotherapy following complete excision of non-osseous sarcomas. *J Clin Oncol* 1984; **2:** 1390–6.
17. Glenn J, Kinsella T, Glatstein E et al, A randomized prospective trial of adjuvant chemotherapy in adults with soft tissue sarcomas of the head and neck, breast and trunk. *Cancer* 1985; **55:** 1206–14.
18. Chang AE, Kinsella T, Glatstein E et al, Adjuvant chemotherapy for patients with high grade soft tissue sarcomas of the extremity. *J Clin Oncol* 1988; **6:** 1491–500.
19. Bramwell V, Rouëssé J, Steward J et al, Five year results of CYVADIC adjuvant chemotherapy for soft tissue sarcoma: an EORTC randomized trial (abst) *Eur J Cancer* 1991; **27**(Suppl 2): S161.
20. Ravaud A, Bui NB, Coindre JM et al, Adjuvant chemotherapy with CYVADIC in high risk soft tissue sarcoma: a randomized prospective trial. In: *Adjuvant Therapy of Cancer VI* (Salmon SE, ed). WB Saunders: Philadelphia, 1990: 556–66.
21. Kleinerman ES, Erickson KL, Schroit AJ et al, Activation of tumoricidal properties in human blood monocytes by liposomes containing lipophilic muramyl tripeptide. *Cancer Res* 1983; **43:** 2010–14.
22. Asano T, Kleinerman ES, Liposome-encapsu-

lated MTP–PE: a novel biologic agent for cancer therapy. *J Immunother* 1993; **14:** 286–92.

23. Kleinerman ES, Meyers PA, Raymond AK et al, Combination therapy with ifosfamide and liposome-encapsulated muramyl-tripeptide: tolerability, toxicity and immune stimulation. *J Immunother* 1995; **17:** 181–93.

24. Gaynor JJ, Tan CC, Casper ES et al, Refinement of clinicopathologic staging for localized soft tissue sarcoma of the extremity: a study of 423 adults. *J Clin Oncol* 1992; **10:** 1317–27.

25. Suit HD, Tepper JE, Impact of improved local control on survival in patients with soft tissue sarcoma. *Int J Radiat Oncol Biol Phys* 1986; **12:** 699–700.

26. Brennan MF, Shiu MH, Collin C et al, Extremity soft tissue sarcomas. *Cancer Treat Symp* 1985; **3:** 71–81.

27. Potter DA, Kinsella D, Gladstein E et al, High grade soft tissue sarcomas of the extremities. *Cancer* 1986; **59:** 190–205.

28. Stotter AT, A'Hearn RP, Fisher C et al, The influence of local recurrence of extremity soft tissue sarcoma on metastasis and survival. *Cancer* 1990; **65:** 1119–29.

29. Gustafson P, Rööser B, Rydholm A, Is local recurrence of minor importance for metastases in soft tissue sarcoma? *Cancer* 1991; **67:** 2083–6.

30. Eilber FR, Mirra JJ, Grant T et al, Is amputation necessary for sarcoma: a 7-year experiment with limb salvage. *Ann Surg* 1980; **192:** 431–7.

31. Suit HD, Proppe KH, Mankin HJ, Wood WC, Preoperative radiation therapy for sarcoma of soft tissue. *Cancer* 1981; **47:** 2269–74.

32. Azzarelli A, Quagliuolo V, Audisio A et al, Intraarterial Adriamycin followed by surgery for limb sarcomas. Preliminary report. *Eur J Cancer Clin Oncol* 1983; **19:** 885–90.

33. Mantravadi RVP, Trippon MJ, Patel MK et al, Limb salvage in extremity soft tissue sarcoma: combined modality therapy. *Radiology* 1984; **152:** 423–6.

34. Denton JW, Dunham WK, Salter M et al, Preoperative regional chemotherapy and rapid fractionation for sarcomas of the soft tissue and bone. *Surg Gynecol Obstet* 1985; **158:** 545–51.

35. Goodnight JE, Bargar WL, Voegeli T et al, Limb sparing surgery for extremity sarcomas after preoperative intra-arterial doxorubicin and radiation therapy. *Am J Surg* 1985; **150:** 109–13.

36. Hoekstra HJ, Schraffordt Koops H, Molenaar WM et al, A combination of intraarterial chemotherapy, preoperative and postoperative radiotherapy, and surgery as limb-saving treatment of primary unresectable high grade soft tissue sarcomas of the extremities. *Cancer* 1989; **63:** 59–62.

37. Levine EA, Trippon M, Das Gupta TK, Preoperative multimodality treatment for soft tissue sarcomas. *Cancer* 1993; **71:** 3685–9.

38. Wanebo HJ, Temple WJ, Popp MB et al, Preoperative regional therapy for extremity sarcoma: a tricenter update. *Cancer* 1995; **75:** 2299–306.

39. Eilber F, Eckhardt J, Rosen G et al, Preoperative therapy for soft tissue sarcoma. *Hematol Oncol Clin North Am* 1995; **9:** 817–23.

40. Rouëssé JG, Friedman S, Sevin DM et al, Preoperative induction chemotherapy in the treatment of locally advanced soft tissue sarcomas. *Cancer* 1987; **60:** 296–300.

41. Pezzi CM, Pollock RE, Evans HL et al, Preoperative chemotherapy for soft-tissue sarcomas of the extremities. *Ann Surg* 1990; **211:** 476–81.

42. Shiu M, Hilaris B, Harrison LB, Brennan MF, Brachytherapy and function saving resection of soft-tissue sarcoma arising in the limb. *Int J Radiat Oncol Biol Phys* 1991; **21:** 1485–92.

43. Creech OJ, Krementz ET, Ryan RF, Winblad JN, Chemotherapy of cancer: regional perfusion utilizing an extracorporeal circuit. *Ann Surg* 1958; **148:** 616–32.

44. Benckhuijsen C, Kroon BBR, Van Geel AN, Wieberdink J, Regional perfusion treatment with melphalan for melanoma in a limb: evaluation of drug kinetics. *Eur J Surg Oncol* 1988; **14:** 157–63.

45. Thompson JF, Gianoutsos MP, Isolated limb perfusion for melanoma: effectiveness and toxicity of cisplatin compared with that of melphalan and other drugs. *World J Surg* 1992; **61:** 227–33.

46. Krementz ET, Carter RD, Sutherland CM, Hutton I, Chemotherapy of sarcomas of the limbs by regional perfusion. *Ann Surg* 1977; **185:** 555–64.

47. Muchmore JH, Carter RD, Krementz ET, Regional perfusion for malignant melanoma and soft tissue sarcoma: a review. *Cancer Invest* 1985; **3:** 129–43.

48. Filippo FD, Giannarelli D, Botti C et al, Hyperthermic antiblastic perfusion for the treatment of soft tissue limb sarcomas. *Ann Oncol* 1992; **3:** S71–4.

49. Pommier RF, Moseley HS, Cohen J et al, Pharmacokinetics, toxicity, and short-term results of cisplatin hyperthermic isolated limb perfusion for soft tissue sarcoma and melanoma of the extremities. *Am J Surg* 1988; **155:** 667–71.

50. Klaase JM, Kroon BBR, Benckhuysen C et al, Results of regional isolation perfusion with cytostatics in patients with soft tissue tumors of the extremities. *Cancer* 1989; **64:** 616–21.

51. Rossi CR, Vecchiato A, Foletto M et al, Phase II study on neoadjuvant hyperthermic–antiblastic perfusion with doxorubicin in patients with intermediate of high grade limb sarcomas. *Cancer* 1994; **73:** 2140–6.

52. McBride CM, Sarcomas of the limbs: result of adjuvant chemotherapy using isolation perfusion. *Arch Surg* 1974; **109:** 304–8.

53. Stehlin JS, de Ipolyi PD, Giovanella BC et al, Soft tissue sarcomas of the extremity: multidisciplinary therapy employing hyperthermic perfusion. *Am J Surg* 1975; **130:** 643–6.

54. Lethi PM, Stephens MH, Janoff K et al, Improved survival for soft tissue sarcoma of the extremities by regional hyperthermic perfusion, local excision and radiation therapy. *Surg Gynecol Obstet* 1986; **162:** 149–52.

55. Hoekstra HJ, Schraffordt Koops H, Molenaar WM, Oldhoff J, Results of isoalted regional perfusion in the treatment of malignant soft tissue tumors of the extremities. *Cancer* 1987; **60:** 1703–7.

56. Haranaka K, Satomi N, Sukarai A, Antitumor activity of murine tumor necrosis factor against transplanted murine tumors and heterotransplanted human tumors in nude mice. *Int J Cancer* 1984; **34:** 263–7.

57. Creasy AA, Reynolds TR, Laird W, Cures and partial remissions of murine and human tumors by recombinant tumor necrosis factor. *Cancer Res* 1986; **46:** 5687–90.

58. Balkwill FR, Lee A, Aldham G et al, Human tumor xenografts treated with recombinant human tumor necrosis factor alone or in combination with interferons. *Cancer Res* 1986; **46:** 3990–3.

59. Asher AL, Mule JJ, Reichert CM et al, Studies of the antitumor efficacy of systemically administered recombinant tumor necrosis factor against several murine tumors in vivo. *J Immunol* 1987; **138:** 963–74.

60. Carswell EA, Old LJ, Kassel RL et al, An endotoxin induced serum factor that causes necrosis of tumors. *Proc Natl Acad Sci USA* 1975; **72:** 3666–70.

61. Sugarman BJ, Aggarwal BB, Hass PE et al, Recombinant tumor necrosis factor-alpha: effects on proliferation of normal and transformed cells in vitro. *Science* 1985; **230:** 943–5.

62. Nawroth PP, Stern DM, Modulation of endothelial cell hemostatic properties by tumor necrosis factor. *J Exp Med* 1986; **163:** 740–5.

63. Bevilacqua MP, Pober JS, Majeau GR et al, Recombinant tumor necrosis factor induces procoagulant activity in cultured human vascular endothelium: characterization and comparison with the actions of interleukin-1. *Proc Natl Acad Sci USA* 1986; **83:** 4533–7.

64. Blick M, Sherwin SA, Rosenblum M, Gutterman, Phase I study of recombinant tumor necrosis factor in cancer patients. *Cancer Res* 1987; **47:** 2986–9.

65. Selby P, Hobbs S, Viner C et al, Tumor necrosis factor in man: clinical and biological observations. *Br J Cancer* 1987; **56:** 803–8.

66. Gamm H, Lindemann A, Mertelsmann R, Herrmann F, Phase I trial of recombinant tumor necrosis factor-alpha in patients with advanced malignancy. *Eur J Cancer* 1991; **7:** 856–63.

67. Fiedler W, Zeller W, Peimann CJ et al, A phase II combination trial with recombinant tumor necrosis factor and gamma interferon in patients with colorectal cancer. *Klin Wochenschr* 1991; **69:** 261–8.

68. Spriggs DR, Sherman ML, Michie H et al, Recombinant human tumor necrosis factor administered as a 24 h intravenous infusion. A phase I and pharmacologic study. *J Natl Cancer Inst* 1988; **80:** 1039–44.

69. Creaven PJ, Plager JE, Dupere S et al, Phase I trial of recombinant human tumor necrosis factor. *Cancer Chemother Pharmacol* 1987; **20:** 137–44.

70. Blick MB, Sherwin SA, Rosenblum M et al, A phase I trial of recombinant human tumor necrosis factor in cancer patients. *Cancer Res* 1987; **47:** 2986–9.

71. Kimura K, Taguchi T, Urushizaki I et al, Phase I study of recombinant human tumor necrosis factor. *Cancer Chemother Pharmacol* 1987; **20:** 223–9.

72. Chapman PB, Lester TJ, Casper ES et al, Clinical pharmacology of recombinant human tumor necrosis factor in patients with advanced cancer. *J Clin Oncol* 1987; **5:** 1942–51.

73. Feinberg B, Kurzrock R, Talpaz M et al, A phase I trial of intravenously administered recombi-

nant tumor necrosis factor alpha in cancer patients. *J Clin Oncol* 1988; **6**: 1328–34.

74. Bartsch H, Pfizenmaier K, Schroeder M et al, Intralesional application of recombinant human tumor necrosis factor alpha induces local tumor regression in patients with advanced malignancies. *Eur J Cancer Clin Oncol* 1989; **25**: 287–91.

75. Regenass U, Muller M, Curschellas E, Matter A, Anti-tumor effects of tumor necrosis factor in combination with chemotherapeutic agents. *Int J Cancer* 1987; **39**: 266–73.

76. Krosnick JA, Mule JJ, McIntosh JK, Rosenberg SA, Augmentation of antitumor efficacy by the combination of tumor necrosis factor and chemotherapeutic agents in vivo. *Cancer Res* 1989; **49**: 3729–33.

77. Haranaka K, Sakurai A, Satomi N, Anti-tumor activity of recombinant human tumor necrosis factor in combination with hyperthermia, chemotherapy or immunotherapy. *J Biol Response Modif* 1987; **6**: 3790–1.

78. Watanabe N, Niitsu Y, Umeno H et al, Synergistic cytotoxic and antitumor effects of recombinant human tumor necrosis factor and hyperthermia. *Cancer Res* 1988; **48**: 650–3.

79. Niitsu Y, Watanabe, Umeno H et al, Synergistic effects of recombinant human tumor necrosis factor and hyperthermia on in vitro cytotoxicity and artificial metastasis. *Cancer Res* 1988; **48**: 654–7.

80. Hill S, Fawcett WJ, Sheldon J et al, Low-dose tumour necrosis factor α and melphalan in hyperthermic isolated limb perfusion. *Br J Surg* 1993; **80**: 995–7.

81. Vaglini M, Azzarrelli A, Carraro O et al, Preliminary results of alpha-TNF + L-PAM in stage IIIA–IIIAB melanoma and non resectable soft tissue sarcomas of extremities. *Proc Am Soc Clin Oncol* 1995; **14**: A1323.

82. Lejeune FJ, Liénard D, Leyvraz S, Mirimanoff RO, Regional therapy of melanoma. *Eur J Cancer* 1993; **29A**: 606–12.

83. Liénard D, Eggermont AMM, Schraffordt Koops H et al, TNF in isolated limb perfusion for treatment of locally advanced melanoma. *Eur Cytokine Netw* 1996; **7**: 299.

84. Sijens PE, Eggermont AMM, Van Dijk P, Oudkerk M, ^{31}P magnetic resonance spectroscopy as predictor for clinical response in human extremity sarcomas treated by single dose TNFα + melphalan isolated limb perfusion. *NMR in Biomed* 1995; **18**: 215–24.

85. Renard N, Liénard D, Lespagnard L et al, Early endothelium activation and polymorphonu-
clear cell invasion precede specific necrosis of human melanoma and sarcoma treated by intravascular high-dose tumour necrosis factor alpha (TNFα). *Int J Cancer* 1994; **57**: 656–63.

86. Renard N, Nooijen PTGA, Schalkwijk L et al, VWF release and platelet aggregation in human melanoma after perfusion with TNFα. *J Pathol* 1995; **176**: 279–87.

87. Nooijen PTGA, Eggermont AMM, Verbeek MM et al, Transient induction of E-selectin expression following TNF-based isolated limb perfusion in melanoma and sarcoma patients is not tumor specific. *J Immunother* 1996; **19**: 33–44.

88. Watanabe N, Niitsu Y, Umeno H et al, Toxic effect of TNF on tumor vasculature in mice. *Cancer Res* 1988; **49**: 2179–83.

89. Nawroth P, Handley D, Matsueda G et al, TNF/cachectin-induced intravascular fibrin formation in Meth-A fibrosarcomas. *J Exp Med* 1988; **168**: 637–47.

90. Manusama ER, Nooijen PTGA, Stavast J et al, Synergistic antitumour effect of recombinant human tumour necrosis factor a with melphalan in isolated limb perfusion in the rat. *Br J Surg* 1996; **83**: 551–5.

91. Manusama ER, Stavast J, Durante NMC et al, Isolated limb perfusion in a rat osteosarcoma model: a new anti-tumour approach. *Eur J Surg Oncol* 1996; **22**: 152–7.

92. Nooijen PTGA, Manusama ER, Eggermont AMM et al, Synergistic effects of TNFα and melphalan in an isolated limb perfusion model of rat sarcoma. *Br J Cancer* 1996; **74**: 1908–15.

93. Manda T, Nishigaki F, Mukumoto S et al, The efficacy of combined treatment with recombinant human tumor necrosis factor-α and 5-fluorouracil is dependent on the development of capillaries in tumor. *Eur J Cancer* 1990; **26**: 93–9.

94. Mule JJ, Asher A, McIntosh J et al, Antitumor effect of recombinant tumor necrosis factor-α against murine sarcomas at visceral sites: tumor size influences the response to therapy. *Cancer Immunol Immunother* 1988; **26**: 202–8.

95. Manusama ER, Durante NMC, Marquet RL, Eggermont AMM, Ischemia promotes the antitumor effect of tumor necrosis factor alpha (TNFα) in isolated limb perfusion in the rat. *Reg Cancer Treat* 1994; **7**: 155–9.

96. Schiller JH, Bittner G, Storer B, Wilson JKV, Synergistic antitumor effects of tumor necrosis factor α and gamma-interferon on human colon carcinoma cell lines. *Cancer Res* 1987; **47**: 2809–13.

97. Brouckaert PGG, Leroux-Rouls GG, Guisez Y et al, In vivo anti-tumor activity of recombinant human and murine TNF, alone and in combination with IFN-gamma on a syngeneic murine melanoma. *Int J Cancer* 1986; **38**: 763–9.

98. Manusama ER, De Wilt JHW, Marquet RL, Eggermont AMM, IFNγ does not enhance the antitumor effects but enhances regional toxicity in a rat tumor isolated limb perfusion model. *Oncol Rep* 1999; **6**: 173–7.

99. Manusama ER, Nooijen PTGA, Stavast J et al, Assessment of the role of neutrophils on the antitumor effect of TNFα in an in vivo isolated limb perfusion model in sarcoma bearing Brown Norway rats. *J Surg Res* 1998; **78**: 169–75.

100. Manusama ER, Durante NMC, Marquet RL, Eggermont AMM, Nitric oxide inhibition enhances the antitumor effects of TNFα in an isolated limb perfusion (ILP) model in the rat. *Eur J Surg Res* 1995; **27**(S1): 79(abst).

101. Prograbniak HW, Witt CJ, Terrill R et al, Isolated lung perfusion with tumor necrosis factor: a swine model in preparation of human trials. *Ann Thorac Surg* 1994; **57**: 1477–83.

102. Fraker DL, Alexander HR, Thom AK, Use of tumor necrosis factor in isolated hepatic perfusion. *Circulatory Shock* 1994; **44**: 45–50.

103. Borel-Rinkes IHM, Vries de MR, Jonker AM et al, Isolated hepatic perfusion with TNFα, with and without melphalan in the pig. *Br J Cancer* 1997; **75**: 1447–53.

104. Veen van de AH, Manusama ER, Kampen van CA et al, Tumor necrosis factor-α (TNFα) in isolated kidney perfusions in rats: toxicity and antitumor effects. *Eur J Surg Oncol* 1994; **20**: 404–5.

105. Veen van der AH, ten Hagen TLM, Marquet RL, Eggermont AMM, Treatment of solid limb tumors with liposome-encapsulated tumor necrosis factor-α in the rat. *Proc Am Assoc Cancer Res* 1996; **37**: 483(abst).

Index

Abbreviations: BMT, bone marrow transplantation; MAb/MAbs, monoclonal antibody/antibodies.